THE FOOD TREE

HOLISTIC NUTRITION & WELLNESS CURRICULUM

A Mind, Body, Soul Approach to Teaching Kids How to Eat Well and Be Healthy

JILL TRODERMAN, N.C.

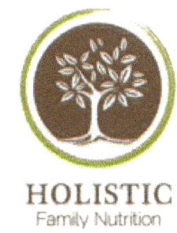

HOLISTIC
Family Nutrition

All rights reserved. No part of the publication may be reproduced, distributed, or transmitted in any form or by any means, including photocopying, recording, or other electronic or mechanical methods without the prior written permission of the publisher except in the case of brief quotations embodied in critical reviews and certain other non-commercial uses permitted by copyright law. For permission requests write to the publisher.

Limited permission is granted to the purchasing party to photocopy only those pages of this book that bear the notice "permission to photocopy granted" for use with his or her student during the use of The Food Tree Holistic Nutrition and Wellness Curriculum. Permission to reproduce: 70, 92, 125, 143, 153, 175, 176, 177, 181, 182, 183, 184, 185, 186, 197,198, 199, 228, 229

ISBN: 978-1-7349107-04 (Paperback Edition)

ISBN: 978-1-7349107-1-1 (ebook Edition)

Library of Congress

Food Tree art, graphic and characters: Michael Sherman

Curriculum and Content Contributors: Samantha Palmer; Tami Pippin

Editors: Doris Katz; Abby Klein; Lisa Radding; Kariman Pierce; Tyler Pierce; Barbara Schirmer

Design and layout: Christina Gaugler

For Dylan and Max

PREFACE

I was asked almost a decade ago about what future projects I might want to create. I spontaneously said, "write a book." I surprised myself when the words popped out of my mouth. But now, more than ten years later, this curriculum has grown in me, through me (on a mostly organic diet), and is now ready to bear its fruit. It has been a long time coming and I am so excited to share with you my philosophy about eating a healthy and environmentally friendly diet.

I grew up in a family that loves to eat and celebrate with delicious foods, so the topic of nutrition and healthy eating was a deep passion of mine for as long as I can remember. Yet over the years, I saw the ubiquitous lack of quality food in others' lives. I saw the connection to the destruction of our modern food system and the negative impact it has on our planet and, subsequently, on the health of the animals and people.

The necessary act of eating took on more meaning and significance than only how to get nourishment and pleasure from food. My decisions emerged from an understanding that the choices I made about food could make a difference in more than just my life but make a difference in the world.

I witnessed first-hand the positive impact of eating from our garden and fruit trees had on my children. I saw this simple, natural act as a human right. A right that every single person deserves to have. It is my vision and belief that we can create a world we want to live in—a world where there is abundance and all are well-nourished. To make that happen, we need a paradigm shift. We need to alter our path as a society. And I see it already happening. We know that all positive changes start with ourselves. The choice to be healthy and thrive is right at our fingertips and our mouths.

The health and wellness of the next generations are simply about providing them with the motivation and championing that they deserve. *The Food Tree Holistic Nutrition and Wellness Curriculum* offers the supportive guidance needed for that change. It is my highest wish that this book becomes a well-used tool to educate, empower, and inspire others to live to their highest potential.

I love this quote by Mahatma Gandhi. These words often guide the choices I make in my life. Perhaps you will resonate with them as well.

> *"Your beliefs become your thoughts, Your thoughts become your words,*
> *Your words become your actions, Your actions become your habits,*
> *Your habits become your values, Your values become your destiny."*

With peace and love in my heart,

Jill Troderman

Soquel, California USA
December 13, 2019

ACKNOWLEDGEMENTS

I was able to write this curriculum and guide knowing I had the endless support and encouragement from my amazing family, friends and colleagues. Parents, I thank you for believing in me even when I took the uncharted path into the unknown. Dad, 11:11. Mom, thanks for modeling how to stop work and make time to play through your love of Mah Jongg. To my children, my muses, Dylan and Max, who brought forth in me a deep passion to create this body of work. Thank you both for your wisdom and humor, I love you guys! Thanks to my brother Jeff for always feeding me, and I really wish I had your excellent kitchen skills. To my sister, Tami, I am so grateful for helping me paddle when the wind died down and for being such a great sounding board during this journey. To my extended family and my dearest friends, I am blessed to have all of you in my life. I listened to each of you cheering me on, even when I wanted to give up. Thanks finally to all of my business colleagues and the wise folks at the National Association of Nutrition Professionals for supporting me and my work.

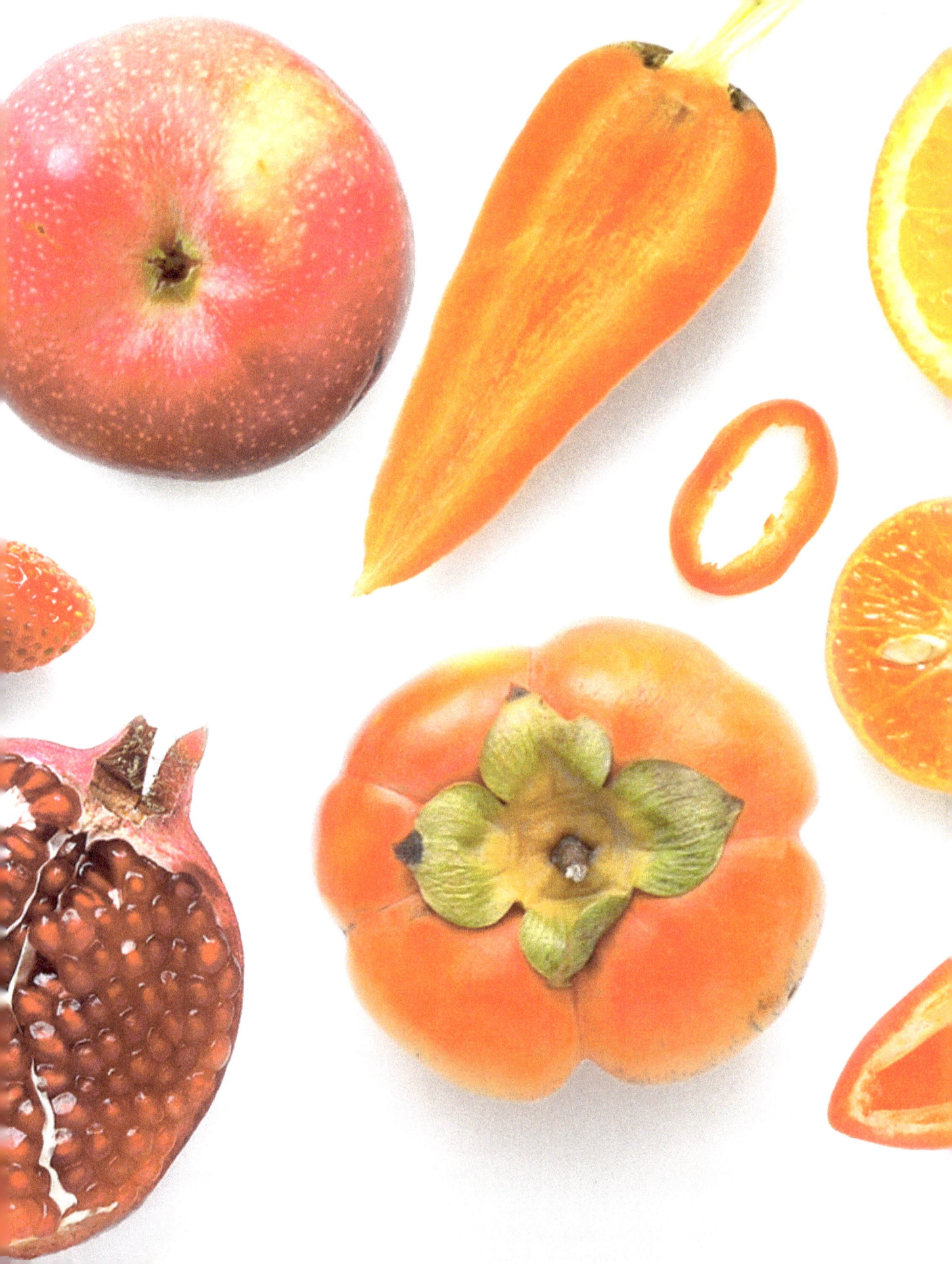

TABLE OF CONTENTS

xi User Guide to The Food Tree Holistic Nutrition and Wellness Curriculum

INTRODUCTION TO THE FOOD TREE HOLISTIC NUTRITION AND WELLNESS CURRICULUM • 1

- 1 Graphic—Eat Like a Tree
- 2 Holistic Nutrition and The Mind, Body, and Soul Connection
- 4 The Food Tree Holistic Nutrition Curriculum
- 8 The Food Tree Analogy
- 9 *You as A Tree* Visualization
- 10 The Food Tree Characters

THE FIVE FOOD GROUPS—CREATE A DIET AS UNIQUE AS YOU! • 12

13 INTRODUCTION TO THE PROTEINS FOOD GROUP

- 14 Lesson: Getting to Know Proteins—Plant-Based and Animal-Based
- 16 Lesson: Serving Sizes and Daily Recommendations for Proteins
- 20 Lesson: Benefits and Functions of Protein Foods
- 21 Classification of Amino Acids
- 23 Lesson: Exploring Plant-Based, Vegetarian, Vegan Diets and Lifestyles
- 28 Lesson: Protein Deficiencies
- 30 Lesson: Protein Foods to Avoid
- 32 Lesson: Protein Calculations

33 INTRODUCTION TO THE WHOLE GRAINS FOOD GROUP

- 34 Lesson: Getting to Know Grains—Whole and Refined
- 39 Lesson: Serving Sizes and Daily Recommendations for Grains
- 41 Lesson: Benefits and Functions of Whole Grains
- 43 Lesson: Take a Poll on Grain Diversity
- 45 Lesson: The Cost of Grain in the Marketplace
- 47 Lesson: History and Trade of Grains in The United States

49 INTRODUCTION TO THE FATS FOOD GROUP

- 50 Lesson: Getting to Know Fats
- 54 Lesson: Serving Sizes and Daily Recommendations for Fats
- 57 Lesson: Benefits and Functions of Fats
- 61 Lesson: Benefits of Essential Fatty Acids Omega 3 and Omega 6
- 64 Lesson: Problems Associated with Eating Damaged Fats and Hydrogenated Oils
- 68 Fat Calculations: Fat gram and calorie calculations for optimal daily nutrition
- 69 Classification of Fats and Oils

71 INTRODUCTION TO THE VEGETABLES FOOD GROUP

    72 *Lesson: Getting to Know Vegetables*

    75 *Lesson: Serving Sizes and Daily Recommendations for Vegetables*

    78 *Lesson: Benefits and Functions of Vegetables*

    80 *Lesson: Problems Related to Low Dietary Intake of Vegetables*

83 INTRODUCTION TO THE FRUITS FOOD GROUP

    84 *Lesson: Getting to Know Fruit*

    86 *Lesson: Serving Sizes and Daily Recommendations of Fruit*

    89 *Lesson: Benefits and Functions of Fruits*

    91 *Lesson: Cost Analysis of Fruits*

    93 *Lesson: Eat Locally Grown and In-Season Fruit*

95 SUPPORT LESSONS

    95 *Lesson: Rainbow Food Phytonutrients and Antioxidants*

    101 *Lesson: Focus on Fiber*

    104 *Lesson: The Delicate Dynamic Digestive Tract*

    107 *Lesson: Developing Critical Thinking Skills—Food, Diet, Eating, and the Media*

    111 *Lesson: How to Read Nutrition Facts Panel and Package Labeling*

113 NUTRITION VAMPIRES

    114 *Lesson: The Nine Nutrition Vampires*

    117 *Lesson: Too Much Sugar!*

    122 *Lesson: Nutrition Vampires and FDA Approval*

    124 *Activity: Nutrition Vampire Snack Attack*

PHYSICAL ACTIVITIES • 126

    127 *Lesson: Introduction to Physical Activities*

    129 *Cardiovascular Aerobic Exercises and Activities*

    130 *Strength Training and Resistance Exercises*

    133 *Stretching Moves*

    135 *Yoga Poses*

    138 *Grounding, Earthing, and Walking Barefoot*

    140 *Mirror Reflection Exercises*

MINDFULNESS ACTIVITIES • 144

    146 *Mindfulness Affirmations, Mantras, and Meditations*

    149 *Mindful and Intuitive Eating*

    152 *Gratitude Journals and Ideas*

    153 *Gratitude Journal Template*

    154 *The "I Wonder" Exercise*

    155 *The Scale of Human Consciousness*

    157 *Hand Mudras*

    160 *Alternate Nostril Breathing—Nadi Shodhana*

ACTIVITIES: ARTS, CRAFTS, AND SCIENCE EXPERIMENTS • 162

    163 *Indian Corn Jewelry*

    164 *Make Lavender Wands*

    165 *DIY Plant Dyes*

    168 *Papier Mâché Fruit and Bowls*

    169 *Do It Yourself Playdough*

    170 *Positive Word Cloud*

    172 *Thank a Farmer, Baker, and Cheese Maker*

    172 *Draw, Sketch, Paint, and Illustrate Fruits and Vegetables*

    173 *Food Tree Decoupage Collage*

174 Taste the Rainbow
175 Taste the Rainbow Taste Test
176 Taste the Rainbow Taste Test
177 The Five Food Group's Match-up
178 Observing Oxidation
179 Milk Color Burst Experiment
181 Word Search Power Proteins
182 Word Search Nutritious Nuts and Scrumptious Seeds
183 Word Search Hello Whole Grains
184 Word Search Fabulous Fats
185 Word Search Fruits and Vegetables
186 Plant Part Matching Worksheet
187 DIY pH Papers
190 Grow Plants from Kitchen Scraps
193 DIY: Sprouts and Microgreens
194 Bazillions of Beans
196 Take A School Field Trip
197 Scientific Method Sheet
198 Recipe For Health Worksheet
199 Food Journal

RECIPES • 198

202 Tamari Toasted Pepitas
203 Toasted Nori Sheets
204 Roasted Chickpeas
205 Kale Chips
206 Brussels Sprouts Chips
207 Power Nut Balls
208 Dill Pickles
209 Nut and Seed Butters
210 Steel Cut and Rolled Oat Oatmeal
210 Quinoa Hot Cereal
211 Broccoli Soup
212 Lentil and Greens Soup
212 Cheddar Cheese Whole Wheat Muffins
213 Watermelon and Arugula Salad
214 Corn Tortillas
215 Broccoli with Garlic and Walnuts
215 Nutty Raw Soft Tacos
216 Most Excellent Refried Beans
217 Rainbow Rolls
218 Vegetable Sushi Rolls
220 Tofu Scramble
221 Curried Sweet Potato Latkes
222 Frozen Ice Pop Favorites
223 Herbal Infused Water
224 Stevia Lemonade
224 Coconut Turmeric Smoothie

CALCULATIONS • 225

226 Macronutrient Calorie, Percentage, and Gram Calculations
228 MACRONUTRIENTS—What percentage is best for you?
230 BMI
231 BMR
232 Ideal Daily Water Intake

APPENDIX • 233

233 The Food Tree Nutrient Scroll
235 Girls BMI Percentiles
236 Boys BMI Percentiles
227 Body Mass Index Chart for Adults
238 References
246 About the Author

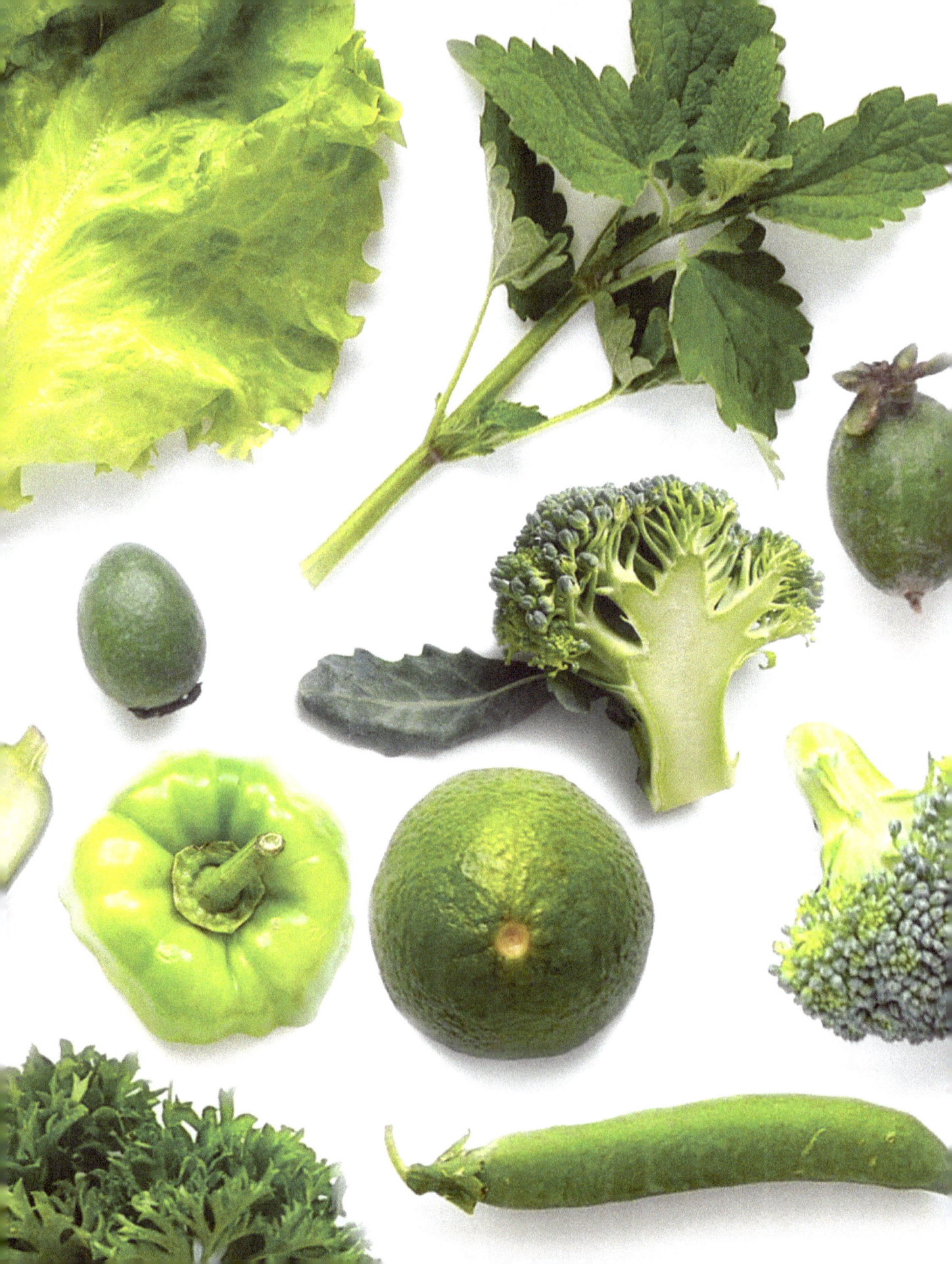

USER GUIDE TO THE FOOD TREE HOLISTIC NUTRITION AND WELLNESS CURRICULUM

The Food Tree Holistic Nutrition and Wellness Curriculum is designed to address the fundamentals of holistic nutrition in an easy to use format. I offer foundational lessons in holistic nutrition while providing more advanced materials for those who want to explore this topic on a deeper level. Each section is crafted with the utmost intention so that you can bring to your students a more engaging experience in learning about holistic nutrition.

The instructor can mix and match lessons from all of the sections, create intensive modules focusing on a specific area or topic, or teach the entirety of the materials over a more extended period of time.

GETTING STARTED

The Food Tree Curriculum has eight main sections that include:

1. The Introduction
2. The Five Food Groups
3. The Nine Nutrition Vampires
4. Physical Activities
5. Mindfulness Activities
6. Activities: Arts, Crafts, and Science Experiments
7. Recipes
8. Nutrient Calculations

Section 1 The Introduction

Read this section first to familiarize yourself with The Food Tree philosophy.

Section 2 The Five Food Groups

The lessons are categorized as being:

- Foundational—Just the basics
- Discovery—A little more in-depth
- Comprehensive—More advanced materials

The following sections are found in each lesson:

- Materials
- Goal(s)
- Objective(s)
- Activating Prior Knowledge
- Background Information
- Procedure(s)/Exercises
- Assessment(s)

Section 3 Nutrition Vampires

The Nutrition Vampire section focuses on nine specific ingredients or applications found in our food system that negatively impacts many, if not most, people's lives in some way. As such, it may be the most important of all the sections in The Food Tree Curriculum.

Section 4 Physical Activities

The Physical Activities Section focuses on physical activities that build a healthy body. The lessons and activities focus on restorative, strength training, and aerobic exercises.

Section 5 Mindfulness Activities

The Mindfulness Activities Section provides mindfulness-based practices, like writing in a gratitude journal, to enhance the lives of your students, their learning experience, and their well-being.

Section 6 Activities: Arts, Crafts, and Science Experiments

This section activates creativity, wonder, and exploration with its activities and will surely add to the fun and joy of learning about holistic nutrition.

Section 7 Recipes

Get tasting in the kitchen with this fun collection of plant-based, kid-tested, nutritious and delicious recipes.

Section 8 Calculations

This section is fun for the math enthusiast. Even if playing with numbers isn't your thing, the equations I have included are still useful and informative. They can be used with those students who are proficient at basic math, multiplication and division. Older students can engage more with using the BMI and BMR.

SAMPLE UNIT AND LESSON SEQUENCES

Unit 1 Introduction to The Food Tree and The Five Food Groups

The Food Tree Standards

The Food Tree Analogy

The Food Tree Visualization

Unit 2 Proteins Food Group

Introduction to the Proteins Food Group

Lesson: Getting to Know Proteins

Lesson: Serving Sizes and Daily Recommendations for Proteins

Lesson: Benefits and Function of Proteins

SUPPORT ACTIVITIES

Strength Training and Resistance Exercises

The Food Tree Decoupage Collage

Word Search—Power Proteins

Word Search—Nuts and Seeds

The "I Wonder" Exercise

Unit 3 Whole Grains Food Group

Introduction to the Whole Grains Food Group

Lesson: Getting to Know Grains

Lesson: Serving Sizes and Daily Recommendations for Whole Grains

Lesson: Benefits and Functions of Whole Grains

SUPPORT ACTIVITIES

Cardio/Aerobic Exercises

Word Search—Hello Whole Grains

Indian Corn Jewelry

Mirror Reflection Exercises

Grow Plants from Kitchen Scraps

Unit 4 Fats Food Group

Introduction to the Fats Food Group

Lesson: Getting to Know Fats

Lesson: Serving Sizes and Daily Recommendations for Fats

Lesson: Benefits and Functions of Fats

SUPPORT ACTIVITIES

Stretching Moves

Word Search—Fabulous Fats

Milk Color Burst Experiment

Positive Word Cloud

Unit 5 Vegetables Food Group

Introduction to the Vegetables Food Group

Lesson: Getting to Know Vegetables

Lesson: Serving Sizes and Daily Recommendations for Vegetables

Lesson: Benefits and Functions of Vegetables

SUPPORT ACTIVITIES

Yoga Poses

Word Search—Fruits and Vegetables

Grow Your Own Sprouts and Micro Greens

Plant Part Matching

Gratitude Journals and Ideas

Unit 6 Fruits Food Group

Introduction to the Fruits Food Group

Lesson: Getting to Know Fruits

Lesson: Serving Sizes and Daily Recommendations for Fruits

Lesson: Benefits and Functions of Fruits

SUPPORT ACTIVITIES

Grounding, Earthing, and Walking Barefoot

Draw, Sketch, Paint, and Illustrate Fruits and Vegetables

Taste the Rainbow Taste Test

Observing Oxidation

Thank a Farmer, Baker, and Cheese Maker

Unit 7 Nutrition Vampires

Introduction to The Nine Nutrition Vampires

Nutrition Vampires and FDA Approval

SUPPORT ACTIVITY

Nutrition Vampire Snack Attack

INTRODUCTION to THE FOOD TREE HOLISTIC NUTRITION and WELLNESS CURRICULUM

EAT LIKE A TREE!

Daily Recommended Servings

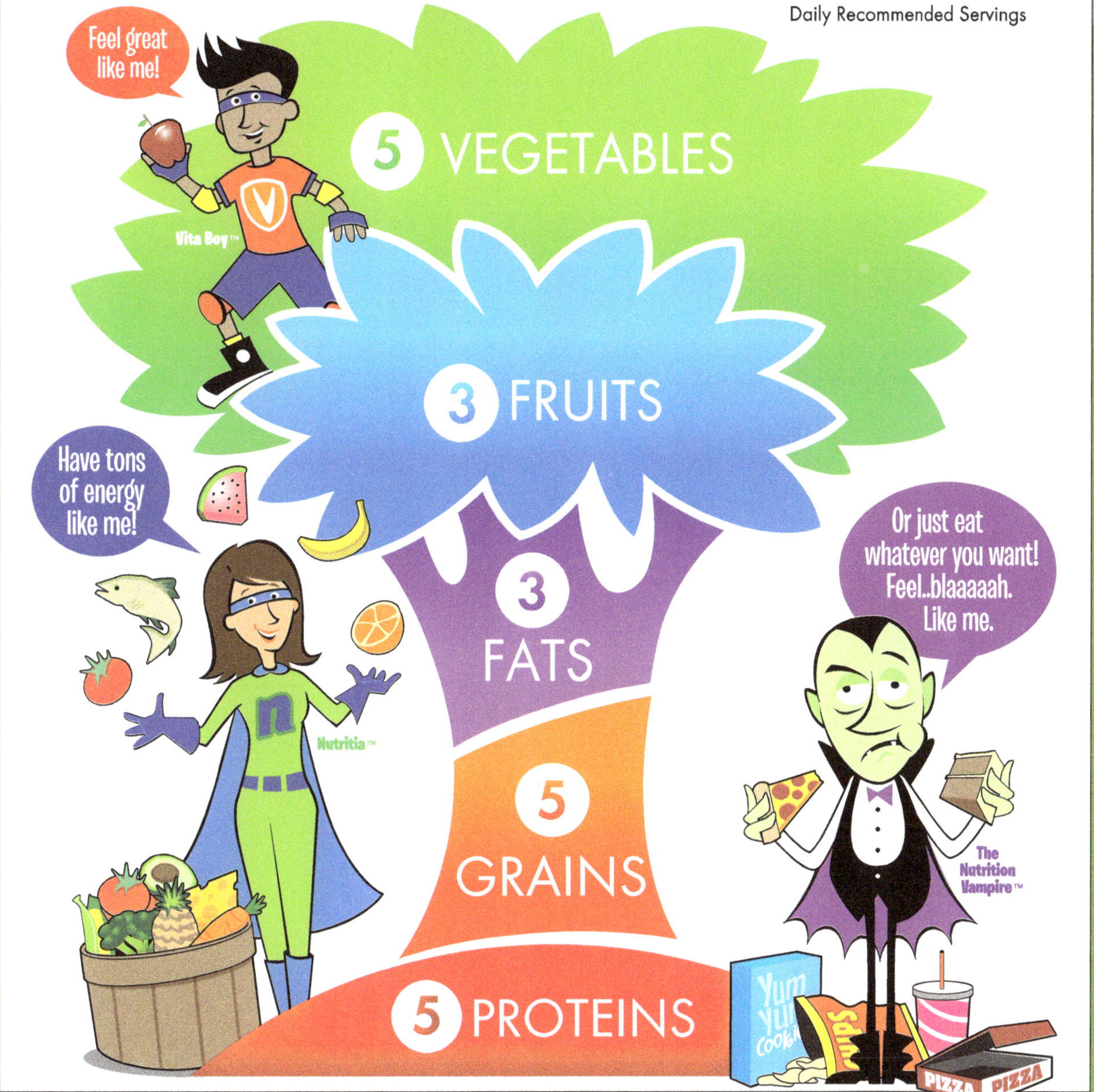

- 5 VEGETABLES
- 3 FRUITS
- 3 FATS
- 5 GRAINS
- 5 PROTEINS

Feel great like me! — Vita Boy™

Have tons of energy like me! — Nutritia™

Or just eat whatever you want! Feel..blaaaaah. Like me. — The Nutrition Vampire™

A GUIDE TO HOLISTIC NUTRITION FOR THE ENTIRE FAMILY

VEGETABLES
asparagus, artichokes, beets, broccoli, brussels sprouts, carrots, celery, collards, cucumber, eggplant, herbs, kale, onion, peas, peppers, potatoes, salad greens, sea vegetables, spinach, squash, tomatoes, yams

FRUITS
apples, bananas, blueberries, cherries, kiwi, lemons, mango, nectarines, oranges, papaya, peaches, pears, pineapple, plums, strawberries, watermelon

FATS
nuts/seeds; flax, walnut, pumpkin, fruit/oils; olive, avocado, coconut, dairy; butter, cheese, animal fats, fish/fish oil, eggs

GRAINS
amaranth (gf), barley, buckwheat (gf), corn (gf), millet (gf), oats, rice (gf), rye, quinoa (gf), spelt, sorghum, teff (gf), triticale, wheat (gf = gluten free)

PROTEINS
beans, legumes, nuts, seeds, dairy, meat, blue gree algae

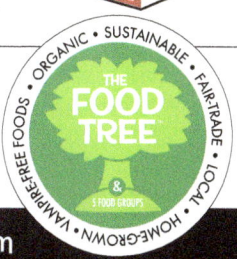

THE FOOD TREE & 5 FOOD GROUPS
ORGANIC · SUSTAINABLE · FAIR-TRADE · LOCAL · HOMEGROWN · VAMPIRE-FREE FOODS

Learn all about how to "Eat Like a Tree" to stay healthy at healthyfoodtree.com

HOLISTIC NUTRITION AND THE MIND, BODY, AND SOUL CONNECTION
Three Ingredients Needed for Optimal Health

The core of The Food Tree Holistic Nutrition philosophy bases itself on the foundation of Holistic Nutrition and the role the Mind, Body, and Soul have in a person's life. According to The National Association of Nutrition Professionals, the governing body for Certified Holistic Nutrition Practitioners:

> *"The philosophy of Holistic Nutrition is that one's health is an expression of the complex interplay between the physical and chemical, mental and emotional, as well as spiritual and environmental aspects of one's life and being."*

It is through this lens that allows people to gain perspective on the interconnectedness we have to our food, to the earth, and each other.

The Mind—Educate

The Mind approach supports an individual's quest for knowledge and intellectual understanding of their world around them. As such, I encourage you to stretch your students' minds for them to explore the fascinating world of food and holistic nutrition through their mental and cognitive aspects of themselves. The mind is the keeper of knowledge. And we know being knowledgeable is powerful! The Food Tree encourages children to make their own food choices. A solid background in nutrition will help people understand how diet, food-related issues, and human physiology impacts and affects their lives. A child educated in nutrition boosts their ability, possibility, and potential to be healthy and to thrive.

I encourage children to become critical thinkers. I want kids to be able to trust themselves in the decisions they make around food and eating. Because we know making choices about food is one of the most important decisions a person can make for themselves, when children get involved and take an interest in their diet, they will make the most educated choices! Even if that means eating the brownie!

By developing critical thinking skills, children become confident in how to eat delicious, quality, clean, and nutrient-dense foods. They learn how to navigate around the insidious amounts of junk and toxic foods, while not being manipulated by corrupt ads in media, in the world, or even through peer or family norms and pressure. We want our kids to ask themselves who they trust for information about food instead of being passive about their food choices.

Considering that more than 50 percent of America's youth suffer from some form of physical, mental, or chronic illness, I believe it is past time to shed light and create a viable path to correct this unfortunate trend.

- Children exercise less and have more screen time than ever before. The average American child experiences more than twenty-nine hours of screen time a week.
- The junk food industry spends over two billion dollars a year on advertising and marketing to young people.
- Children view more than 11,000 junk food commercials a year, which reinforce false, misleading, confusing information and messages. (1)

- Ninety-eight percent of packaged foods, high in salt, damaged fat, sugar, and artificial chemicals, are designed to be highly addictive.
- Exposing children as young as age three to packaged foods have a lasting negative impact on their brains, studies show. It is essential to retrain the brain and your taste buds away from the addictive flavors and chemicals found in processed foods.
- Forty percent of an American child's diet, and almost half of their daily calories, come from fast food. (2, 3)
- Only 1 in 5, or 20%, of children, eat the daily recommended amount of fruits and vegetables. (4)

The Body—Empower

Let's face it; we are physical beings. Whether we want to or not, we humans get just one chance to take care of this amazing earth vessel. The Physical Activities Section provides lessons that are all about empowering young students to engage in more physical activity in their lives. Not because they HAVE to, but because they find that connection to themselves makes them WANT to.

The Food Tree emphasizes one essential aspect of being physically active is to have fun. Knowing how to have fun is the easiest way to keep the body fit for life. Being in the sunshine every day is also important for growth and physical development. The Food Tree recognizes there are limitations to all living situations, so be creative and say yes to the possibility of being active.

The Food Tree focuses on three main areas of physical exercises: Strength Training, Cardio/Aerobic Exercise, and Restorative Activities and Exercises.

The Food Tree teaches how to listen to what the body needs. Counting calories and measuring food is one way to figure out what you need to eat. But a more long-term and natural way to figure that out is to combine your mind science-based knowledge while listening to the signals your body sends you. As an example, a craving is your body telling you that you need something. And what you crave might not always be food. It could be you need water, fresh air, personal connection, or sleep.

Other activities of being physical include the growing and cooking of food. That means encouraging kids to get busy in the kitchen and garden. Learning how to cook and grow food is a gift that will last a lifetime. These invaluable life skills are all excellent ways to empower your students to have a sense of joy and sacredness in the act of eating, growing, buying, preparing, and cooking food.

The Soul—Inspire

In the Mindfulness Activities Section, I explore the necessity of humans to be able to connect to their inner life. The Food Tree supports the importance of having quiet time during the day, especially for children. Having quiet time will develop in children the skill of being able to listen and to trust themselves. Then when they trust themselves, they learn that they are quite capable of making beneficial life choices that nobody else can decide for them. The Food Tree provides inspiring lessons that model every person is a gift to the world and that you are enough!

Also included are lessons on how people fit into and are all part of a larger ecosystem in the broader earth landscape. Knowing this is a way we can model for children how to think about more than just themselves. That what they do, and the choices they make, impact planetary health, wellbeing, and healing.

As well, I share the proven health benefits of expressing gratitude in ones' life. The Food Tree offers lessons on how to cultivate being more grateful, giving thanks, and giving back.

THE FOOD TREE HOLISTIC NUTRITION CURRICULUM
Philosophy, Guidelines, and Standards

CREATE A DIET AS UNIQUE AS YOU
CLIMB THE FOOD TREE
GATHER YOUR NUTRIENTS

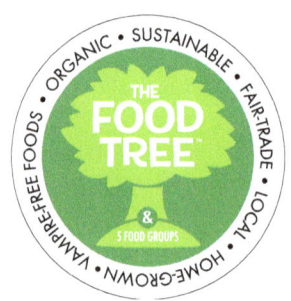

The Food Tree Holistic Nutrition Curriculum and Wellness Guide intends to be an educational, empowering, and inspiring tool. Its design supports an individual's unique diet, food preferences, and nutritional needs. The foundation of The Food Tree is rooted in the fact that you can create a unique diet based on acquiring the necessary nutrients vital for human survival from the three macronutrients: proteins, carbohydrates, and fats. From that base, you can choose to eat as a vegan, vegetarian, omnivore, gluten-free, or any combination of diets as needed to support your optimal health.

The Three Macronutrients

Proteins—Animal and Plant-Based Proteins

Carbohydrates—Fruits, Vegetables, Whole Grains, Legumes

Fats – Fat-containing Foods, Fats, and Oils

The Food Tree breaks the macronutrients down into Five Food Groups that are easy to remember because it's based on the image of a tree. The Food Tree!

The Food Tree's Five Food Groups

The Fruit: Fruits

The Leaves: Vegetables

The Branches: Healthy Fats

The Trunk: Whole Grains

The Roots: Proteins

Food Literacy

The Food Tree encourages and teaches children to become aware of the who, what, where, how, why, and when, of foods and how these relate to their life and life around them. And as a part of this, The Food Tree recommends that we make conscious decisions and choices around food. The Food Tree teaches the importance of knowing how and having the tools to take care of oneself and the environment. And thus, we have standards.

The Food Tree Standards

Most everyone has standards they strive to live by. The Food Tree Guide has standards, as well. These standards reflect the utmost respect for you, the earth, and our quest to create a healthy future. Yes, idealistic. Yes, optimistic. Yes, I believe we must create the world in which we want to live.

The Food Tree standards suggest you buy, grow, prepare, and eat as best as you can and as often as possible organic, sustainable, fair-trade, local, homemade, and Nutrition Vampire-free foods. What does that mean?

ORGANIC

The USDA (United States Department of Agriculture) Organic is a term used to label food set around specific strict standards. Farms and fields can also be certified organic by other authorized verifying agents and labeling organizations like California Certified Organic Farms and Oregon Tilth. Farms and agricultural operations go through a rigorous process to prove they adhere to conserving biodiversity, which includes using only approved treatments and protecting natural resources. (1)

For instance, it is prohibited for an organic farmer to use genetic engineering or genetically modified organisms as a seed or feed. (2) Non-GMO Project Verified is a non-GMO certification organization that farms work with to adhere to their standards. To be certified organic, the product must be produced using the National List of Allowed and Prohibited Substances that comply with USDA organic regulations. (3)

As an example, farmers raise poultry without the use of antibiotics. It is not permitted to treat milk and dairy cows with growth hormones, rBGH, nor can their diet contain animal byproducts. Fruits and vegetables use natural fertilizers and pest management techniques. For organic meat, the label would say "USDA Processed Verified Grass-Fed" or "Grass-fed Approved."

SUSTAINABLE

The word sustainable means "capable of being maintained at a steady level without exhausting natural resources or causing severe ecological damage." Therefore, I encourage people to take into consideration the impact their food choices and purchasing habits have on their local communities, as well as the impact they may make on a larger global scale.

FAIR TRADE

Fair Trade was set up as a global business practice that aims to support responsible companies, empower farmers, support workers, especially in developing countries, support fishers, and protect the environment. In the United States, you can apply for a Fair Trade Certificate from a third-party certification process. This agency sets standards and adheres to guidelines for the way crops are produced and goods sold. (4)

According to TransFair USA, a fair-trade labeling firm, fair trade practices are:

- Fair prices for farmers and decent working and living conditions for workers
- Engaged in direct trade with farmers, bypassing intermediaries
- A free association of workers and co-ops, with structures for democratic decision-making
- Having access to capital
- Sustainable agricultural practices including restricted use of agrochemicals

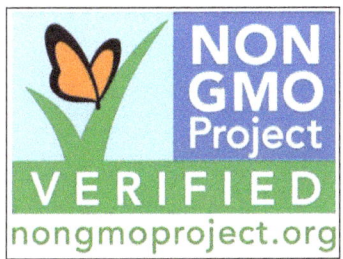
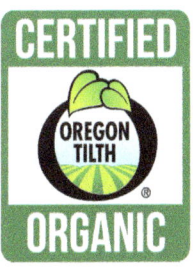
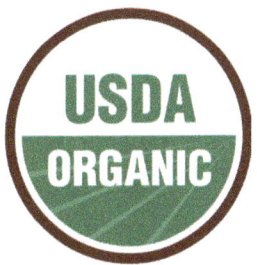
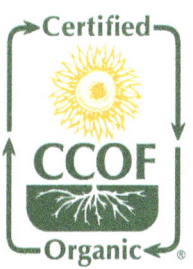

LOCAL

The local concept refers to buying your food as close to where you live and work as possible. For some people, they strive to shop and support local farms and growers from within a 100-mile radius of where they live. The concept of local also includes the notion of eating in season. For instance, if you live on the east coast in the United States, forgo buying tomatoes in the middle of winter from Mexico.

It is easy to go local. Some ways of eating more locally include:

- Growing a kitchen garden at your school, work, or home
- Joining a CSA (Community Supported Agriculture) program
- Shopping at your local farm stand and farmers market
- Buying from local grocery stores or national chains that support local farms and vendors

HOMEMADE

Homemade is a term that means exactly as it sounds. The idea is for people to learn how to make food from scratch and to start cooking at home again. Yes, like back in the old days. *The really old days.* We do encourage you and your students to engage in the art of cooking, baking, sprouting, and fermenting. Learning to make your own bread, pasta, salad dressing, fermented vegetables, sprouts, and jams are all incredibly empowering activities to know how to do. Gather the cooking skills you already have and expand upon them. Most often, food is healthier when made at home or school with pure, wholesome, and natural ingredients.

Nutrition Vampire-Free Foods

The Food Tree teaches kids early on about foods that may contain harmful ingredients and the health consequences of eating them. There is no sense in hiding the truth about the ingredients that are in food from our children. Talking about Nutrition Vampire Foods can seem like you are telling them about the latest horror movie you just saw, especially when discussing the meat industry's factory farm practices. So, use discretion on the age appropriateness of certain topics.

I have found that children WANT to eat healthy, nutritious foods. At least most of the time! Kids who are poorly nourished don't feel well. When kids improve their diets and start to feel better, there is no turning them back. Oftentimes older children or young adults may feel sad about the years lost being unhealthy from eating a Standard American Diet.

THE NINE NUTRITION VAMPIRES

The Food Tree identifies NINE Nutrition Vampires that can be omitted entirely from our food system and your diets. See the Nutrition Vampire section for a more in-depth look into these vampires.

1. Artificial Colors
2. Artificial Flavors
3. Preservatives
4. Processed, Refined, and Artificial Sugars
5. Partially Hydrogenated Oils and Damaged Fats
6. Genetically Modified Organisms (GMOs)
7. Herbicides, Fungicides, and Pesticides (Glyphosates)
8. Impure, Chlorinated, and Fluoridated Water
9. Your Vampire (particular food, thoughts, action, behavior)

USE THIS ACROSTIC AS A POINT OF MOTIVATION.

V	**Void of Nutritional Value**—nutrient-poor foods
A	**Adulterated**—foods altered from their natural DNA form
M	**Manufactured**—foods packaged, canned, or frozen using unhealthy ingredients
P	**Processed**—foods made with chemical ingredients or changed by chemical processing
I	**Impulsive**—foods and ingredients that trigger cravings like sugar and salt
R	**Robs Health**—foods that steal, deplete, and take nutrients away from the body
E	**Empty**—foods that leave you feeling dissatisfied, guilty, and regretful

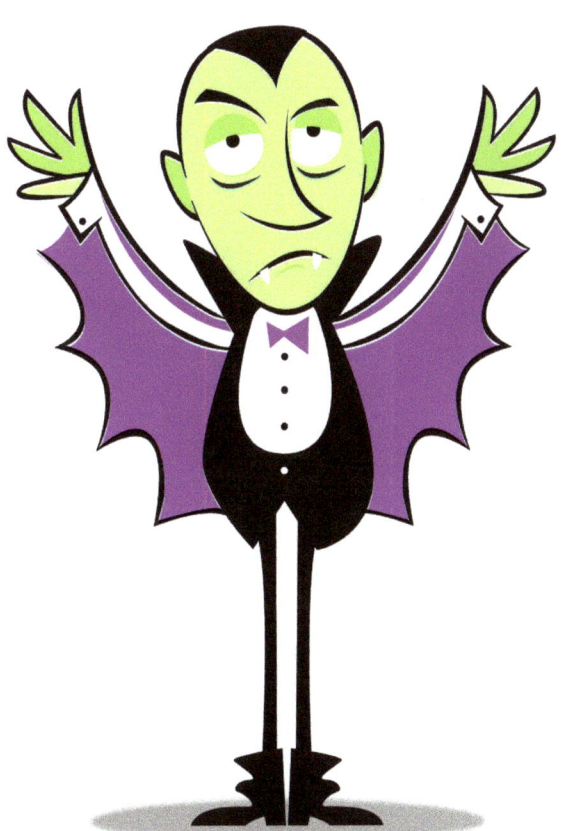

THE FOOD TREE ANALOGY

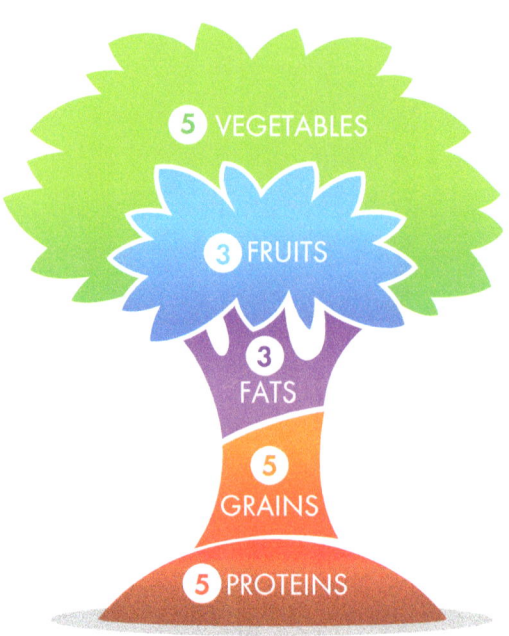

The Food Tree Guide uses the image of a tree as its teaching model because all people can identify with a tree. It is most notably relatable as it is a living thing. I encourage you and your students to imagine yourself like a tree when learning about the Five Food Groups.

Proteins—The Roots

The Roots represent the Protein Food Group on The Food Tree. The roots of a healthy tree are grounded securely in the earth. Stable and secure, roots keep a whole tree standing firmly. Imagine that eating protein foods are like the roots of a tree as they both create the foundation of a physical structure.

Whole Grains—The Trunk

The Trunk represents the Whole Grain Food Group on The Food Tree. Imagine symbolically that the tree trunk is like the trunk of your body. Eating whole grains keeps the trunk of our body flexible but always standing strong and well balanced.

Healthy Fats—The Branches

The Branches represent the Fats Food Group on The Food Tree. Imagine that the fats you eat are like the branches of a big tree. The branches reach out far and wide, creating the structure for the whole canopy. Branches bring nutrients to the leaves and the fruit, and are like fats that make up every cell in the body and provide nutrients to every cell in our body.

Vegetables—The Leaves

The Leaves represent the Vegetables on The Food Tree. The shiny, healthy leaves reflect a well-nourished tree and its vital life-giving energy like the health and vitality a person will receive when eating a diet rich in vegetables.

Fruit—The Fruit

The Fruit represents the Fruit Food Group on the Food Tree. Metaphorically, fruit is symbolic of fertility. Fruit bear seeds that make new plants and trees. Like fruit, fully nourished people have enough to share with their families, communities, and the world. Fruits represent being creative, generous, and abundant.

YOU AS A TREE VISUALIZATION

Guide your students on a journey to visit their tree. Ask your students to sit down and get into a comfortable position. Ask them to close their eyes and take a few, slow, deep, and relaxing cleansing breaths.

A Vision Walk to Your Tree

Say to them...

Imagine you are walking down a wide dirt path. The path is lined with trees. There is a warm breeze gently blowing. Up ahead, you see a wood fence. You walk towards the fence and you see a gate. You reach for the gate. You open the gate and walk under an archway covered with flowering vines. You walk into this space that feels so comfortable and welcoming. You feel safe and at home. You start to notice the surroundings. It is a beautiful place.

What do you see?

Are there mountains? A valley? A lake? A desert? An ocean? A backyard? A hill?

You look around and right in front of you see a tree, a healthy and vibrant tree. It is a one-of-a-kind, unique, and extraordinary tree.

What does this tree look like? What kinds of leaves does it have? Are they large and shiny, or are they small and make dappled shade? What sort of trunk does it have? Is the tree deeply rooted? Can you see the roots extending from the ground? What about the branches, do they reach out far, or do they hang gently and sway in the breeze? Does this tree bear abundant, deliciously sweet fruit? Or nuts? Does it have flowers? Is it tall? Can it bend easily in the wind? Does this tree prefer sunshine or does it prefer shade? Does it stand alone or is it part of a grove? Notice all the trees are different from one another. Even the ones in the same family are different. There are no two trees alike. Just like you! No one is exactly like you.

Say hello to the tree and give it a big hug. As you stand next to the tree, imagine yourself as a "Tree." With deeply grounded roots, a strong, flexible trunk, far-reaching branches, shiny leaves, and abundant fruit. Now imagine that you are this tree, and you are healthy and thriving just like it is. Like the tree, you come with your own set of unique needs. Your tree is a reminder to be kind to yourself, to take care of yourself, and to love yourself. You feel that this tree is deeply connected to its surrounding environment. This tree belongs to the whole community and feels unconditionally loved.

Take a few deep breaths with your tree.

In and out.
In and out.
In and out.

Now it is time to say goodbye to your tree. Start walking back towards the fence, and back under the archway and through the gate, and back down the path dotted with trees.

Your tree is always with you.

You can return to your tree any time you need to.

Now slowly open your eyes.

*Connect the "You as A Tree" Visualization to The Food Trees' Five Food Groups Analogy.

THE FOOD TREE CHARACTERS

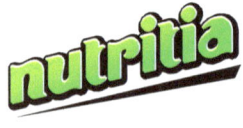

Nutritia is a strong-willed young woman who is on a mission to share nutrition knowledge with kids and families. She and her family live in a friendly community where they crash-landed from another planet. They all love growing, cooking, and eating delicious, nutritious, healthy food. Her family commits to living a green lifestyle on planet Earth. While her parents are busy being nerdy scientists geeking out on how amazing Planet Earth is, Nutritia is engaged in her endeavors. She befriended a neighborhood boy named Vita Boy. Well, his real name is Kevin. They love to hang out and go on all kinds of fascinating adventures and are always getting into all sorts of exciting antics, usually related to food and eating.

Vita Boy loves spending his Sundays cooking with his Abuela, grandmother. He enjoys the rest of his time being curious about nature and taking care of the environment. He is a scientist like Nutritia's parents. His life was altered forever when Nutritia and her family moved in next door. Or, actually, landed next door, you could say!

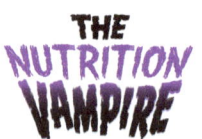

The Nutrition Vampire is madly in love with junk food. He can't get enough and, as such, he is always getting in his own way. He is moody. He is clumsy. He is silly. He often suffers with belly aches from his lousy food and lifestyle choices. So sometimes he is grumpy. But Nutrition Vampire does love to chuckle when he plays with his pet ant who eats the crumbs he leaves behind. He lives in an empty cereal box on a hill on the outskirts of town with empty soda cans and chip bags littering his yard.

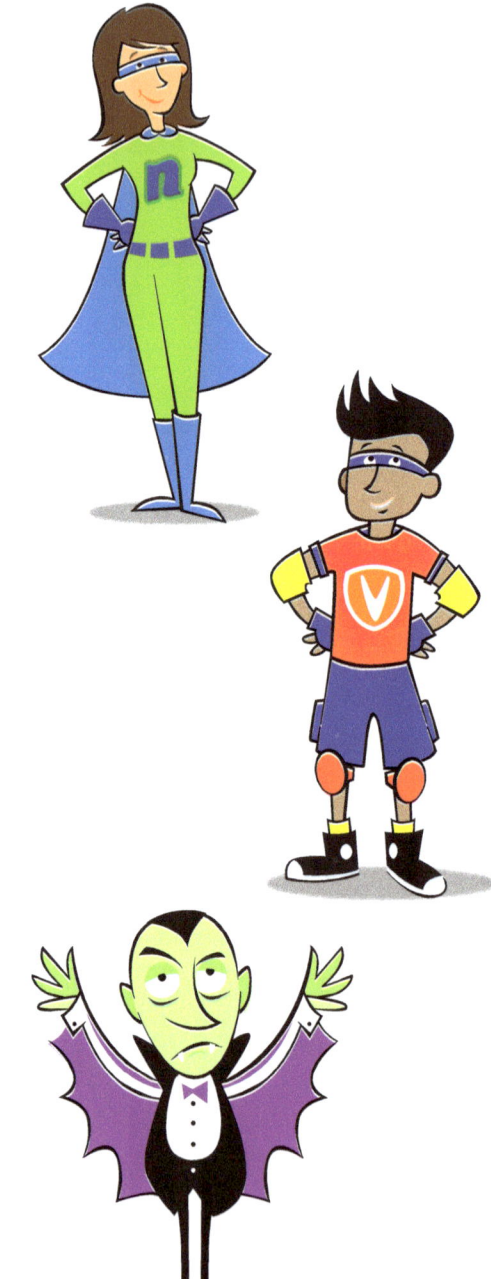

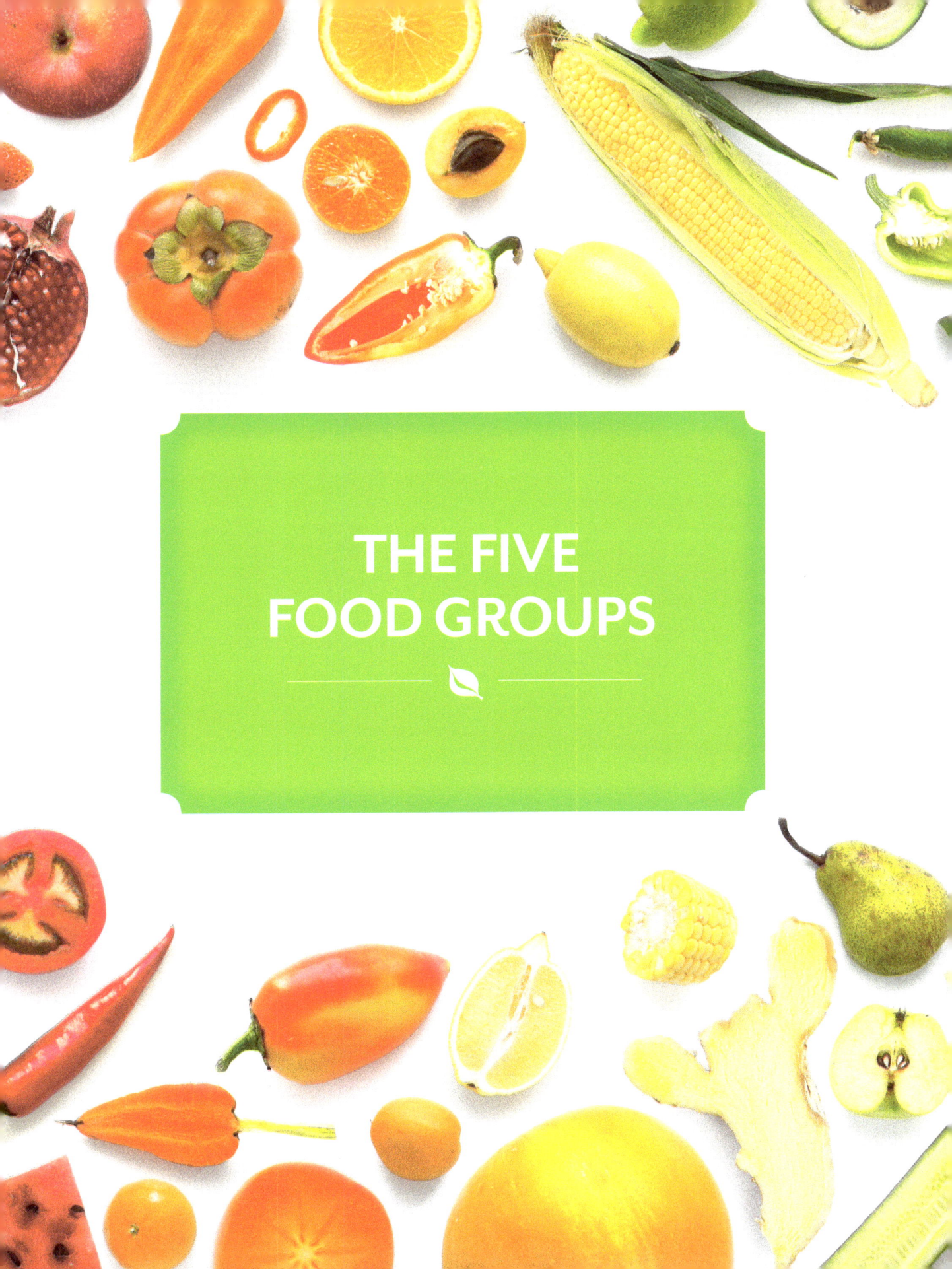

THE FIVE FOOD GROUPS

CREATE A DIET AS UNIQUE AS YOU!

The foundational philosophy of The Food Tree is rooted in the fact that people must gather all of the necessary nutrients they need from the three macronutrients.

The Three Macronutrients

Proteins—Animal and Plant-based Proteins

Carbohydrates—Fruits, Vegetables, Whole Grains, Legumes

Fats—Fat-containing Foods and Oils

The Food Tree takes the three macronutrient groups and breaks them down into Five Food Groups. It is easy to remember the food groups because it is based on the image of a tree. The Food Tree! The Food Tree is unique because we celebrate eating from all of The Five Food Groups. Each of The Five Food Groups offers different and essential nutrients, phytonutrients, fiber, vitamins, and minerals that are important to include in a well-balanced diet.

Please take into consideration the nutritional needs of an individual change often, usually daily and weekly, and most certainly over an entire lifetime. The diet for sure will change during the year, during periods of illness or stress, during sports training, while traveling, in growth spurts, recovering from an injury, while pregnant and nursing, and in puberty or old age. So, The Food Tree supports and encourages a person to eat according to their unique needs.

Please note that The Food Tree reflects the understanding that not everyone likes every type of food. People have preferences, likes, and dislikes. That is why one of my goals is to encourage people to "Create A Diet as Unique as You!"

THE FOOD TREE'S FIVE FOOD GROUPS

	DAILY SERVING SUGGESTION	% OF DAILY CALORIES
The Fruit: Fruits	3	10%
The Leaves: Vegetables	5	20%
The Branches: Healthy Fats	3	25%
The Trunk: Whole Grains	5	20%
The Roots: Proteins	5	25%

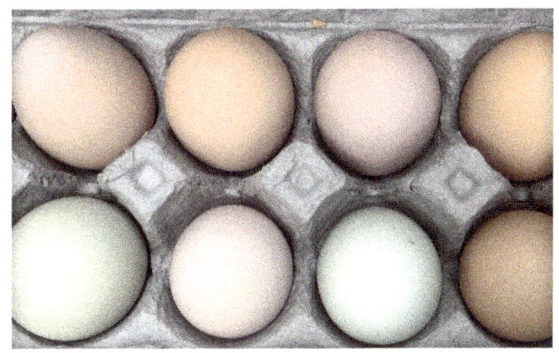

INTRODUCTION TO THE PROTEINS FOOD GROUP
The Building Blocks of Life

THE FOOD TREE ANALOGY
The Roots represent the Proteins Food Group on The Food Tree. The roots of a healthy tree are grounded securely in the Earth. Stable and secure, roots to keep a whole tree standing firmly. Imagine that eating protein foods are like the roots of a tree as they both create the foundation of a physical structure.

DAILY RECOMMENDED SERVING SUGGESTION: 5
25%–30% of daily calories
Energy source, protein, four calories per gram

SOURCES OF PROTEIN FOODS
Eat a combination of the following:
Beans, Peas, and Lentils ~ 2-3 servings a day
Nuts and Seeds ~ 1-2 servings a day
Animal Proteins ~ 0-3 servings a day

WHAT ARE PROTEINS?

Proteins are one of the three macronutrients that are found in plant and animal foods. The other two macronutrients are carbohydrates and fats. Proteins are essential to include in a healthy human diet.

There are two types of protein foods: plant-based proteins and animal-based proteins. Protein containing foods come from a variety of sources and are made up of different chemicals called amino acids. There are 22 types of amino acids. Eight of the amino acids are referred to as essential amino acids because you must eat and obtain them from the foods you eat. (1) The body can make the other 14 amino acids.

Proteins execute vitally crucial tasks and are critical components for performing dozens of actions including creating the body's physical structure, the building of the immune system, and the formation of your thoughts, emotions, and moods. (2)

FOUNDATIONAL

Lesson: Getting to Know Proteins— Plant-Based and Animal-Based

➤ MATERIALS
- Food Tree Magnetic Board
- Examples of protein foods. Use real food, food packaging, or pictures.
- Food Tree Nutrient Scroll, located in the appendix

➤ GOALS
Learn about the variety of protein sources and understand the health benefits of eating a diet rich in quality protein food.

➤ OBJECTIVES
- To identify three types of proteins foods
- To determine if a protein food comes from an animal or plant-based source

➤ ACTIVATING PRIOR KNOWLEDGE
Ask your students if they can name different kinds of protein foods. Ask your students to name the ones they eat the most. Ask your students if they think including protein foods in their diet is essential. Why or why not? Do they eat both animal-based and plant-based protein foods?

BACKGROUND INFORMATION

Protein Food Sources
Proteins are available from both animal and plant sources.

Plant-Based Proteins
- Beans: adzuki bean, black bean, garbanzo bean, kidney bean, pinto bean, soybean (tofu, tempeh, milk)
- Lentils: brown, green, red, orange
- Peas: green peas; either dried or split peas
- Nuts: almonds, Brazil nuts, cashews, peanuts, filberts, macadamia nuts, pine nuts, pistachio nuts, walnuts
- Seeds: flax seeds, hemp seeds, pumpkin seeds, sesame seeds, sunflower seeds
- Whole grains: corn, oats, millet, quinoa, rice, seitan (wheat gluten)
- Vegetables—trace amounts
- Micro-proteins: microalgae, spirulina, chlorella, blue-green algae, bee pollen, barley greens, whey, nutritional yeast, cereal grasses

Animal-Based Proteins
- Eggs
- Dairy: milk, cheese, yogurt, kefir, cottage cheese, sour cream
- Fermented dairy
- Meat: beef, pork, bison, goat, lamb, elk, venison
- Poultry/Foul: chicken, duck, turkey, quail, Cornish hen
- Fish and seafood: salmon, haddock, cod, tuna, mackerel, sardines, shrimp, scallops, clams

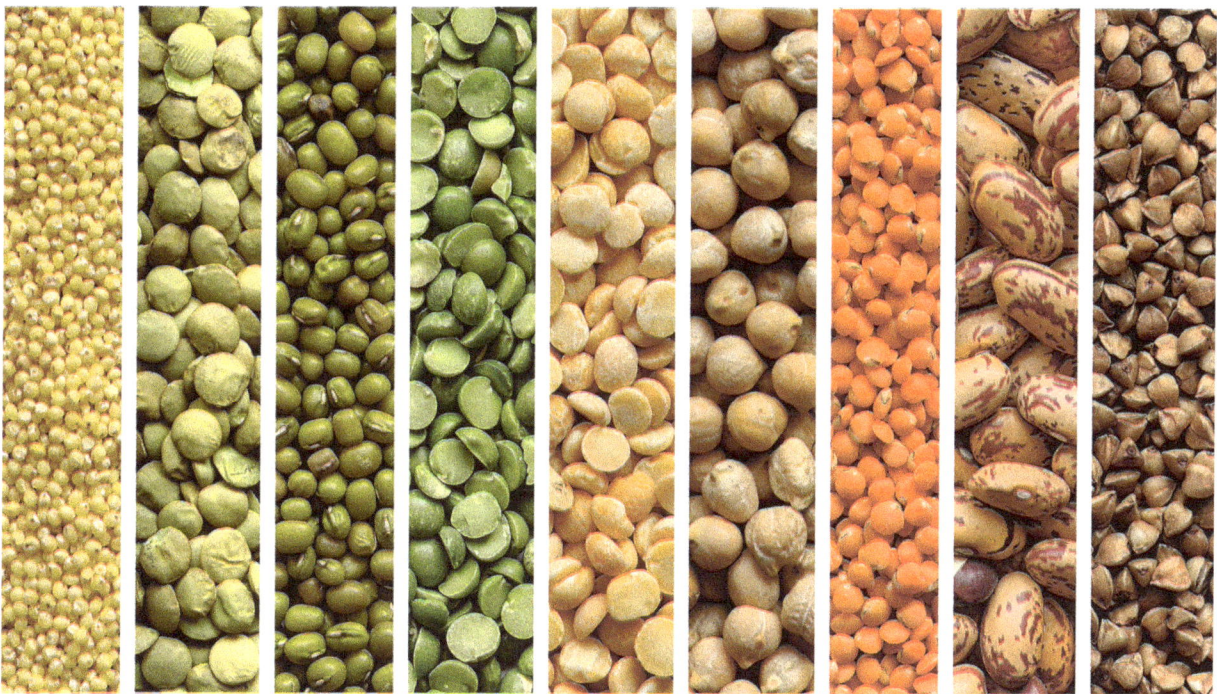

➤ Procedure 1
SORTING

1. Distribute a variety of protein food props to groups of students. Use empty food containers, pictures from magazines, or images from the internet.
2. Ask if the picture shows a plant or animal-based protein.

➤ Procedure 2
LABELING

Provide students with a Food Tree template handout. Ask them to label the roots with protein and color the roots red.

1. Ask the following question. "What is an example of a protein?"
2. Display the chart with animal protein and plant protein. Ask the following question. "Which category would _____ go in?" Refer to the list of protein foods.
3. Give students a list of the animal and plant protein food examples. Students are to identify three plant and three animal protein examples from the list and write it on their Food Tree handout.

Assessment

Discuss the insights your students have about categorizing proteins.

FOUNDATIONAL

Lesson: Serving Sizes and Daily Recommendations for Proteins

➤ **MATERIALS**
- The Food Tree Magnetic Board
- Examples of protein foods. Use real food, food packaging, or pictures.
- Measuring tools
- Protein Log Sheet
- The Food Tree Daily Food Journal, located in the Activities Section
- The Food Tree Nutrient Scroll, located in the Calculations section

➤ **GOAL**

Understand what the serving sizes and daily recommendations are for proteins.

➤ **OBJECTIVE**
- To explain what the appropriate serving sizes are for proteins
- To demonstrate an ability to choose proper portions of plant-based and animal-based protein foods according to an individuals' unique dietary needs

➤ **ACTIVATING PRIOR KNOWLEDGE**

Ask students what they think a portion size looks like and how many portions of proteins are recommended to eat in one day.

Action Item! Show The Food Tree Nutrient Scroll.

BACKGROUND INFORMATION

The Food Tree Protein Recommendations

DAILY SERVING SUGGESTION: 5

25%-30% of daily calories

Energy source, macronutrient protein, four calories per gram

The five servings will be a combination of the following:

- Beans, Peas, and Lentils ~ 2-3 servings a day
- Nuts and Seeds ~ 1-2 servings a day
- Animal Proteins ~ 0-3 servings a day (adjust to suit your philosophy and health needs)

Take into account the actual amount of protein foods eaten as well as a person's height, weight, age, caloric needs, and activity level. (1)

Other factors to consider in choosing your protein food include:

- The balance of Essential Amino Acids (EAA) to Non-Essential Amino Acids (NEAA)
- The quantity and quality of protein eaten
- The efficiency of absorption in the digestive tract
- Person's daily physical and mental activity levels
- The season
- Illness or sickness
- Pregnant, breastfeeding, menses
- Before and after surgery
- During periods of stress—psychological or physical

Choose Quality Plant-Based Proteins

NUTS AND SEEDS

Eat one serving of nuts and seeds a day. Add nuts and seeds to your pasta and salads. Almond butter and peanut butter are hearty protein foods that are easy to incorporate into many snacks and meals.

- Make nut butters and almond milk.

BEANS

Try to eat at least one serving of beans a day. Put hummus on crackers or celery. Try black bean soup or minestrone soup using garbanzo beans and navy beans. Make it a habit to buy beans in the bulk food section and make them from scratch.

SOY FOODS

Soy foods, like tofu and fermented tempeh and miso, can be an incredibly healthy foods to include in your diet, especially if you are vegan or vegetarian. In particular, fermented soy offers many positive health benefits. Fermented foods feed the beneficial bacteria in the gut and will support the microbiome ecosystem.

However, 93% of soy grown in the U.S. is GMO soy. Studies show that GMOs are linked with adverse health effects. Risks associated with GMOs are heightened because farmers use the genetically engineered RoundUp Ready soybean that is resistant to the highly carcinogenic and disease-causing glyphosate. (3) To some, genetic engineering uses sound science, but those at The Food Tree prefer to use the Precautionary Principle, "avoid until proven safe."

- Add tofu and soy milk to your meals.
- Enjoy fermented soy products like tempeh, miso, and natto.
- Add baked tofu to a sandwich.

SUPERFOODS CHLORELLA AND SPIRULINA

Superfoods such as blue-green algae that have notable amounts of protein, are a rich source of minerals. A super way to incorporate this superfood into your day is simply to add a teaspoon or two to your water.

Choose Quality Meat and Dairy Foods

- Keep hard-boiled eggs in the fridge.
- Enjoy fermented dairy, like kefir and yogurt, to support gut health.
- Buy grass-fed and pasture-raised meat, chickens, and eggs.

When it comes to eating and buying meat or any animal products, I encourage students to pay attention to the quality of the product and to avoid meat, egg, and dairy foods with preservatives, hormones, additives, curing chemicals, and pesticides used in it. Thankfully, there are many quality and healthy types of meat and dairy to choose from. I suggest purchasing from ranchers and farmers who are doing the right thing by raising and slaughtering their animals in the healthiest way possible.

Someone who has been doing just that, using grass-based farming practices for over four decades, is Joel Salatin, owner of Polyface Farms. Not only is Farmer Salatin a leader in the field of sustainable animal husbandry, but he is also an educator who inspires others to raise their awareness of the environmental and health impact of eating meat and how to do it responsibly.

For the safest meat, always choose grass-fed beef over grain-fed beef. Cattle fed natural grass offers more omega 3 essential fatty acids. A typical diet for commercially raised beef fed in a massive feed-lot are grains and soy. A grain-based diet is associated with an increase in weight in humans and having a higher exposure to the toxic herbicide, glyphosate, found in RoundUp. Herbicides like glyphosates are sprayed on the grains that are fed to the animals. (2)

Dairy cows are also injected with rBGH (recombinant Bovine Growth Hormone) to increase their milk supply. The increase in milk often causes mastitis, an infection, which leads the cows needing anti-biotics. Choose only organic, rBGH (recombinant Bovine Growth Hormone)-free dairy products.

What other ideas do students have on getting the best and healthiest sources of protein foods? Share your thoughts with your classmates and your community.

➤ Procedure 1
SERVING SIZES

1. Reveal and discuss the list of the recommended serving sizes of protein foods.
2. Show examples of protein servings sizes. Use real food, models, or pictures.
3. For instance, show your students what a serving size of walnuts looks like in a bowl. Or explain a serving of black beans, tofu, eggs, chicken, meat, or fish.

How does this compare to the number of protein foods a student would typically eat?

➤ Procedure 2
MEAL PLANNING—POWERFUL PROTEINS!

Have students create a day's worth of what eating five servings of proteins looks like on a meal planning sheet. Students write down how they will prepare each serving. Have students include recipes and nutrition facts for an extra challenge.

Or have students use an outline of The Food Tree. Students can write the foods on The Roots of the Food Tree image. Students can also draw or cut and paste pictures from food magazines and glue onto The Food Tree.

Sample Meal Plan Ideas: Five servings of protein foods a day

Breakfast—Tofu scramble

Snack—Walnuts

Lunch—Yogurt, chicken

Snack—Hard-boiled eggs

Dinner—Pinto bean burrito

SERVING SIZE EXAMPLES FOR PROTEINS

For serving size estimates for children, use the size of their palm as a serving.

BEANS, PEAS, AND LENTILS ~ 2–3 SERVINGS A DAY

Serving examples:
- ½ cup cooked dried beans, peas, or lentils
- ¼ cup hummus
- 1 cup or 2–3 oz. baked, sautéed, fresh tofu
- 1 cup of soy milk
- 3 ounces or ½ cup tempeh
- ⅓ cup seitan

NUTS AND SEEDS ~ 1–2 SERVINGS A DAY

Serving examples:
- 2 tablespoons–¼ cup walnuts, almonds, sunflower seeds
- 2 tablespoons nut or seed butter (almond, cashew, peanut, tahini)
- 1 cup almond milk, rice milk
- 1 cup hemp milk

ANIMAL-BASED PROTEINS ~ 0–3 SERVINGS A DAY

Serving examples:
- 3–4 ounces meat, chicken, fish (check Seafood Watch for the latest safety and sustainability information)
- ½–1 can tuna (once a month or less)
- 1 cup of milk
- 1 cup of yogurt
- ¾ cup cottage cheese
- ½ cup shredded cheese
- 2 whole eggs

*Vegetables and grains do contain small amounts of amino acids.

➤ Procedure 3

KEEP A PROTEIN FOOD JOURNAL

Provide students with a Protein Log Sheet. On the log write across the top: "Date, Plant-Based Protein, Animal-Based Protein, Serving Size, From Home, From School, From a Restaurant." Down the left side, write a list of protein foods. Ask students to keep the journal for one week. Explore data findings: What were the most common sources of proteins eaten? Record the student responses on a big wall chart. You can do this anonymously to protect the children's privacy.

Assessment

- What have students learned from looking at their diets compared to The Food Tree recommendations? Students can take this lesson a step further and calculate the number of proteins (in grams) that they are eating every day.

- Have students look at the list of protein foods they wrote down at the beginning of the lesson. Ask the following question: Are you eating plant-based or more quality animal proteins more often? Are you eating appropriate serving sizes? What changes have you, or can you make to your diets?

- Record the responses on the chart.

- Ask students to write down the changes they could make. Challenge them to implement these changes, even if it's just one meal at a time.

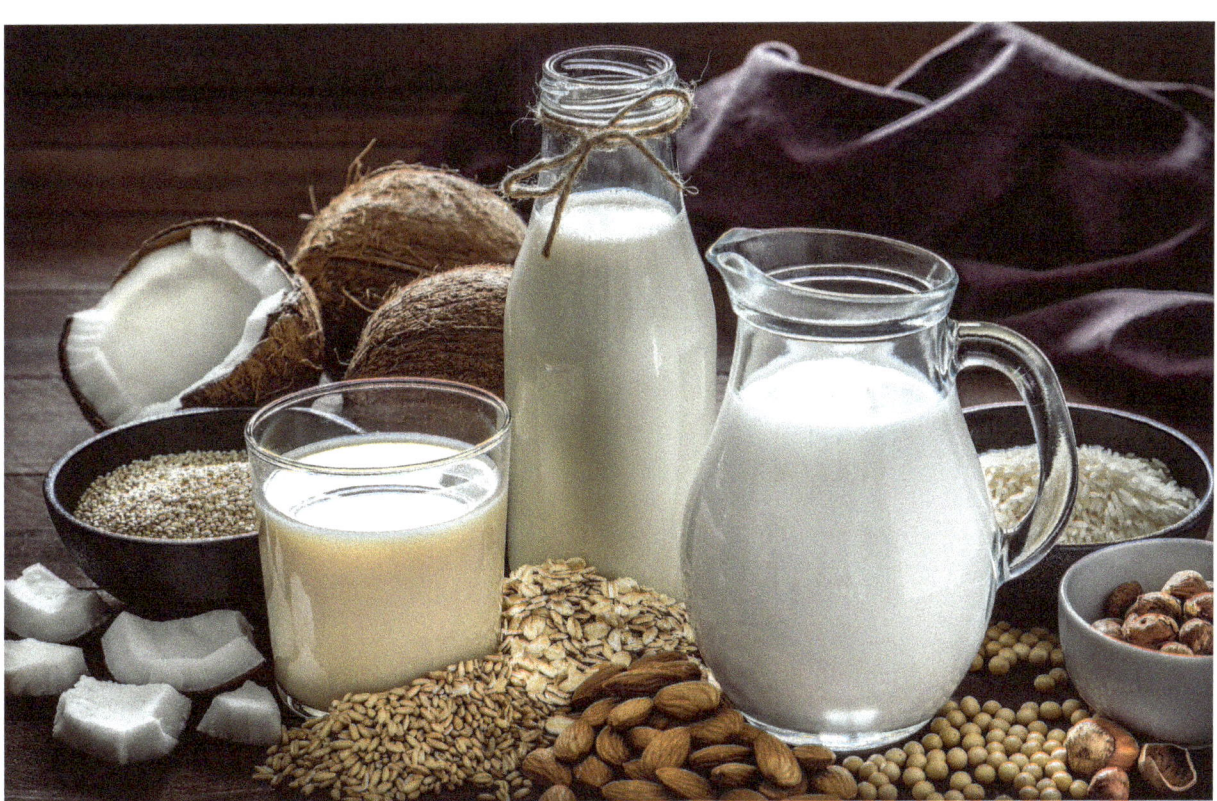

FOUNDATIONAL

Lesson: Benefits and Functions of Protein Foods

➤ MATERIALS
- Food Tree Magnetic Board
- Images or a model showing human muscles

➤ GOAL
Understand the many health benefits of eating a diet rich in quality protein foods.

➤ OBJECTIVE
- To explain three benefits and functions protein foods provide the body

➤ ACTIVATING PRIOR KNOWLEDGE
Ask students how and why they think protein foods are helpful and necessary for good health.

BACKGROUND INFORMATION

Talk with students about the role protein foods have in their health. The Food Tree recommends eating five servings of protein foods a day.

Benefits and Functions of Protein Foods

Proteins are hard-working, high-demand nutrients that are used continually for dozens of critical processes. They nourish, support, build, and provide for us in innumerable ways. The range of protein functions spans form nourishing, supporting, and building the foundation of the human body to supporting the formation of a person's thoughts, emotions, and moods. (1)

Proteins break down during digestion into smaller parts called amino acids. Amino acid molecules are absorbed directly into the bloodstream via the gut or small intestine.

GROWTH, DEVELOPMENT, AND REPAIR OF ALL BODY TISSUE

Proteins are responsible for the construction, repair, and maintenance of all body tissue. Protein provides the structure of the skin, nails, cell membranes, blood, organs, tendons, ligaments, bones, joints, and muscles.

Proteins are needed to maintain strength, muscle tone, skin elasticity, mobility, joint integrity, and physical endurance. (2) For example, collagen, an element necessary for the formation of skin, needs the amino acids lysine and proline, plus vitamin C to work.

ORGAN SUPPORT

Proteins and amino acids restore and nourish the organs such as the liver, heart, and the kidneys. For example, the amino acid l-glutamine is known for its restorative effects on the stomach lining.

MAKE ENZYMES

Enzymes act as a catalyst to make many functions in the body happen. For instance, the pancreas produces digestive enzymes like protease that assists in protein digestion.

BUILDING BLOCKS FOR BLOOD

Proteins are involved in red blood cell production. Specifically, hemoglobin a protein that carries oxygen from the lungs to all tissue in the body and then transports the carbon dioxide out.

IMMUNE SUPPORT

Proteins provide support to the immune system. Proteins make up the antibodies, like immunoglobulins, that are known as the fighter cells that attack germs and viruses in our body.

HORMONE SUPPORT

Proteins support and nourish glands that make hormones. Healthy hormones do actions like manage sugar in the blood, provide energy, help regulate sleep, and work towards fostering good mental health by helping to maintain emotional balance and stability.

Proteins make the hormones insulin and glucagon in the pancreas that regulate blood sugar. Hormones are impacted based on what, when, and how much you eat so start paying attention to the correlation between mood, energy, and food eaten. For example, hormone imbalances stemming from the adrenal, and thyroid glands can cause cravings and mood swings. (3)

NEUROTRANSMITTER SUPPORT

Proteins contribute to the formation of neurotransmitters. Neurotransmitters are chemical messengers important for brain health. They are made up of specific amino acids that feed the communication system in the brain. Neurotransmitters are responsible for influencing moods, feelings, outlook, motivation, pain, calm, alertness, stress levels, agitation, and focus. (4)

A healthy and well-nourished brain will have better messaging, support happier moods, create sharper focus, provide a sense of well-being, and give a better response to stress. Scientists are now discovering neurotransmitters throughout cells in the entire body. For instance, there are cell receptor sites found in the gut that make serotonin. Serotonin is your body's feel-good neurotransmitter produced from the amino acid tryptophan, your happy mood-making amino acid.

The integrative medical community would suggest that it is possible to restore, replenish, and nourish neurotransmitters with food, nutrients, herbal therapies, and healing the gut. These natural, cost-effective, low impact approaches are incredibly promising for children, adolescents, and adults who suffer from anxiety, depression, and other mental health-related issues. (5)

The number of children on antidepressants, ADD/ADHD drugs, and psychotropic drugs is skyrocketing. (6) A 2016 antidepressant study in the British Medical Journal showed that only 1 out of 14 pharmaceutical drugs work and that they may contribute to suicidal thinking. (7, 8)

DETOXIFICATION

Protein foods provide the nutrients that help to detoxify the liver. Liver detoxification utilizes amino acids such as methionine and cysteine. These nutrients work on specific pathways to neutralize toxins and metabolic waste (body processes naturally create waste products).

PRODUCE ENERGY

Proteins contribute to the body's energy source. They provide four calories per gram. In an emergency, only if glucose is not available, your body can harvest amino acids and turn them into sugar to burn as fuel. (9)

➤ Procedure 1

Demonstrate three roles and functions proteins play in our health and well-being.

1. Have students list different parts of their body that protein foods help grow, repair, and maintain.
2. Show the bicep. Use a model or picture of the body's muscles.
3. Ask the question, "How are proteins helping my bicep?"
4. Write down the responses provided by the students.
5. Elicit examples of other parts of the body.

Assessment

As a whole class or in small groups, discuss how protein foods play a role in more than just building muscles.

DISCOVERY
Classification of Amino Acids

There are twenty-two types of amino acids that are all derived from protein-containing foods. Nine of the amino acids are referred to as essential amino acids. People need to eat these different amino acids, unlike the other thirteen amino acids that the body can make on its own. Therefore, no matter what diet you adhere to, all people need to follow the same food rules when it comes to eating proteins.

I classify amino acids into three different categories. The Food Tree refers to this classification as **The Amino Acid Array.** The Amino Acid Array consists of Essential Amino Acids, Non-Essential Amino Acids, and Conditional Amino Acids. (1)

It is essential to eat a variety of protein foods throughout the day and week. Your body can make vitamin B but not vitamin C; your body can make saturated fats but not polyunsaturated fats.

Regarding proteins, your body can make non-essential amino acids but not essential amino acids. Those you need to get specifically from the foods you eat. Thus, you do need to replenish your store of all proteins regularly. It is more important to focus on eating the Amino Acid Array throughout the entire day or over a few days and not be concerned about getting the whole Amino Acid Array at every meal.

THE AMINO ACID ARRAY

Alanine, arginine, asparagine, aspartic acid, cysteine, glutamic acid, glutamine, glycine, histidine, isoleucine, leucine, lysine, methionine, ornithine, phenylalanine, proline, serine, theanine, threonine, tryptophan, tyrosine, valine

ESSENTIAL AMINO ACIDS
Your body is unable to make nine essential amino acids. They must be obtained from the diet.

Histidine, isoleucine, leucine, lysine, methionine, phenylalanine, threonine, tryptophan, valine

CONDITIONAL AMINO ACIDS
Chemicals in the body can manufacture these amino acids. They deplete readily in times of stress and illness. Replenish these regularly.

Arginine, cysteine, glutamine, ornithine, proline, serine, tyrosine

NON-ESSENTIAL AMINO ACIDS
Chemicals in the body can manufacture these amino acids. They do not need to be obtained through food as critically as the others.

Alanine, asparagine, aspartic acid, glutamic acid, glycine, theanine

DISCOVERY

Lesson: Exploring Plant-Based, Vegetarian, Vegan Diets and Lifestyles

➤ MATERIALS
List examples of plant-based protein foods. Ex: Beans, nuts, seeds, whole grains, spirulina, or blue-green algae

➤ GOAL
Understand the fundamentals of eating a plant-based diet.

➤ OBJECTIVES
- To explain the reasons why people may choose not to eat meat or animal foods
- To investigate the trend towards being a vegetarian, vegan, and plant-based eater in your community
- To explain the kinds of food that make a plant-based diet healthy, and the common misconceptions about this kind of diet

➤ ACTIVATING PRIOR KNOWLEDGE
Ask the students what kinds of foods they think vegetarians or vegans may eat. Ask if they know any people who don't eat the meat of animal products. Ask, if appropriate in the setting, if kids in the class are vegetarian or vegan. Remind the class to remain open-minded. Reiterate that it is not okay to judge others based on the foods they choose to eat or not eat.

BACKGROUND INFORMATION

Vegetarians and Vegans

Is it possible to be a healthy vegan or vegetarian? The answer is a resounding YES! Yes, you can be a vegetarian or vegan and be happy and well-nourished. The Food Tree advocates for eating a primarily plant-based diet as a general rule.

There are more than 375 million people around the world who identify as someone who eats a plant-based, vegan, or vegetarian diet (1). According to PETA, The People for Ethical Treatment of Animals, 5% of Americans are vegetarians, and another 2.5% identify as vegans. In India, approximately 40% are considered vegetarian (2).

The Food Tree guide supports a variety of diets and advocates for personal choice as long as it is ethical and humane. Food choice is an individual right all people have. However, that said, The Food Tree recommends, in general, eating a plant-based diet. And let me tell you why. Eating vegetarian or vegan for a good part of your week or life can be beneficial for all kinds of reasons. It benefits your overall health, your wallet, and even the Earth.

People around the world live long, healthy lives without eating meat. History and research has shown that it is absolutely 100% possible to create a healthy and thriving diet for you and your family based purely on plant foods and still be well nourished.

One of the fathers of the vegetarian movement, John Robbins, author of the classic *Diet for a New America*, professes that people from cultures all around the world can live well into their hundreds on a plant-based diet. (3)

The labels we use to identify plant-based eating may mean many different things to many different people. The types of foods, eating habits, cooking styles, and the lifestyle behind it can be as varied and diverse as each person is. In general, vegans choose not to eat any food or food by-products that come from animals. Period. For some, that may include not eating honey, dairy, or eggs, and some may even choose not to wear any leather, whereas vegetarians may incorporate honey, dairy, and eggs. Pescatarians include fish. And there are many more fun names for other dietary combinations of foods that people choose that are plant-based.

Top 10 Countries with the Highest Rates of Vegetarianism

1. India 38%
2. Israel 13%
3. Taiwan 12%
4. Italy 10%
5. Austria 9%
6. Germany 9%
7. United Kingdom 9%
8. Brazil 8%
9. Ireland 6%
10. Australia 5%

World Atlas, 2019 (4)

There often is a misunderstanding that people must include animal food in their diet to meet their protein nutritional requirements. They may believe that it is not possible for a person to receive all of their nutrients from eating only plant foods, which is a false conclusion.

It IS entirely possible to be well-nourished and thrive on a vegetarian or vegan diet. But it IS true, vegans and vegetarians must be mindful of eating proper amounts of proteins to obtain the essential amino acids from the Amino Acid Array. In addition to amino acids, it is critical for vegans and vegetarians to make sure they are getting plenty of vitamin B12. The primary source of B12 is from animal-based foods, with the exception that B12 is high in lacto-fermented foods and in the dietary condiment, nutritional yeast. So, supplementation of vitamin B12 may be necessary for folks who eat an exclusively vegan or vegetarian diet.

It is easy to be inspired nowadays by people who are eating and living according to their higher needs of eating plant foods only. Some of the world's strongest, fastest, and smartest people are vegans and vegetarians. And, also of interest, the world's biggest and fiercest animals are vegan, including elephants, rhinos, and gorillas.

Vegetarian Inspiration

Scott Jurek is a vegan and is also an elite athlete in the sport of ultra-running. He shares his philosophy on food in his book entitled *Eat & Run: My Unlikely Journey to Ultra- marathon Greatness*, where he demonstrates you can become an elite athlete while eating only a plant-based diet.

The Benefits of Eating a Vegetarian, Plant-Based Diet

BETTER HEALTH

Done well, eating a plant-based diet can be incredibly healthy. Vegetarians typically eat more fruits, vegetables, beans, nuts, and seeds that contain antioxidants, fiber, enzymes, and phytonutrients than their meat-eating counterparts. Many vegans and vegetarians eat more home-cooked meals that can be much healthier than restaurant fare. Usually, it is a bit trickier to eat out well as a vegetarian, or for anyone for that matter. For the vegetarian or vegan, the main point would be that it is vital to get all of the essential amino acids (the molecules that make up proteins) into the diet.

IMPROVED ECONOMICS

Going vegetarian is a more economical way to eat. There is no comparing the cost savings that eating a vegetarian vs. meat-based diet will give you.

According to a study published in the Journal of Hunger & Environmental Nutrition, the authors found that purchasing foods for a 2,000-calorie a day diet based on the government recommendations on My Plate vs. a vegetarian diet showed a savings of more than $750 for the plant-based food diet annually. (5)

FAMOUS PLANT-BASED EATERS, PAST AND PRESENT

Pamela Anderson—Actress, animal rights activist

Fiona Apple—Actor

Brigitte Bardot—Animal rights activist, actress

Sandra Bernhardt—Comedian and actress

Ken Bradshaw—Pro Surfer

Orlando Bloom—Actor

Russell Brand—British comedian, actor

Christie Brinkley—Supermodel

Jim Carrey—Actor, stand-up comedian

Cesar Chávez—Civil rights advocate

Bill Clinton—Former U.S. President

Leonardo Da Vinci—Italian painter, inventor

Ellen DeGeneres—Comedian, television host

Leonardo di Caprio—Actor and environmental activist

Thomas Edison—U.S. inventor and entrepreneur

Albert Einstein—Physicist

Ralph Waldo Emerson—Writer and poet

Melissa Etheridge—Musician, singer and songwriter

Benjamin Franklin—Inventor

Michael Franti—Singer of Spearhead

Jane Goodall, Ph.D.—British primatologist/anthropologist

Brian Greene, Ph.D.—U.S. theoretical physicist

Mahatma Gandhi—Indian spiritual, political leader

Al Gore—Former U.S. Vice President, activist

Woody Harrelson—Actor, activist

Faith Hill—Musician, country singer

Samuel L. Jackson—Actor

Steve Jobs—Co-founder, Apple Computer

Scott Jurek—Elite athlete

Franz Kafka—Novelist

Diane Keaton—Actress

John Harvey Kellogg—M.D., U.S. physician

Andy Lally—Race car driver

Phil Lesh—Musician, bass player for The Grateful Dead

Coretta Scott King—Civil rights, women's rights, and anti-war activist

Walter Kowalski—Wrestler

Carl Lewis—Olympic gold medalist track and field

Richard Linklater—U.S. writer-director

Henry J. Heimlich—M.D. and surgeon

Paul McCartney—Singer-songwriter, The Beatles

Rita Moreno—Actress

Alanis Morissette—Singer-songwriter

Morrissey—British vocalist

Martina Navratilova—Tennis star

Sandra Oh—Actress

Yoko Ono—Artist, wife of The Beatles legend John Lennon

Rosa Parks—Civil rights activist

Bill Pearl—U.S. bodybuilder, winner of 4 Mr. Universe titles

Joaquin Phoenix—Award-winning actor

River Phoenix—Actor

Natalie Portman—Academy award-winning actress

Prince—Musician, 2004 Rock & Roll Hall of Fame inductee

John Robbins—Author, Diet for a New America

Ocean Robbins—Author, *The 31-Day Food Revolution*

Rich Roll—U.S. ultra-endurance athlete

Fred Rogers—TV personality, "Mister Rogers"

JD Salinger—American novelist

Jean-Jacques Rousseau—Philosopher

Alicia Silverstone—U.S. actress

George Bernard Shaw—Irish playwright

Russell Simmons—Hip-hop entrepreneur

Upton Sinclair—Pulitzer Prize-winner, author of *The Jungle*

Peter Singer—Australian bioethicist

Ringo Starr—Musician and drummer of The Beatles

Queen Sofia—Queen of Spain

Nikola Tesla—Physicist and inventor

Hannah Teter—U.S. Snowboarder, two-time Olympic medalist

Leo Tolstoy—Russian novelist

Carrie Underwood—Singer, musician

Eddie Vedder—Pearl Jam singer-songwriter

Leonardo da Vinci—Italian painter, inventor

Ricky Williams—Professional football player

Kate Winslet—Actress

CLEANER ENVIRONMENT

Eating a vegetarian or vegan diet is arguably better for the environment. There is no denying that tons of particulate matter and carbon is released into the atmosphere every year from the effects of raising cattle. Documentaries like *Cowspiracy, What the Health* and *Forks Over Knives,* plus many other recent films and TV shows highlight the human cost of raising meat and the impact on human health, animal welfare, and our ecosystem.

> *"Livestock and their byproducts account for at least 32,000 million tons of carbon dioxide (CO2) per year or 51% of all worldwide greenhouse gas emissions."* Cowspiracy (6)

> *"Livestock is responsible for 65% of all human-related emissions of nitrous oxide, a greenhouse gas with 296 times the global warming potential of carbon dioxide, and which stays in the atmosphere for 150 years."* Cowspiracy (6)

So, if you love to eat meat, enjoy it with reverence, because the raising of that meat may have had some serious negative impact on the Earth. Our societal goal should be to reduce greenhouse gas emissions and mitigate climate change.

FARMERS AND ANIMAL RIGHTS

There are innumerable books written about the squalid conditions in which farm animals live. Factory raised chickens, cows, hogs, or lambs live in pretty awful conditions. On the flip side of animal abuse, there are issues related to unsafe working conditions for the farmhands and industry workers. Upton Sinclair wrote in *The Jungle*, about the dangerous and severe conditions in the meatpacking plants in Chicago in the early 1900s. Yes, things have improved, but there are still shadowy issues within the industry.

RELIGION AND SPIRITUALITY

Many world religions share different beliefs and traditions regarding the eating and killing of animals. A person's spiritual practice may not allow for meat or certain preparations of animal foods. For instance, Orthodox Jews follow strict rules called Kashrut that forbid mixing meat and milk during meals. Halal is a Muslim law that governs the treatment of animals. Hinduism, Buddhism, the Quakers, and many other religions suggest forgoing animal foods altogether.

So, whatever *your* reason for eating vegetarian, or eating a mostly vegetarian diet, it's commendable. The Food Tree isn't concerned what you call yourself, enough with the labels. Remember, you are doing it for your sensibilities, and your reasons are legitimate.

*Action Item

Show food awareness related film documentaries like *Cowspiracy, Food Inc., and Forks Over Knives*. There are many other excellent films to view critically. Choose movies for age appropriateness. Some content can be quite disturbing to young and old, so use sensitivity and have a process discussion after seeing each film. Ask each student to share one thing they learned from the documentary.

▶ Procedure 1

1. Students formulate their hypothesis on how many people they think are vegetarian or vegans in their community and postulate the reasons why. The term *community* can refer to a town, school, family, or sports league, for example.

2. Students will design a survey and poll a variety or select group of participants. For example, they can survey friends, family, school students and staff, church members, grocery store staff, and other establishments of interest to the student. A school social media site could be used as well to gather data. Students could also include a survey in the school newspaper.

3. Collect data.

4. Graph the results of the survey.

5. Based on the graph, determine the percentages of people that identify with each type of diet.
6. Find out the reasons why they choose that type of diet. Are the ideas based on concern for the environment, taste, feelings of guilt, financial, religious, or spiritual?
7. Have students summarize their findings with the class and discuss them.

➤ Procedure 2

Are there better or more humane, efficient, and environmentally sustainable ways to raise and consume animals?

1. Calculate the amount of grain, feed, land, and water needed to raise farm animals for human consumption.
2. Choose an animal to analyze like cattle, pigs, lamb, chicken and foul, fish and seafood, buffalo, and venison, for example.
3. Present findings with the class. It can be in the form of a power point, skit, or TV commercial. Let students be creative in the way they present the information.

➤ Procedure 3

Challenge students to eat a plant-based, vegan, or vegetarian diet for one week.

1. Have them explain in a paper or a presentation how the vegetarian/vegan challenge went for them and what they learned.

➤ Procedure 4

Produce a school-wide Vegetarian Day or Vegetarian Week. World Vegetarian Day is observed on October 1st every year. https://worldvegetarianday.navs-online.org/.

➤ Procedure 5

Conduct a field trip to investigate the nearest dairy, feedlot, working farm, or commercial chicken coop. Ask to get a tour of the factory or farm where the animals are kept and raised so students can observe the living and feeding conditions.

➤ Procedure 6

Make some noise! Ask restaurants, parents, schools, and mini-marts to provide more vegan, vegetarian, and plant-based options.

Assessment

Discuss what your students learned about eating a plant-based diet.

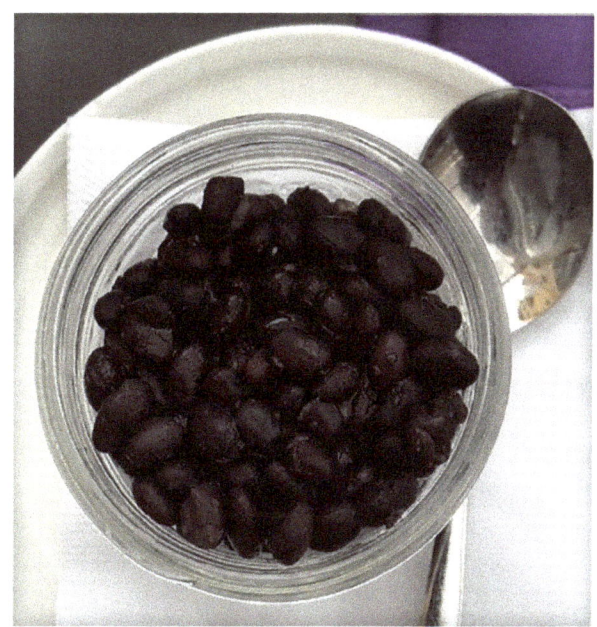

COMPREHENSIVE

Lesson: Protein Deficiencies

➤ MATERIALS
Examples of protein foods: dried beans, yogurt, blue-green algae, eggs, canned tuna, soy milk, a carton of milk, a clean package of meat

➤ GOALS
Understand that a variety of proteins are needed and, like fuel in a car, need to be replenished regularly for proper human functioning.

➤ OBJECTIVES
- To describe situations where people may become deficient in protein foods
- To illustrate the impact protein deficiencies and excesses have on a person's well-being
- To explain the importance of eating proteins regularly, providing two specific examples

➤ ACTIVATING PRIOR KNOWLEDGE
Have the class brainstorm their favorite protein foods. Discuss the types and amounts of protein foods students eat daily.

BACKGROUND INFORMATION

Deficiencies in dietary protein

Protein deficiencies are relatively rare in the United States. However, they may develop under certain conditions. (1) This lesson discusses how eating a diet with inadequate protein or an imbalance of Essential Amino Acids (EAA) to Non-Essential Amino Acids (NEAA) intake can dramatically compromise a person's health.

Deficiencies can create a cascade of health problems. Extreme diets, illness, skipping meals, poor diet choices, high-performance athletes, people recovering from surgery, strict dieters, and those with eating disorders are all vulnerable to inadequate protein intake. Vegans and vegetarians who may be unaware of how to acquire proper nutrition from a plant-based diet are also at risk of imbalance or deficiencies.

The human body is continually breaking down proteins and using them for hundreds of different functions, so people need to eat them regularly. Protein breaks down into smaller components called amino acids. Essential amino acids are the most important to pay attention to because they need to be taken in via the diet.

Most people who consume enough calories from a variety of nutrient sources receive adequate amounts of protein to get their requirement of amino acids (proteins' smaller components).

Amino acids do not store long-term in your body. Different systems and parts of your body use them up continually, so it is essential to replenish them regularly. But as with the other two macronutrients, carbohydrates and fats, it is critical to eat the right amount of protein foods with a variety of amino acids.

Protein deficiencies can occur for many different reasons and can negatively affect body functions.

Even healthy and fit athletes run the risk of a protein imbalance. Athletes, and those who don't eat enough protein to rebuild their body, may experience muscle weakness instead of muscle growth and may become more prone to injury. Protein deficiencies cause cells to die and muscles to break down. Muscle and other tissues fail to receive the protein needed for repair, process metabolic waste, and other purposes. So, pay attention to nutritional needs, especially for those who work out hard, are in extreme sports training like running marathons, biking, surfing, or participate in a competitive athletic program. (2)

Poor diet or food imbalance is easy enough to correct, but it may take some effort and behavior change on your part. If not addressed, these bad eating habits may eventually result in nutrient deficiencies.

Causes of Protein Deficiencies

- Eating an unbalanced diet of macronutrients
- Consuming a low protein diet
- Consuming too much sugar and refined carbohydrates
- Eating a high omega 6 fat vs. omega 3 fat diet (3)
- Eating a restricted diet; skipping meals, extreme dieting
- Having a weak digestive capacity or inadequate absorption
- Experiencing leaky gut, acidosis
- Having cancer or other diseases
- Participating in intense exercise or high physical exertion
- Experiencing chronic stress (4)
- Recovering from surgery
- Making poor diet choices

Symptoms of Protein Deficiencies

- Break down of muscles (5)
- Poor immunity. The body takes amino acids away from feeding the immune system to attend to different needs.
- Impaired digestion
- Slow wound healing
- Thin hair, weak nails, and dull skin
- Unintended weight loss
- Impaired liver detoxification
- Brain chemical and hormone imbalances, mood issues, depression, anger, confusion, sadness
- Susceptibility towards addictions
- Food cravings
- Poor digestion, impaired nutrient absorption
- Fatigue, lethargy, weakness
- Subject to frequent or more severe injury
- Cellular death

➤ Procedure 1

Suggest to your students that they try to eat five servings of proteins every day.

1. Have students use the protein calculation to figure out their daily protein requirements.
2. Have the class brainstorm their favorite protein foods.
3. Ask students to choose examples of what five servings of protein looks like for one day.

➤ Procedure 2

Write a paper explaining situations where people may become deficient in protein or amino acids.

1. Illustrate the impact protein deficiencies and excesses can have on a person's well-being.
2. Explain the importance of eating protein foods regularly, providing two specific examples.

Assessment

Were students motivated to include more protein in their diet if they found they were deficient, or did they decrease the number of protein servings if they felt that they were consuming too much?

COMPREHENSIVE

Lesson: Protein Foods to Avoid

> **MATERIALS**
- Samples of processed luncheon meat packaging and processed meat labels
- Photos or downloads of ingredient lists of processed meat, bacon, luncheon meat

> **GOALS**

Check the ingredients, preservatives, and added chemicals found in processed and cured meat. Know how to purchase high-quality meat products.

> **OBJECTIVES**
- To investigate ingredients found in animal meat products that link to serious health problems including cancer
- To recognize the potential health hazards associated with eating nutrition vampire foods
- To know how to analyze food labels on luncheon meats, cured meats (bacon, sausage), vegetarian proteins, packaged foods
- To defend the right to quality foods in our foods system and especially in our schools

> **ACTIVATING PRIOR KNOWLEDGE**

Hot dogs, luncheon meats, and pepperoni are all foods many people love. Why? They taste good and salty. Ask your students if they ever wonder why they taste so good?

BACKGROUND INFORMATION

What protein foods are best to avoid?

PROCESSED MEATS

Bacon, sausage, hot dogs, salami, and ham are examples of types of processed meats. Not always, but often, these kinds of processed foods contain harmful additives and preservatives. (1) Processed meat products may contain harmful manufacturing chemicals like chlorine and ammonia that are used for cleaning, sterilizing, and sanitizing the meats. (2)

The World Health Organization (WHO) and The International Agency for Research on Cancer (IARC) confirms eating processed meat is "carcinogenic to humans." (2, 3) Many butchers and ranchers produce meat without added preservatives and chemicals. Look for meat products that are approved by the Weston A. Price Foundation, an organization that educates consumers about the preservation of healthy traditional foods.

There are two categories for meat, according to the WHO report.

Processed meat—Meat that has been transformed through salting, curing, fermentation, smoking, or other processes to enhance flavor or improve preservation.

Red meat—Unprocessed mammalian muscle meat such as beef, bison, veal, pork, lamb, mutton, and goat meat

AVOID EATING PROCESSED, BARBECUED, GRILLED, AND CHARBROILED MEATS

Some of the worst protein food offenders are barbecued, grilled, and charbroiled meats. Sorry, everyone who loves those foods. Smoked or cured meat may contain harmful chemicals linked to cancer called nitrates. Nitrates preserve meat from spoilage. The World Health Organization lists sodium nitrate as a carcinogen.

- Processing, curing and smoking meats creates cancer-causing (carcinogenic) chemicals such as N-nitroso-compounds (NOCs) and polycyclic aromatic hydrocarbons (PAHs).
- Scientists discovered a definite link between heme iron found in red meat and the increase in the formation of NOCs, a carcinogenic compound.

Cooking meat at high heat like on an outdoor grill or barbecue turns the fats in the meat into sugary caramelized bits that taste so good. But it also turns that meat into damaged materials called advanced glycation end products, or AGES (4), a carcinogenic substance that contributes to oxidative cellular damage. Oxidative damage occurs when the cells in the body become damaged from the sugars and toxins produced from the high heat.

Cooking foods like fish, chicken, and vegetables on high heat to blacken or char them will turn your food into carbon ash. Charred and burnt by-products contribute to oxidative cellular damage so there is no need to burn your food into a black crisp. (5)

AVOID EATING EXCESS PROTEIN

We are protein obsessed in the United States. What is of concern is not eating too little protein but overeating protein. Excess protein breaks down into by-products and may cause pH imbalance, leading to acidosis. (6) The danger is that the excess may harm kidneys whose job it is to filter out the excess nitrogen wastes. Go easy on overdoing the protein and always go for quality organic whole foods when possible.

➤ Procedure 1
FOOD SNOOP

1. Brainstorm types of processed meat.
2. Investigate all of the ingredients that go into the processing of meat. Sort the chemicals into two groups: those that do comprise human health and those that don't. Refer to the GRAS listings on the USDA website. (7)
3. Have each student choose one processed meat example. Have them research the ingredients to assess the nutritional benefits and potential harmful ingredients that may be found in the product.
4. Write a report on the findings.

➤ Procedure 2
TELL IT LIKE IT IS!

1. Produce a short commercial or film that defends eating and producing cleaner foods with less harmful ingredients. Encourage creativity using parody, comedy, melodrama, or as a documentary.

➤ Procedure 3

1. Research preservatives, additives, flavors, and other chemical ingredients found in processed and cured meats, and any potential health risks associated with them.
2. Use the Environmental Working Group (EWG) website database www.ewg.org or GreenMed.org as resources.

Assessment

Follow up with your students to see the impact the research had on them and how the knowledge they gained impacts them now.

DISCOVERY

Lesson: Protein Calculations

➤ MATERIALS
- Calculators, computers, or brains to compute the math equation
- The Food Tree Daily Food Journal, located in the Activities Section

➤ GOAL
Understand what a daily protein requirement looks like for an individual and that many factors go into determining a person's protein needs for a day.

➤ OBJECTIVES
- To discuss the biological functions happening in the body that determine protein demands
- To be able to calculate a person's protein requirements for the day

➤ ACTIVATING PRIOR KNOWLEDGE
Discuss how a person might calculate how many calories from a macronutrient group they might need. Discuss calories as a way to measure a unit of energy.

BACKGROUND INFORMATION

It is important to consider that many different factors weigh into what a person may need for optimal protein intake. Protein requirements will be unique to each day, week, month, and year. This requirement will fluctuate and vary depending on other factors.

➤ Procedure 1
Students use a standard mathematical formula to estimate the protein needs of a person for a day. Have each student use the calculation below to understand what a daily protein requirement looks like for an individual.

PROTEIN CALCULATION
- Weight in pounds divided by 2.2
- Multiply that number by the person's activity level (.6 -1.5)

    .6 = Sedentary couch potato

    1. = 30 minutes average daily activity

    1.5 = School or professional athlete

The number you get is the recommended number of grams of protein to eat in a day.

➤ Procedure 2
Students calculate their own protein needs for the day.
- Keep track of their foods eaten in a food journal.

Assessment
Have students reflect on their findings.
- Were they surprised at the amount of protein needed? Was it more or less than they thought?
- Ask the class to list the types of protein food they would eat for breakfast, lunch, dinner, and snacks to equal five servings of protein foods for one day.

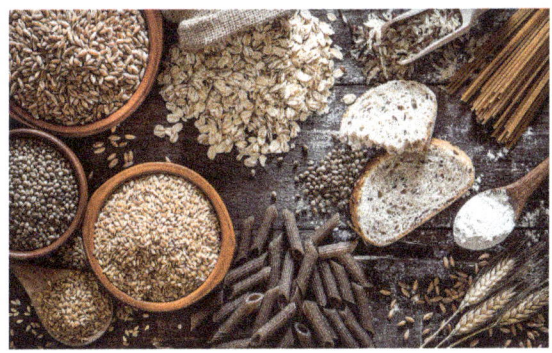

INTRODUCTION TO THE WHOLE GRAINS FOOD GROUP

THE FOOD TREE ANALOGY
The Trunk represents the Whole Grains Food Group on The Food Tree. Imagine symbolically that the tree trunk is like the trunk of your body. Eating whole grains keeps the trunk of our body flexible but always standing strong and well balanced.

DAILY RECOMMENDED SERVING SUGGESTION: 5
20% of daily calories
Energy source, carbohydrate, four calories per gram

SOURCES OF GRAINS
Amaranth, barley, buckwheat (kasha), corn, faro, kamut, millet, oat, rice, rye, quinoa, spelt, sorghum, teff, wheat (bulgur, couscous)

WHOLE UNREFINED GRAINS AND REFINED GRAINS

There are two types of grains that are readily available to eat from our food system: whole, unrefined grains, and refined, processed grains.

- **Whole, Unrefined Grains** are whole foods and considered a complex carbohydrate. (1) They are a single fruit or seed from a plant (grasses), sometimes referred to as a cereal crop. All of the grains' vitamins, minerals, fats, flavor, fiber, and health benefits are still intact in the little grain seed. (2)

- **Refined Grains** are processed and considered to be simple carbohydrates because manufacturers remove the naturally occurring vitamins, fats, and fiber. The white flour, or endosperm, is what is left behind.

There are many benefits to eating whole grains. They are a great source of essential nutrients like vitamins, minerals, trace elements, and fiber that are necessary for optimal health.

FOUNDATIONAL

Lesson: Getting to Know Grains— Whole and Refined

➤ MATERIALS
- Wheat kernel graphic (see appendix)
- Examples of whole grains and refined grains in real form or pictures
- Examples of two different forms of rice
  - White
  - Brown

Or

- Examples of four different forms of oats at various stages of processing
  - Whole oat groats
  - Whole steel cut oats
  - Rolled oats
  - Processed oats (packet of instant oatmeal)

➤ GOAL
Understand that whole and refined grains have differing amounts of nutrients in them.

➤ OBJECTIVES
- To recognize the difference between a whole grain and a processed grain
- To acquire the skills needed to make educated decisions about choosing whole-grain foods and products instead of processed grain foods and products
- To identify five different grains

➤ ACTIVATING PRIOR KNOWLEDGE
Have a conversation with your class about the kinds of bread, rice, or tortillas they typically eat at home or school. Ask what people's favorite grain dishes are. Discuss with your students if they believe eating whole grains in the diet is essential, and why or why not?

Ask if the grain-based foods they eat are whole grains or refined grains. Do they pay attention to the choices they are making with bread and other grain-based foods like pizza, bagels, hot dog/hamburger buns, pastries, crackers and sandwich bread that they eat? Are they eating organic grains? See if your students understand that there are health risks associated with consuming processed nutrient-poor grains, bread, and packaged foods. Read up on the herbicide glyphosate for more information on the importance of eating organic grains.

BACKGROUND INFORMATION

Whole grains can be a nutritious food to include in a balanced diet. However, eating refined and processed grains have the potential to cause serious health issues such as overweight, obesity, insulin sensitivity, and diabetes, (1) even in children.

Different types of grains will contain varying quantities of nutrients, especially when the differences between whole and processed grains are examined. In this lesson, we explore the refining and processing of grains and compare and contrast the different amounts of fiber, vitamins, minerals, amino acids, fatty acids, antioxidants, and phytonutrients found in both whole and refined.

ANATOMY OF A GRAIN

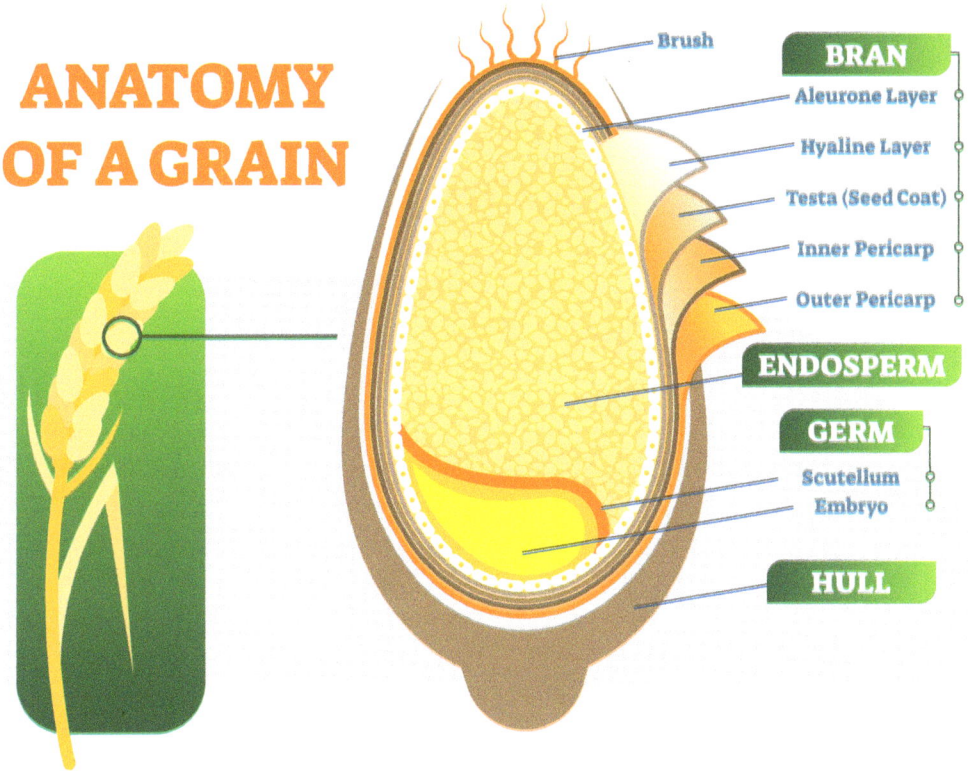

**Action Item—show an illustration of a kernel of wheat

Refer to the illustration of a whole-wheat kernel that identifies the bran, germ, and endosperm.

What Are Whole Grains?

There are two main types of grains that are readily available to eat in our food system: whole, unrefined grains and refined, processed grains.

100% WHOLE GRAINS

Whole Grains are a single fruit or seed from a plant (grasses), sometimes referred to as a cereal crop. They are complex carbohydrates. These include wheat, rice, barley, and oats. They are considered a whole food as, would have been, or is found in nature. Whole grains are intact and therefore retain the naturally occurring bran, germ, and endosperm that provides nutrients like fats, vitamins, minerals, and fiber. (2)

Whole wheat flour is similar to whole grain wheat, except it is missing most of the germ and some of the bran.

Make-up of a Wheat Kernel

The Bran—The outer fibrous layer of the grain

- 14 ½ percent of the weight of the wheat kernel
- Found in whole wheat flour
- Contains proteins, B-vitamins, trace minerals, and fiber

The Endosperm—The middle part of the grain

- 83 percent of the weight of the kernel
- The primary source of white flour, contains protein, carbohydrates B-vitamins, fiber

The Germ—The vitamin E oil-rich part of the grain

- 2 ½ percent of the weight of the kernel
- 10% percent fat, B-vitamins, trace minerals

What Are Refined Processed Grains?

Processed grains are converted from a whole grain and complex carbohydrate to a simple grain and simple carbohydrate. Refining whole grains is a process involving the removal of the tough fibrous outer layer called the bran and the precious oil-containing germ. The white flour is the endosperm, the only remaining part from the original grain. At this stage, most of the nutrients have been removed. The wheat kernel has now become a refined grain.

Refining a wheat kernel removes:

- 70% of the minerals: 50% of iron and 70% of magnesium
- 100% of vitamin E
- 66% of B vitamins
- 19% of protein
- 79% of the fiber

Products using refined grains like white flour, white rice, and white sugar are made into packaged goods like cakes, pastries, granola bars, quick oats, crackers, cookies, pizza dough, donuts, muffins, tortillas, bagels, pasta, and other baked goods. When you eat grains without their naturally occurring nutrients, they are generally less nutritious. (3) Therefore, the USDA requires processed grains to be fortified and enriched with vitamins and minerals.

WHOLE GRAINS FOOD SOURCES

- Amaranth (gf)
- Barley
- Buckwheat (aka kasha)
- Bulgur (wheat)
- Corn (gf)
- Couscous (wheat)
- Faro
- Kamut
- Millet (gf)
- Oats (gf)
- Rice—basmati, black, brown, wild (gf)
- Rye
- Quinoa (gf)
- Spelt
- Sorghum (gf)
- Teff (gf)
- Wheat

gf = gluten-free

Action Item!

Show four different forms of oats at various stages of processing.

- Whole oat groats
- Whole steel cut oats
- Rolled oats
- Processed oats

How did we go from eating mostly complex whole grains to mainly processed grains?

Grains are an utterly delicious food when left whole, so why do food companies go to so much trouble to refine and process them? Food manufactures process and refine grains for many reasons. In baking, white flour makes a sweeter and lighter finished product. Initially, being able to afford refined treats was considered a sign of wealth. People would enjoy eating cakes and candy only on special occasions.

However, in the early part of the 1900s, technology advanced, making refined sweet treats affordable and accessible to almost anyone. Since then, it has become easier than ever before to produce foods in mass and distribute them to every nook and cranny in the world. These products were and are nutritionally inferior, but people became (and still are) hooked.

Refined grains have other advantages for manufacturers. Processing grains was encouraged by the government during the 1930s -1950s to make it more convenient for homemakers. (4) Already prepared, processed packaged foods hit the market with the pitch that they were a time-saving household convenience. The hook was that these products had a long shelf life compared to whole grain bread and baked goods. The naturally occurring fat vitamin E found in wheat was removed during processing because the naturally occurring oils would go rancid with exposure to heat and light and, thereby, ruin the product and decrease the shelf life.

The oils then were replaced with cheap, human-made hydrogenated oils. Cakes, crackers, bread, and pastries made with these processed fats like Crisco shortening can last a very long time on grocery store shelves without spoiling yet they can also lead to a myriad of health problems.

To make it even more interesting, food manufacturers regularly "fortify" processed grain products with added vitamins and minerals. They do this to try to make up for the removal of all of the naturally occurring nutrients found in the original whole grain. (5) As well, the wheat flour may be bleached with chemicals to whiten it.

WHAT TYPES AND KINDS OF GRAINS DO YOU NEED TO AVOID?

Nutritionists advise that it is best to avoid refined and processed grains because they have been stripped of their nutrients like vitamins, minerals, and fiber during processing. It is best to choose organic wheat due to the connection to the toxic link of non-organic wheat from the glyphosate found in RoundUp. (7) Health advocates also highly recommend avoiding grain-fed beef due to the link to higher rates of obesity in humans and the risk of glyphosate exposure.

ABOUT GLYPHOSATE AND GRAINS

The rise of gastrointestinal issues is a huge concern. People around the world know that glyphosate, a toxic chemical in the Monsanto product RoundUp, is sprayed on non-organic wheat and other grain crops as a desiccant (drying) agent days before harvest.

The World Health Organization (WHO) has decided that glyphosate is a carcinogen and is, therefore, harmful to humans. This cancer-causing herbicide, according to Dr. Stephanie Seneff of MIT, is guilty of damaging the intestinal lining in humans. The leaky gut scenario has close links to allergies, gluten intolerance and sensitivity, auto-immune issues, and spectrum disorders.

HEALTH PROBLEMS ARE ARISING IN MASSIVE PROPORTIONS IN PEOPLE EATING TOO MANY PROCESSED GRAINS.

Studies show eating a diet that is high in processed grains contributes to poor health. American children eat too many processed foods, refined wheat foods, fast foods, and soda. Consuming too much refined non-organic white flour bread, bagels, pasta, and white rice can cause digestive issues. Processed flour turns into sugar immediately upon digestion and releases it into the bloodstream. Too much sugar entering the body may cause a spike in blood sugar levels that can lead to insulin sensitivity, metabolic syndrome, or diabetes. (6) The main take-home message about grains is when eating them, choose organic, whole, unrefined, and as unprocessed as possible.

➤ Procedure 1
GRAIN IDENTIFICATION

- Put different grains in jars and pass them around in your class. Let students see, touch, and smell the grains. An example may include corn kernels, cornmeal, wheat germ, wheat flour, wheat kernels.

➤ Procedure 2

Research the nutrients lost during grain processing and the potential health consequences on the consumer.

1. Explore the naturally occurring nutrients found in different grains and compare them to the same grain when it is processed and refined.

2. Have students share their findings with the class.

➤ Procedure 3
EXPLORE A GRAIN

Explore the history and evolution of processing wheat and other grains. Choose one type of grain to explore (corn, rice, millet), research, and investigate how it is used in food production. Ask students to share their research and opinions on today's changing food system.

1. Have students present the information on

a poster board, PowerPoint, or another medium.

2. Answer these or other thought-provoking questions:

   - How was the grain eaten 10, 100, and 1000 years ago?
   - How is the grain eaten today?
   - What part of the world did the grain come from?
   - How was it traded or sold?
   - Where are the crops grown now?
   - How are wheat or other grains manufactured and stored?
   - What percentage of the grain sold on the market is in processed foods?
   - What percentage of whole bulk food (including packaged whole organic wheat flour and wheat kernels) is sold at local and chain grocery stores?
   - Do you notice any trends changing towards people and children eating more whole-grain foods? What evidence have you discovered to support your claim?

➤ Procedure 4

Create a commercial, advertisement, or some media pitch about the benefits of eating whole grain products. Or create one about the potential health risks of eating processed, refined grains. Present it as a parody, comedy, or spoof.

Assessment

- Were your students surprised at how differently our modern society eats grains compared to our ancestors? What was the most shocking difference?

- Do you feel empowered to ask your local bakery, school cafeteria, pizza parlor, taqueria, or Chinese restaurant to offer whole organic grains on the menu? What action steps can you take to make a difference in your home? Your community?

FOUNDATIONAL

Lesson: Serving Sizes and Daily Recommendations for Grains

➤ MATERIALS
- The Food Tree Magnetic Board
- Examples of whole grain foods or foods that contain whole grains in them. Use real food, food packaging, or pictures.
- Measuring tools
- Grain Log Sheet
- The Food Tree Daily Food Journal, located in the Activities Section
- The Food Tree Nutrient Scroll, located in the appendix

➤ GOALS
Understand the importance of eating healthy portion sizes and amounts of whole grains.

➤ OBJECTIVE
- To identify the servings needed of whole grains required to maintain a healthy daily diet

➤ ACTIVATING PRIOR KNOWLEDGE
Check-in with your students about how many servings of grains they think they eat, on average, every day. Explore what they believe would be healthy portions sizes.

BACKGROUND INFORMATION

The Food Tree Whole Grain Recommendations

DAILY SERVING SUGGESTION: 5

20% of daily calories

Energy source, macronutrient carbohydrate, four calories per gram

The Food Tree recommends an average healthy person can eat five servings of whole grains every day. However, like all things, it depends on the person and your unique requirements. In general, the serving size can and will vary for each person depending on height, weight, and nutrient needs.

The Food Tree suggests eating a variety of organic whole grains and grains that are minimally processed. Whole grains are healthier than refined, processed grains. (1) Remember to strive to eat in season, locally, fair trade, homegrown, and organic whenever possible.

Choose whole grains as your first preference. For example, make a switch to whole brown rice instead of the usual white rice in Asian food and go for a whole wheat tortilla instead of a white tortilla in Mexican cuisine. Simple switches will go a long way towards improved health.

Serving Size Examples for Whole Grains

CORN, BARLEY, BROWN RICE, QUINOA, AMARANTH, MILLET, WHOLE WHEAT, OATS

1 ounce cooked cereal

¾ cup dried cereal

½ cup cooked rice, pasta, or grain

1 slice bread

1 slice pita

¾ cup dried cereal

1 oz. of dry, ready-to-eat cereal

½ bagel, English muffin

1 tortilla

➤ Procedure 1
KEEP A FOOD JOURNAL

Ask the class to keep a food journal to track what they eat during the day. Keep the journal for at least a week. Pay extra attention to the amount of whole grains and refined grains eaten at each meal. Reading labels is a must.

➤ Procedure 2
CREATE A MEAL PLAN

Create a meal plan for one day, highlighting the types of grain needed to fulfill a person's daily requirements. Group two or three students together. Have them collaborate on one or up to a week's worth of daily meal plans. The students will use the meal plan they each created individually as part of the meal plan that they create for an entire week.

Assessment

Ask the students, what whole grains are you willing to add to your daily meals and snacks? Are you able to curb eating processed grains? Why or why not?

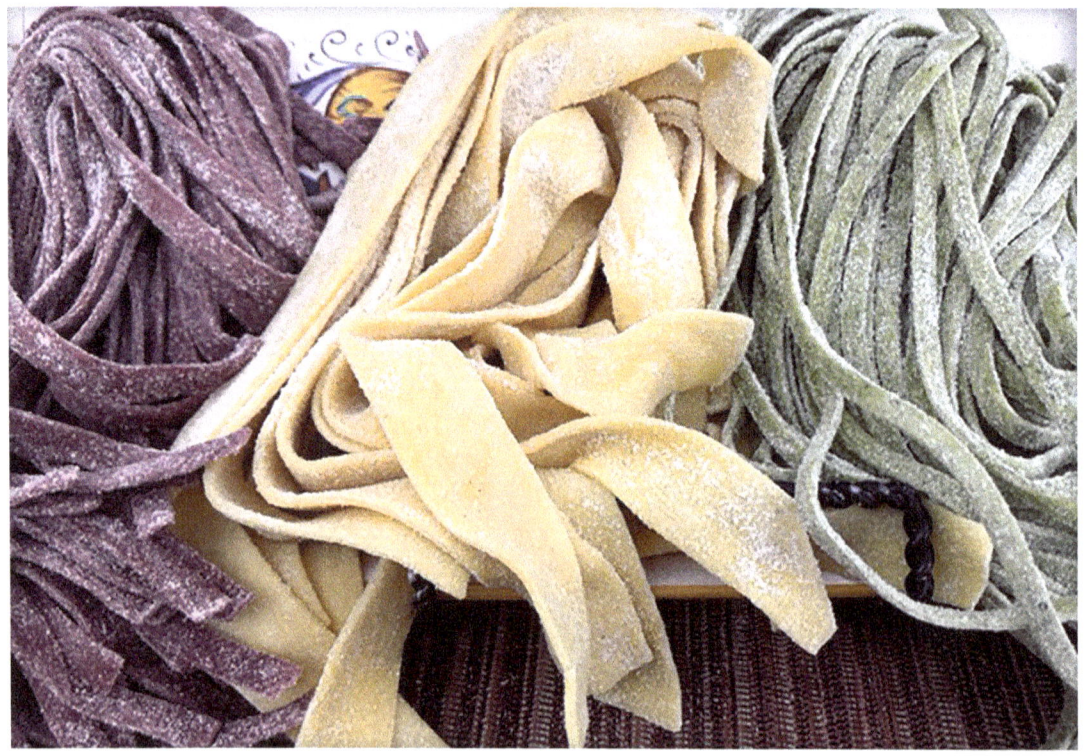

FOUNDATIONAL

Lesson: Benefits and Functions of Whole Grains

➤ MATERIALS
- Food Tree Magnetic Board
- Examples of whole grain foods, either real or pictures from magazines, the internet

➤ GOALS
Understand the health benefits of eating a diet rich in quality whole grains.

➤ OBJECTIVES
- To state the number of servings of whole grains needed to be eaten daily for optimal health
- To explain two health benefits of eating whole grains

➤ ACTIVATING PRIOR KNOWLEDGE
Discuss the students' favorite whole grains. Ask why and how they like to eat them.

BACKGROUND INFORMATION

Whole grains are plant-based foods that are part of the macronutrient group, carbohydrates, one of the three macronutrients. Macronutrients are the food sources from which people receive their primary nutrients. Whole grains are a great source of essential vitamins, minerals, trace elements, and fiber that are all necessary for your health and wellbeing.

Benefits and Functions of Eating Whole Grains

PROVIDE ENERGY SOURCE
Whole grains provide four calories per gram of food that provide long-lasting energy in the form of complex carbohydrates. Whole grains break down quickly into sugars, called glucose, during digestion. The primary source of energy that fuels the body, especially the brain, is glucose or sugar.

PROVIDE NUTRIENTS
Whole grains provide essential nutrients, such as many of the B vitamin family including thiamin (vitamin B1), riboflavin (vitamin B2), niacin (vitamin B3), pantothenic acid (vitamin B5), pyridoxine (vitamin B6) choline, folate (vitamin B9), vitamin E, and minerals like iron, magnesium, manganese, phosphorus, potassium, and zinc. And they are rich in many antioxidants, including phytonutrient carotenoids lutein and zeaxanthin. (1)

PROVIDE VARIETY OF TASTES
There are dozens of different grain varieties. How wonderful that they all have unique flavors, textures, and culinary potential.

SOURCE OF FIBER
One of the best reasons to eat whole grains is that they are rich in fiber. An average adult needs between twenty-five and forty grams of fiber daily. However, most Americans get far less in the diet. Fiber is also found in beans, legumes, fruits, and vegetables.

Since they are a rich source of fiber, whole grains will help regulate blood sugar levels. Whole grains will slow digestion and release sugars steadily into the bloodstream. (2) Fiber-rich foods keep energy steady with fewer energy bursts and slumps. Fiber is essential for a healthy intestinal tract and is necessary for digestive wellness. It promotes the growth of beneficial intestinal bacteria. Fiber helps maintain a healthy weight and is known to help reduce the incidence of colon disease. Fiber helps to eliminate waste, including carcinogens and excess hormones, and prevents re-absorption in the colon, thereby avoiding certain cancers. (3)

Fiber Benefits:

- Promotes healthy digestion and keeps your intestines healthy
- Helps maintain a healthy weight
- Creates a variety of taste
- Attributed to reducing colon disease and cancer
- Promotes the growth of beneficial intestinal bacteria
- Eliminates waste, including carcinogens and excess hormones, and prevents reabsorption in the colon
- Slows digestion and releases sugars steadily into the bloodstream (4)
- Good for the heart
- Prevents certain cancers

▶ Procedure 1
WHOLE GRAIN HIGHLIGHT

Have students create a paper, presentation, or poster board featuring the benefit of whole grains. Include its vitamins, minerals, and fiber content. Discuss any unique qualities or health benefits. For added fun, have students share a recipe or do a cooking demonstration featuring their grain.

▶ Procedure 2
GET YOUR WHOLE GRAINS HERE!

Have groups of students prepare a commercial selling the benefits of eating whole grains. Get as creative as you want. Use video, print, song, jingle, or a skit.

Assessment

Were the students surprised at how beneficial eating whole grains can be to their health?

DISCOVERY

Lesson: Take a Poll on Grain Diversity

➤ MATERIALS
- Paper
- Writing utensils, markers, paint
- Poster board

➤ GOALS
Investigate the types and amounts of grains people eat in the community.

➤ OBJECTIVES
- To examine the kinds of grains offered in the school cafeteria, at home, and in restaurants
- To impart change in the people around them, including their school, restaurants, community organizations, camps, sports clubs, home, family and friends
- To develop a plan for making an excellent grain change in their dietary habits
- To inspire students to eat more whole grains in place of processed grains
- To share research data with their class and school paper

➤ ACTIVATING PRIOR KNOWLEDGE
Ask students what kinds of grains they typically eat during the day. Discuss the benefits of eating a variety of grains. Ask kids to share their favorite grains and why. Prompt them by asking about what they had for breakfast this morning or for dinner last night. Was it pasta? Then ask how often during the week do they think they eat pasta. Do they always have wheat pasta, or have they tried rice or quinoa pasta? Do they choose whole grains over refined grains?

BACKGROUND KNOWLEDGE

Eating processed grains, especially white-wheat based grain foods and products, has significantly contributed to the decline in health in our youth and society at large. (1) We must start paying attention to this health crisis and demand more access to whole grains in our food supply, restaurants, grocery stores, and especially our schools.

This lesson allows your student an opportunity to explore what kinds of grains are most present in their community while sharing with their community the importance of eating whole grains. For instance, I recommend to always buy organic grains due to pesticides. Especially avoid grains sprayed with the highly toxic glyphosate that may damage gut health. (2)

➤ Procedure 1
Ask your students to take a poll of people in their communities to gather real-life information about the different types of grains people eat. Have your students investigate people's knowledge about grain diversity.

1. As individuals, groups, or as a class, have students decide on which communities they would like to focus.
   - Example communities: one class, an entire grade, the whole school, sports team, drama club, church/spiritual group, family.

2. Brainstorm questions to ask people, depending on what kinds of things students want to learn. The class can all ask the same set of questions, students can come up with their own set of questions, or students can do a mix of both. Example questions:

   - What kinds of grains do you typically eat? Would you eat them if they were in a whole grain form? Why or why not? Have you ever tried _____ as a whole grain? (i.e., bagels, pancakes, pizza dough, cookies, crackers, bread, tortillas).
   - Do you tend to eat the same grains, or do you enjoy eating a wide variety of grains? Do you change types of grains for different meals? Or do you tend to eat the same thing for days on end?
   - On average, how many different grains do you eat daily?
   - What are your favorite types of grains? In what form do you like to eat them?
   - Do you eat the same grains as your friends? As your family?

3. Have students carry out their poll, either as a written or oral questionnaire.
4. Have students organize their results in a comprehensive written report or graphics display.
5. Share their research data with their class and school paper.
6. What patterns did students notice from their survey? What surprised them? What was not surprising? Compare results between groups. Did all students have similar results from their polls?
7. Did people tend to eat differently depending on different factors like cultural background, age, gender, work hours, family life, etc.?

▶ Procedure 2
WHOLE GRAIN CHANGE

Inspire students to add more whole organic grains instead of processed refined grains into their diet.

- Have students develop a personal plan for making a whole grain change in their dietary habits. Have them present a list of ideas for making positive changes, make a collage of healthy whole grain foods and meals, or do a cooking demonstration featuring a whole grain.

▶ Procedure 3

Challenge your students to examine the kinds of grains that are offered in the school cafeteria, at home, and in restaurants. Are there whole, organic or gluten free options available?

- See if they can come up with a plan to make a whole grain change on the people around them by encouraging their school, restaurants, community organizations, camps, sports clubs, home, family, and friends to eat more healthy whole organic grains.

Assessment

- Ask students to think about why their eating habits are the way they are. Ask them to identify the most effective ways they can positively impact their community's eating habits? It is highly likely that each community will require different action steps to change the way they eat grains.
- Encourage students to put in the work and take those action steps to improve the grains offered in their town, school, and home.

COMPREHENSIVE

Lesson: The Cost of Grain in the Marketplace

> **MATERIALS**
- Calculators
- Graph paper
- Charts, graphs, Excel spreadsheets

> **GOALS**

Learn the actual costs of buying packaged foods versus homemade bread and baked goods.

> **OBJECTIVES**
- To calculate the price of different grains bought in the bulk food section of grocery stores
- To analyze the difference in store-bought products like crackers, bread, pizza dough, or tortillas and the cost of making homemade crackers, bread, pizza dough, or tortillas
- To compare taste and convenience between store-bought and homemade baked foods

> **ACTIVATING PRIOR KNOWLEDGE**

Do you or anyone in your family bake their bread or pasta? Many people grow their foods and make and bake their bread. Homesteaders, home gardeners, your neighbor, your mom or dad, grandparents, friends, schools, restaurants, hotels, resorts, and cafés are some examples. Is baking and making food from scratch a lost art? How important is it to know how to make your food from scratch?

BACKGROUND INFORMATION

Grain is a widely traded commodity sold on a global scale. In this lesson, go deep in exploring how we eat, procure, and pay for grains today compared to past generations. Today, most Americans depend on grocery stores and restaurants to provide them with food. But does that make the food more cost-effective, nutritious, or tastier? Or is it just the opposite? Students will dive into the real financial costs of making bread from scratch compared to buying it in the store. Ask your students to share their findings.

> Procedure 1

Calculate, compare, contrast, and analyze the cost of commercially sold crackers, bread, pizza dough, or tortillas vs. baked at home vs. what you would get at an independently owned bakery.

1. Make a list of factors that go into the cost of baking bread—whether made at home or as a commercially prepared food product.
   - Ingredients
   - Labor
   - Transportation
   - Food distributors
   - Storage facilities
   - Packaging
   - Waste

2. Calculate the price of different grains in the bulk food section of grocery stores.

3. For instance, if 25 lbs of long-grain rice costs $37.50, that equals $1.25 a pound. How much is one cup of rice? There are 2 ½ cups of rice in one pound, so figure out how much one cup of rice would cost.

4. Compare taste, cost, and convenience between store-bought and homemade baked foods.

5. Have students identify the ingredients found in bread that would be baked at home and then have them figure out what the cost of those ingredients would be per loaf of bread.

Assessment

- Ask students what inspired them about this lesson?
- Are they more or less motivated to bake and make food from scratch at home or school?
- Is it worth the effort financially, timewise, healthwise, and environmentally to grow, make, bake, and cook food?

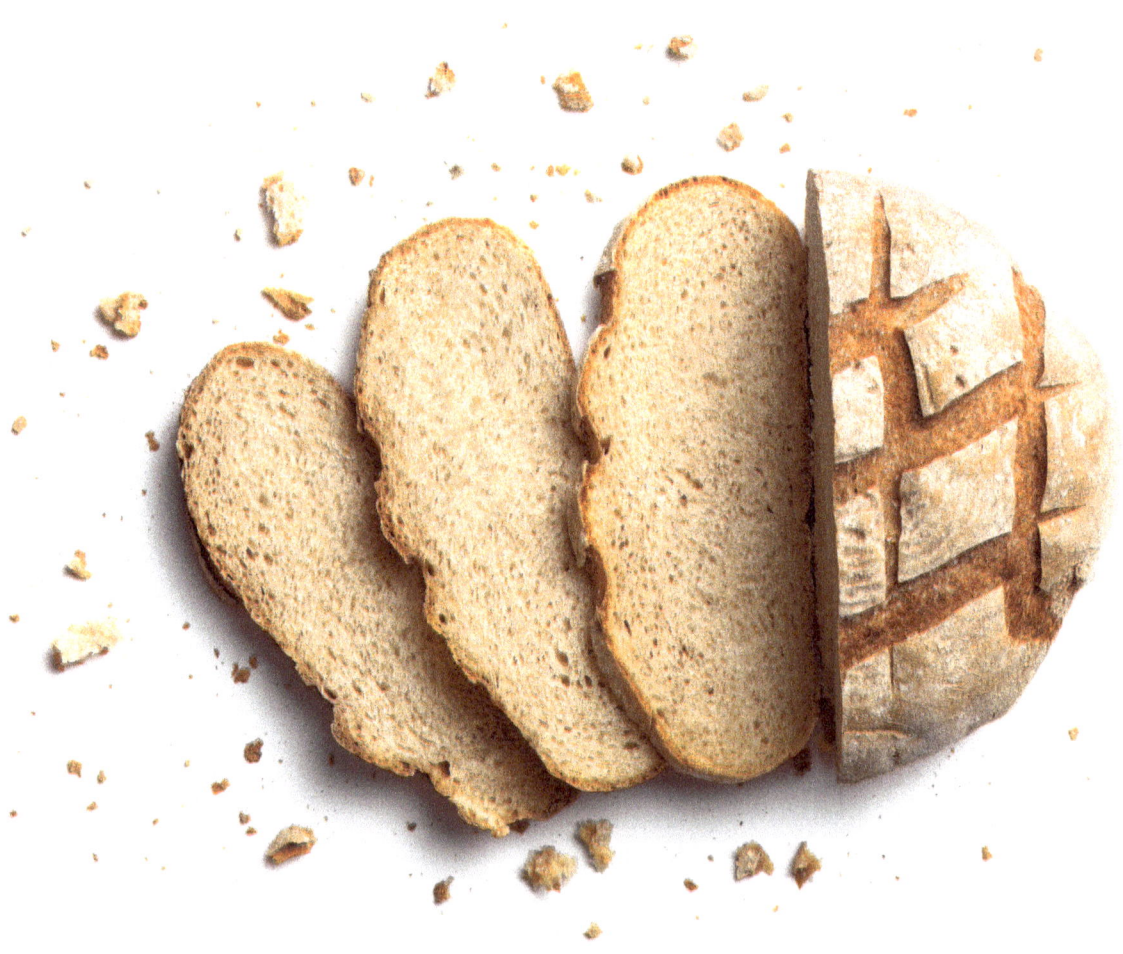

COMPREHENSIVE

Lesson: History and Trade of Grains in The United States

➤ MATERIALS
- Textbooks and access to the Internet
- Poster boards
- Maps

➤ GOAL
Explore the wide variety of grains that we eat.

➤ OBJECTIVES
- To compare the size, taste, growing conditions, and variety of grains grown hundreds or thousands of years ago to today's modern grains
- To list countries that produce or trade grains

➤ ACTIVATING PRIOR KNOWLEDGE
Engage students in a discussion about the grains they typically eat. Discuss the countries or continents of origin and the trade routes that got them onto our plates. Press them to see if they know where those grains originated. Explore wheat, corn, and quinoa, for example.

BACKGROUND INFORMATION

Grains are a favorite food eaten around the world. They also happen to be a massive part of the American diet. But do you know where these grains (i.e., wheat, rice, corn) originally came from? The grains we eat today have originated from all over the world. People have traded grains across continents for thousands of years, and now it is easier than ever, thanks to the advancement of transportation.

FOCUS ON SORGHUM
Sorghum was found near the Egyptian-Sudanese border dating back to 8,000 B.C. From there, it spread across Africa then to India, China, and Australia. It made its way to the United States in the 1700s, where it was used in making brooms, according to the writings of Benjamin Franklin. (1)

Grain List
- Amaranth
- Barley
- Buckwheat (aka kasha)
- Bulgur (wheat)
- Corn
- Couscous (wheat)
- Faro
- Kamut
- Millet
- Oats
- Rice- basmati, black, brown, wild
- Rye
- Quinoa
- Spelt
- Sorghum
- Teff
- Wheat

▶ Procedure 1
GETTING REAL WITH GRAINS

Discover more about the grains you eat regularly as well as those with which you are not so familiar. Have students research one type of grain. Have students focus on the history, origins, trade routes, growing conditions, agricultural uses, cultural roots, and how and when the grain found its way to the U.S. Discuss the size, color, taste, growing conditions, farming and cultivation practices that may have changed since humans first started eating or growing it.

Address the concept of heirloom grains, varieties, and cultivars.

▶ Procedure 2
TRADE ROUTES OF GRAINS

Have students prepare a paper about:

- Countries that grow or trade grains with the United States.
- Distinguish if the grains are fairly traded, sustainably harvested, or organically grown. What grains are endemic (native) to the continental United States? Hawaii? Alaska? Puerto Rico? What grain crops are grown in the U.S. today?

Assessment

- Ask students if they were surprised by the outcomes of their research projects.
- Ask if this lesson made them more appreciative of where their food originates.
- Were your students interested in the long history grains have played in our diets and our traditional foods?

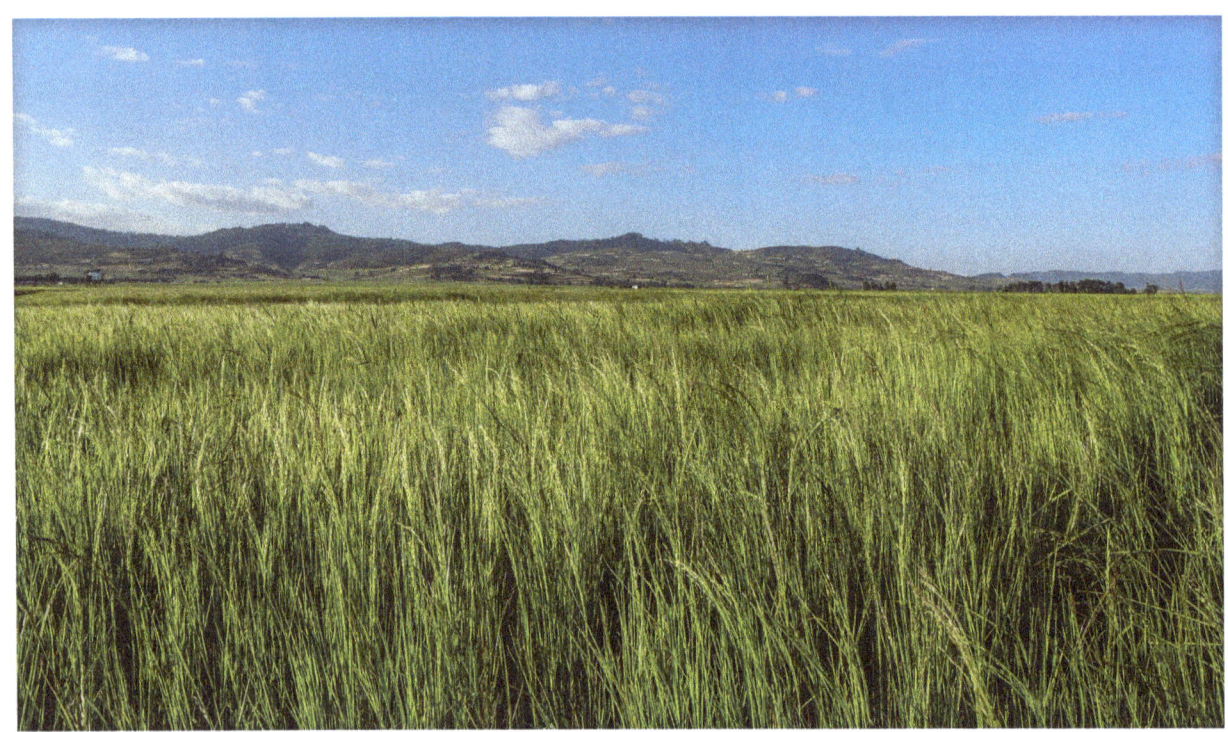

Teff field in Ethiopia

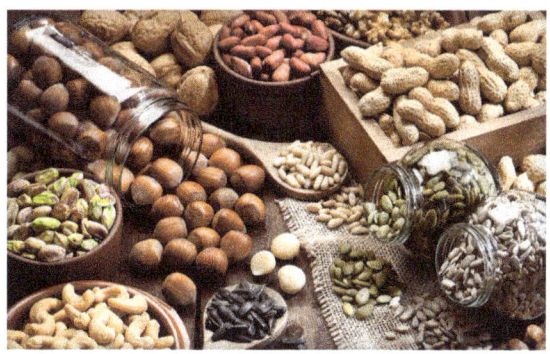

INTRODUCTION TO THE FATS FOOD GROUP

THE FOOD TREE ANALOGY
The Branches represent the Fats Food Group on The Food Tree. Imagine that the fats you eat are like the branches of a big tree. The branches reach out far and wide, creating the structure for the whole canopy. Branches bring nutrients to the leaves and the fruit. They are like the fats that make up every cell in the body and provide nutrients to every cell in our body.

DAILY RECOMMENDED SERVING SUGGESTION: 3
25% of daily calories
Energy source, fat, nine calories per gram

PLANT-BASED AND ANIMAL-BASED FAT FOOD SOURCES
Plant-Based Fat Food Sources

- Nuts and seeds as a whole food; milk, oil, or butter; grains and legumes and their oils
- Seaweeds, seaweed oil
- Blue-green algae

Animal-Based Fats

- Meats, dairy, fish, poultry

WHAT ARE FATS?

Fats are one of the three macronutrients found in plant and animal foods. Fats are made up of fatty acids that fit into three subgroups called Polyunsaturated Fatty Acids (PUFAs), Monounsaturated Fatty Acids (MUFAs), and Saturated Fatty Acids (SFAs). The Polyunsaturated Fatty Acids (PUFA's) are made up of Omega 3 essential fatty acids and Omega 6 essential fatty acids.

FOUNDATIONAL

Lesson: Getting to Know Fats

➤ MATERIALS
- Examples of different types of fats and oils found in foods or oils, either real or from books, pictures, magazines, or online
- The Food Tree Daily Food Journal, located in the Activities section
- The Food Tree Nutrient Scroll, located in the Appendix
- Fatty Acid Chart, located at the end of the Fats Chapter
- Frequency of Eating Fatty Foods and Oils handout, located at the end of the Fats Chapter.

➤ GOALS
- Understand both animal and plant foods have fats and oils.
- Know that all fats and oils contain a variety of fatty acids.

➤ OBJECTIVES
- To name five different types of fat-containing foods and oils
- To classify different foods and their fatty acids into the three fat sub-groups: polyunsaturated, monounsaturated, and saturated fats
- To compare different fatty acids and the ratios found from three different kinds of fat-containing oils or food

➤ ACTIVATING PRIOR KNOWLEDGE
Fats and oils are found abundantly in many foods, including, for example, avocado, butter, nuts, and fish. Ask students to discuss the types of foods with fats or oils they usually eat or that they are familiar with. Discuss with your class if they think eating fats in their diet is essential, and why or why not? Do they believe that fats get a bad rap?

BACKGROUND INFORMATION

In this lesson, you will become familiar with different types of fats and oils. Then, you will look carefully at how fats are classified to see how the fat subgroups are broken down, as well as to demystify them.

Over the last 50 years, at least, there has been unrelenting confusion about what types of fats are good or bad for you. I will do my best to recommend what is the most current and up to date scientifically researched information to support optimal nutrition. (1)

Food Source of Fats
People may receive fats from two different kinds of food, plant-based or animal-based. For instance, a person can obtain saturated fats from either a plant-based source, like coconut oil, or from an animal-based source, such as butter.

Almost all fats and oils contain all three types of fat subgroups in them, with varying percentages of these fatty acids. For example, olive oil is made up of a bit of saturated fat, omega 3, and omega 6 PUFA's and the majority is made up of monounsaturated fatty acids, whereas salmon has a majority of omega 3 PUFA's, some MUFA's, and a bit of saturated fat. (2)

Plant-Based Fat Food Sources
FRUITS, WHOLE NUTS, SEEDS, BEANS, GRAINS, AND OILS

Nuts and seeds in their whole food form, as a milk, in oil form, or as a butter

Almond, avocado, blue-green algae, Brazil nut, cashew nut, chestnut, chia seed, coconut, corn, flaxseed, grape seed oil, hazelnut, hemp seed, macadamia nut, palm oil, peanut, pecan, pine nut, pistachio nut, poppyseed, pumpkin seed, rice bran oil, safflower oil, sesame seed (tahini), soybeans, sunflower seed, olive, walnut

Avoid eating and purchasing packaged foods that contain unsustainably grown and harvested palm oil for ecological reasons.

SEAWEEDS, SEAWEED OIL, AND BLUE-GREEN ALGAE

Seaweeds and algae are highly nutritious superfoods. They contain polyunsaturated fats, including EPA and DHA Omega 3 EFAs (essential fatty acids).

Arame, bladderwrack, chlorella, dulce, gim, gracilaria, hijiki, Irish moss, kelp, kombu, laver, nori, sea lettuce, sea palm, wakame

Animal-Based Fats

Meats: beef/tallow, bison, wild game

Dairy: milk, buttermilk, butter, kefir, ghee, sour cream, yogurt

Fish and seafood: anchovy, mackerel, herring, wild salmon (avoid farm-raised), shrimp, trout, tuna

Poultry: chicken, chicken fat, chicken eggs, duck, duck fat, duck eggs, quail, turkey

Fats and oils are categorized based on their make-up of chemicals, called fatty acids. They are classified into three groups:

Polyunsaturated fatty acid (PUFA)

Monounsaturated fatty acid (MUFA)

Saturated fatty acid (SFA)

Refer to the Classification of Fats and Oils, following this lesson, that demonstrates the distribution of fatty acids found in the different types of fats and oils.

The Food Tree believes that good health depends on consuming a variety of fats from all three fat groups and in specific amounts. Then, from there, an individual can decide which food to eat to get the nutrients they need and desire.

➤ Procedure 1
KEEP A FOOD JOURNAL

1. Students keep a food journal for one week.
2. Identify the type of fat found in each food.

➤ Procedure 2
TAKE A POLL ON DIETARY FATS INTAKE DIVERSITY IN YOUR COMMUNITY

Interview or survey 5-10 people to research the diversity of dietary fat intake in their diet. Use

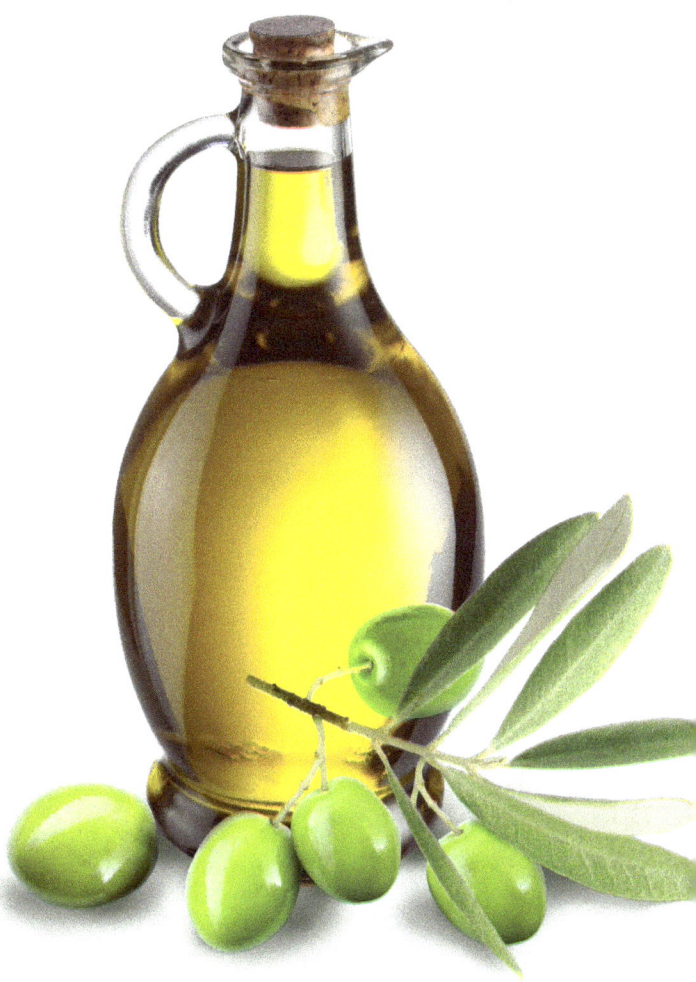

CLASSIFICATION OF FATS AND OILS

Fats and fatty acids are categorized by their molecular structure involving the degree of saturation of hydrogen molecules on the carbon chain.

POLYUNSATURATED FATTY ACIDS (PUFAs)

Recommend 40% of your daily fat intake

Polyunsaturated fats are made up of essential fats- omega 3 essential fatty acid and omega 6 essential fatty acid.

OMEGA 3 ESSENTIAL FATTY ACID (EFAS) (PUFA)
Recommend 10% of your daily polyunsaturated fat intake

- ALA (Alpha-Linolenic Acid)
- EPA (Eicosapentaenoic Acid)
- DHA (Docosahexaenoic Acid)

Sources of Omega 3s

- Nuts and Seeds: chia, hemp seeds, walnuts
- Dark leafy greens: collards and kale
- Fish: anchovies, cod liver, herring, mackerel, salmon, rainbow trout, pollock, tuna
- Meat: beef, grass-fed, chicken
- Seaweed
- Blue-green algae, spirulina

OMEGA-6 ESSENTIAL FATTY ACID (EFAs)(PUFA)
Recommend 30% of your daily polyunsaturated fat intake

- LA (Linoleic acid)
- GLA (Gamma-Linolenic Acid)
- ARA (Arachidonic Acid)
- CLA (Conjugated Linoleic Acid)

It is best to get these types of fatty acids in food form, if possible, instead of vegetable cooking oils

- Borage oil
- Canola oil
- Corn/oil
- Evening primrose oil
- Grapeseed oil
- Hemp seeds/oil
- Peanuts/oil
- Poppyseed oil
- Rice bran oil
- Safflower oil
- Sesame seeds/oil
- Soybeans/oil
- Spirulina
- Sunflower seeds/oil
- Walnuts/oil
- Poultry, fish, eggs

*Only use organic corn, soybean oil, and canola oil due to GMOs. (1) Canola oil is generally not recommended.
*Always buy bovine growth hormone free dairy and meat and choose organic, pasture raised grass-fed animals.

MONOUNSATURATED FATS OMEGA 9

Recommend 30%—40% of your daily fat intake

Oleic acid

Sources of Omega 9's

- Nuts, nut butter: peanuts/oil
- Avocado oil
- Corn/oil
- Canola oil
- Soybeans/oil
- Dark leafy greens: kale
- Olives/oil
- Poultry fat
- Lard (pork)

*Only use organic corn, soybean oil, and canola oil due to GMOs.

SATURATED FATS

Recommend 20%—30% of your daily fat intake

Lauric acid, stearic acid, palmitic acid, myristic acid, capric acid, caprylic acid

Sources of Saturated Fats

- Coconut oil: coconut butter, coconut milk
- Dairy Fats: butter, milk, yogurt, beef/tallow

*Palm oil is to be avoided due to the destruction of the rainforest and orangutan habitat.

the Frequency of Eating Fatty Foods and Oils handout or the students can create their own. Come up with a list as long as you desire of foods containing fats. Use your reporter's mic, video recorder, or smartphone and interview friends, parents, teachers, and neighbors about their views and understanding of dietary fats. Present your findings later to the class.

1. Take a poll at your school, your local library, a grocery store, or some local place in your community to get a better understanding of people's eating habits regarding fats.
2. Get a glimpse of how much people know about the variety of health benefits of eating all types of fatty acids.
3. Create a list of basic questions to ask. Record the answers.

Here is a list of sample questions. Have students come up with questions on their own as well.

- What is saturated fat, and in what foods are they found?
- Do you think saturated fats are healthy to eat?
- What quantity of saturated fat should a person eat in one day?
- What types of attitudes and opinions do you have about eating fats in your diet?
- What foods are EFAs found in?

Reflections

- Do you think people eat vastly different from each other? Or more similar? Does eating different types of fats vary between races, ages, working status, or economics?
- How often do people switch up the fats they eat daily? For different meals?

▶ Procedure 3
DIVE INTO THE CHEMISTRY OF FATTY ACIDS

This activity explores the chemistry of fatty acids that make up the Fatty Acid Spectrum- Saturated, Monounsaturated, and Polyunsaturated Fats.

1. Create a poster describing in detail the chemical composition and benefits of one of the fatty acids.

   OR

2. Compare and contrast the nutrition profiles of different fat-containing foods or fatty acids.

Assessment

Reframe what the students learned about fat containing foods and oils and the fatty acids found in fats and oils. Appraise their level of understanding.

FOUNDATIONAL

Lesson: Serving Sizes and Daily Recommendations for Fats

➤ MATERIALS
- The Food Tree Magnetic Board
- Examples of cooking oils and foods that contain fat: avocado, a bag of nuts, a jar of coconut oil, butter packaging
- Measuring spoons
- Fat Log Sheet
- The Food Tree Food Journal found in the Activities Section

➤ GOAL
Understand serving sizes and daily recommendations for fats.

➤ OBJECTIVES
- To state daily serving sizes and the percentages of each fat group needed to maintain a healthy diet
- To demonstrate an appropriate serving size of fats
- To learn and identify three different types of healthy fats and oils to include in a person's diet
- To make clear and educated decisions about the kinds and amounts of fats needed in a daily diet

➤ ACTIVATING PRIOR KNOWLEDGE
Engage students in a conversation about the different types and amounts of fats found in the foods they commonly eat. Examples may include foods like nuts or seeds, butter, and olive oil. Ask how much fat-containing foods they think they should eat every day.

BACKGROUND INFORMATION

I recommend eating three servings a day of a variety of fats and oils from all of the fat groups.

The Food Tree Fats Recommendations

Daily Recommended Serving Suggestion: 3

25% of our daily calories, energy source, macronutrient fats, nine calories per gram

However, like all things, how much fat you need depends on the person and your unique requirements. Adjust the actual amount eaten to take into account a person's height, weight, age, caloric needs, and activity level.

Dietary Daily Recommendations of Fats and Oils

Polyunsaturated: 40% total of your daily fat intake
 Omega 3: 10% of PUFA total
 Omega 6: 30% of PUFA total

Monounsaturated Fats: 30%–40% of your daily fat intake

Saturated Fats: 20%—30% of your daily fat intake

There are many delicious, nutritious ways to incorporate healthy fats into your diet. But almost more important than the amount of fat eaten is the type of fat eaten, the quality of the fat eaten, and the ratio consumed. Eat a variety of fats and oils to obtain all the necessary fatty acids from each of the three fat group: polyunsaturated, monounsaturated, and saturated fats. Most people can always afford to add more omega-3 EFAs into their diets to create a better ratio to omega 6s. (1, 2)

Explore more ways of getting beneficial fats into your diet.

If your diet preferences agree, eat a variety of fats from both animal and plant-based sources. Or, it is entirely possible to get all of your necessary nutrients from eating only plant-based fat sources.

- Have a serving of a PUFA, a MUFA, and a saturated fat every day.
- Make your own salad dressing.
- Put flax oil (never heat flax oil) on your homemade popcorn.
- Add avocado to toast.
- Eat nuts and seeds every day as a snack.
- Add olives to a salad.
- Eat and drink full fat dairy and milk products.
- Use soy milk instead of water in hot cereals.
- Add coconut milk to soups.
- Put almond, cashew, or peanut butter on celery or apples.
- Eat the right proportions of fats.

What other ideas do students have? Share your thoughts with your classmates and your community!

Choose Quality Fats and Oils

Strive to eat The Food Tree way: in-season, locally, sustainably, fair trade, homegrown, and organic whenever possible. And, just like with animal-based proteins, make sure that you choose hormone-free dairy and animal fats. Watch out for Nutrition Vampires, and read labels. Pay careful attention to avoid partially hydrogenated oils and bovine growth hormones. Big business will have you believe dairy products from cows injected with growth hormones are safe to drink. But studies show otherwise.

These hormones are linked to many serious health concerns, not only in the animals that are treated but to us humans as well.

Samuel Epstein, MD from the Cancer Prevention Coalition recently released a press statement about the European Commission report on rBGH which concluded that excess hormone (growth factor) poses a serious risk of breast and prostate cancer. The EC has banned the use of Monstanto's products since 1999. Look for the rBGH-free label on food labels.

Serving Size Examples for Fats

The serving size can and will vary for each person depending on height, weight, and nutrient needs.

1 or 2 tablespoons walnuts or sunflower seeds

2 tablespoons nut butter or seed butters

2 tablespoons coconut milk

1 tablespoon coconut oil, butter, or cold-pressed vegetable oil

1/8–1/4 avocado

8-10 medium olives

1-2 eggs

3 ounces salmon, salmon jerky, sardines, mackerel, herring

1 tablespoon butter

1 ounce cheese

▶ Procedure 1
SERVING SIZES

Discuss the list of the recommended serving sizes of fats.

- Show examples of fat servings sizes. Use real food, models, or pictures. For instance, show your students a serving size of salad dressing, nuts, or butter on toast. How does this compare to what they usually would eat?

▶ Procedure 2
MEAL PLANNING—FATS, WE LOVE YOU!

Have students create a day's worth of what eating three servings of fats looks like on a meal planning sheet.

1. Create a meal plan for one day and up to one week, highlighting the types of fats needed to fulfill a person's daily requirements. Have them do this exercise as an individual or group two or three students together to collaborate on one to seven daily meal plans.
2. Students write down how each serving would be prepared.
3. Have students include recipes and nutrition facts for an extra challenge.
4. Or, have students use an outline of The Food Tree and write the fat foods and oils on The Branches of The Food Tree image. Students can also draw or cut and paste pictures from food magazines and glue onto The Food Tree.

SAMPLE MEAL PLAN IDEAS: THREE SERVINGS OF FATS A DAY

Breakfast 2 scrambled eggs

Snack 2 tablespoons toasted sunflower seeds with tamari

Lunch 1 tablespoon flax oil salad dressing over a green salad

Snack ½ cup guacamole

Dinner 3 ounces of wild-caught salmon

▶ Procedure 3
KEEP A FATS FOOD JOURNAL

Young students can keep a simple food journal, and older students can keep a more comprehensive journal.

▶ Procedure 4
EXTRA JOURNAL CHALLENGE: FAT LOG SHEET

1. Keep track and classify the fats as fatty acids you eat—Polyunsaturated, Monounsaturated, Saturated.
2. In the log, write across the top: "Date, Polyunsaturated, Monounsaturated, Saturated, Serving Size, From Home, From School, From a Restaurant."
3. Down the left side, write a list of fat-containing foods.
4. Ask students to keep the journal for one week. Explore data findings:
5. What were the most common sources of fats eaten?
6. You can record student responses on a big wall chart or do anonymously to protect the student's privacy.

Assessment

- What have students learned from looking at their diets compared to The Food Tree recommendations?
- Students can take this lesson a step further and calculate the variety and serving intake that they are eating every day. Explore the Fatty Acid Spectrum for a more in-depth look at fats and how they are categorized.
- Consider what new variety of fats and oils students are willing to try in their diets. For instance, challenge them to use homemade salad dressings in the family home and in the school cafeteria instead of eating highly processed fats and oils. Ask students to write down the changes they could make.
- Challenge them to implement these changes, even if it's just one meal at a time.

FOUNDATIONAL

Lesson: Benefits and Functions of Fats

➤ **MATERIALS**

Fatty Acid Spectrum Chart, located at the end of the Fats Chapter

➤ **GOAL**

Educate students on the myriad of benefits that comes from eating a diet rich in healthy fats.

➤ **OBJECTIVES**

- To identify and describe at least three functions and benefits that eating healthy fats play in a person's health and well-being
- To foster awareness of the health impact of deficiencies and excesses of fats in the diet

➤ **ACTIVATING PRIOR KNOWLEDGE**

Ask students to discuss why they believe eating fat in the diet may be useful for them. It may be a good time to talk about the taboo of fats in the diet world, as age appropriate.

BACKGROUND INFORMATION

In the past few decades, fats have gotten a bad rap, but the truth is all types of fats, naturally occurring, of course, are essential to your health. Pay attention to the types, amounts, and quality of the fat you are eating.

Benefits and Functions of Fats

Fats do amazing things. They are critical nutrients that facilitate hundreds of different functions in your body. Here are some of the highlights that fats are responsible for:

PROVIDE ENERGY SOURCE

Fats provide nine calories per gram that supply long-lasting, stable energy. Unused fats are stored in cells for later usage.

PROVIDE NUTRIENTS

Fats provide valuable nutrients in the form of fatty acids. Examples of fatty acids include lauric acid found in coconut oil and oleic acid found in olive oil.

BUILD CELL STRUCTURE

Fats are critical components of the body's composition. The outer membrane of every cell in the body is made up of fats. The brain is made up of 60% fat. (1)

PROVIDE PROTECTION

Fats surround, protect, and insulate vital organs and nerves. A cushioning enables the nerves to perform faster messaging. Fats keep organs in place and act as a buffer preventing them from injury.

HORMONE PRODUCTION

Fatty acids help make many different chemical messengers called hormones that are critical to physical and emotional processes. A proper fatty acid balance will help keep a person in a good mood and will help to lower stress levels.

MANAGE INFLAMMATION

Fatty acids make chemicals called prostaglandins that regulate important body functions like inflammation. (2)

FACILITATE NUTRIENT ABSORPTION

Specific vitamins called fat-soluble vitamins need fat for absorption into the body. These vitamins are vitamin A, vitamin D, vitamin E, and vitamin K. These vitamins can only be absorbed and used by the body with the help of fat.

PROVIDE WARMTH
Fats will keep the body warm and regulate body temperature.

CREATE SATIETY
Fats help create that full feeling. They burn more slowly and provide more calories than their counterpart macronutrients. So, they tend to create a full sensation that has a more long-lasting effect.

ENJOY THE TASTE!
People like the taste of fats. Whether it's butter on a biscuit, olive oil drizzled over pasta, or a flax oil salad dressing, we naturally crave fats in our diet. Fats add a complex dimension to food, making foods and dishes more nutritious, tasty, and satisfying.

The Forms and Functions of Different Types of Fats

Fats come in different forms and perform various functions. They include:

TRIGLYCERIDES
Triglycerides make up ninety-five percent of the fat we eat and make up ninety-five percent of the fat that is in our bodies. They are made up of three (tri) fatty-acid chains attached to a glycerol (sugar) molecule. Our body breaks off the sugar molecule from the fatty acids to use as nutrients.

FATTY ACIDS
Fat foods and oils, like coconut oil and olive oil, contain different ratios of fatty acids. The three main groups are Polyunsaturated Fatty Acids, Monounsaturated Fatty Acids, and Saturated Fatty Acids. Fatty acids do thousands of important tasks for our human functioning. It is crucial to understand that ALL fat-containing foods have a mix of all of the fatty acids in them but different ratios. Eating a diet rich in a range of natural fats found in all of the fat groups is critical for optimal health.

POLYUNSATURATED ESSENTIAL FATTY ACID FUNCTIONS—HIGHLIGHTING THE BENEFITS OF OMEGA 3 ESSENTIAL FATTY ACIDS
Omega 3 Essential Fatty Acids are called "essential" because the body cannot make them. The same goes for omega 6s, but deficiencies in those fatty acids are not as common. Omega 3s EFAs are found in cold water fish, walnuts, flax oil, and hemp seeds.

Omega 3s EFAs

- Improve learning attention span and cognitive functions in children and the elderly (3)
- Necessary for brain development and function
- Elevate mood, decrease depression
- Calm the body's stress defenses
- Promote healthy skin
- Improve heart health, reduce heart disease
- Lower cholesterol by up to 25%
- Lower triglycerides by up to 65%
- Improve vision, especially night vision
- Improve metabolic rate (energy)
- Reduce inflammation
- Convert to prostaglandins (PGE 3)
- Help maintain healthy weight
- Help produce hemoglobin in the blood
- Help muscles recover from fatigue
- Keep blood thinner and healthier

HIGHLIGHTING THE BENEFITS OF OMEGA 6 ESSENTIAL FATTY ACID

- Promote hormone balance
- Alleviate PMS symptoms
- Improve rheumatoid arthritis
- Improve ADHD symptoms

EFAs helped preserve learning ability and cognitive function in the face of emotional stress. In a study in the International Journal of Neuroscience, researchers found when "laboratory rodents that consumed an EFA mixture before being administered either cortisol or saline to induce 'cold stress' their cortisol and cholesterol levels did not rise as much in response. Additionally, their ability to maneuver a maze was not impaired by stress inducers." (4)

Monounsaturated Fatty Acid Functions Omega 9s

- Improve the quality and health of the skin
- Reduce the risk of heart disease and stroke
- Increase availability of energy

Saturated Fatty Acid Functions

- Regulate body temperature
- Promote heart health
- Solid or semi-solid at room temperature
- Heat stable

PHOSPHOLIPIDS

Phospholipids are the main component making up every cell membrane in the body. They form a bilayer containing cholesterol that behaves as a barrier between the outer physical environment and the cell. Their molecular structure contains two fatty acids, a glycerol molecule, and a phosphate group, all attached. They keep cells soft and supple. They carry fatty materials across cell membranes. They may be beneficial for brain health and memory. Lecithin is a common phospholipid found in egg yolk and soybeans. It is made up of phosphatidylcholine and phosphatidylserine. (5)

LIPOPROTEINS

HDL (High-Density Lipoproteins)—HDL carries cholesterol from the body's tissues to the liver for excretion, thereby being protective against heart disease. It is critical in the break-down of fat cells.

LDL (Low-Density Lipoproteins)—LDL transports cholesterol and triglycerides from the liver and small intestine to cells and tissues.

VLDL (Very Low-Density Lipoproteins)—VLDL are made in the liver. They bring cholesterol and triglycerides from the liver and small intestine to cells.

CHOLESTEROL

Cholesterol is a waxy alcohol-based chemical substance that is made in the liver and in most cells, as needed, for human functioning.

- Aids in the manufacturing of bile necessary for fat digestion
- Is the precursor for the synthesis of Vitamin D
- Necessary for steroidal hormone production, like the adrenal hormones and the sex hormones, estrogen and testosterone
- Used in the vascular system to soothe inflammation
- Makes the cells more flexible and permeable
- Carried through the bloodstream by lipoproteins
- Carried out of the body when attached to fiber

Cholesterol is often tagged as the number one culprit in cardiovascular disease. However, Dr. Stephan Sinatra, author of *The Cholesterol Myth*, suggests that current data show that inflammation is the real link to heart disease. Inflammation caused by drugs, poor diet, and stress can create wounds in the blood vessels. The job of cholesterol in this case is to act as a soothing agent, balm, or band-aide on the site of the inflammation. Cholesterol is only doing its job. Your body will make cholesterol as needed depending on how much or how little is in the diet. The point is to figure out what is causing the inflammation and to reduce it. (6)

Metabolism of Fats and Oils

- Digestion—requires enzymes and bile salts
- Absorption—thru lymph, size of fatty acid matters

- Assimilation—making energy from triglycerides
- Distribution—lipoproteins carry fats thru the body
- Storage—if not used as fuel, triglycerides are stored in adipose tissue

Deficiencies in fatty acids may occur if a person does not eat enough fat-containing foods and oils or has the wrong kinds of balance. The health problems that may arise can be numerous and might include poor skin condition, sex hormone imbalances, depression and mood issues, heart issues, cognitive issues, digestive issues, and issues related to inflammation. (7)

➤ Procedure 1
SELL IT!

Students will identify and research at least three functions healthy fats play in a person's health and wellbeing. They can present their findings via a class presentation, skit, commercial, rap, poster board display, or paper.

➤ Procedure 2
FAT MYTHS

Create an informational sheet, graph, poster, or trifold depicting Ten Myths and Truths about dietary fat.

Common Fat Myths

- All fats are bad for you.
- A fat-free diet is a crucial part of a weight loss program.
- Cardiovascular Disease (CVD) is linked to the consumption of fats and induces high cholesterol.
- Hydrogenated and partially hydrogenated fats keep food fresh longer and are therefore healthy.
- Olive oil is the best type of fat and provides all of the nutrients I need.

➤ Procedure 3
Q & A HEALTH PANEL

Create a panel of two to five students to field questions from the rest of the class on the topic of fats. Explore ideas regarding different health trends and how people perceive fats in their diets. Switch around as needed to accommodate your class size so that everyone gets a turn to be on the panel to answer a question.

Assessment

- Discuss with your students how their attitudes towards eating fats have changed.
- Have a follow-up talk on the importance of eating a variety of fats to support a healthy diet.
- What was one surprising fact learned about the functions of fats in this lesson?

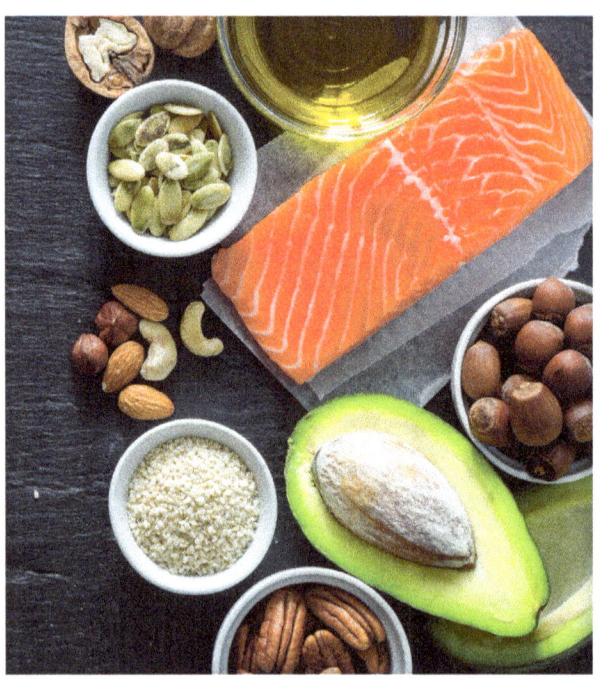

DISCOVERY

Lesson: Benefits of Essential Fatty Acids Omega 3 and Omega 6

➤ MATERIALS
- Foods that contain omega 3 and omega 6 essential fatty acids: flax seeds, walnut, hemp seeds, sardines, salmon, blue-green algae

➤ GOAL
Learn the health benefits of foods that provide polyunsaturated omega 3 and omega 6 essential fatty acids.

➤ OBJECTIVES
- To identify three different types of essential omega 3 fats and three types of essential omega 6 fats
- To demonstrate one's understanding of the important role polyunsaturated essential omega 3 and omega 6 fats play in the body
- To identify at least three functions essential fatty acids' play in our health and wellbeing

➤ ACTIVATING PRIOR KNOWLEDGE
Discuss what the word *essential* means. Provide examples of things that are essential for survival. For example, trees need sunlight. Humans need to breathe air. Then, talk about the types of fats students might eat during the day. Do they think fats could possibly be essential to their health?

BACKGROUND INFORMATION

Polyunsaturated fats are one of three sub-groups of how fatty acids, or lipids, are classified. The other two groups are monounsaturated fats and saturated fats. Polyunsaturated omega 3 and omega 6 essential fatty acids are essential because the body cannot make them, unlike saturated and monounsaturated fats that can be made by the body if and when needed. Therefore, it is critically important that people consume essential fats because a lack of them in a person's diet could lead to health issues.

It's all about balance with these two types of fats. Most Americans are deficient in omega 3 EFAs and are too high in omega 6 EFAs. A healthy ratio to eat would be 1:3 omega 3 to omega 6 essential fatty acid (EFA). It is common in the United States for people to eat a ratio of 1:20 omega 3s to omega 6s. (1) An imbalance like this is a result of eating too many heavily processed and packaged foods that use omega 6 oils in their products.

Examples of foods with high omega 6 oils are crackers, pastries, salad dressings, and bread. Eating a poor ratio of EFAs can contribute to inflammation, aches, and pains from igniting our bodies' inflammatory pathway.

Food Sources of Omega 3 EFAs
Flax seeds, flax seed oil, hemp seeds, hemp seed oil, walnuts, walnut oil, soybeans, soybean oil, wheat germ, dark leafy greens, pumpkin seeds, seaweed, cold water fish, salmon, sardines, mackerel, herring, eggs, grass-fed beef

*Never heat or cook flax seeds or flax oil due to its low heat point

Food Sources of Omega 6 EFAs

Borage oil, blackcurrant oil, corn, hemp seeds, soybeans, safflower oil, sunflower seed/oil

Benefits and Functions Omega 3 and Omega 6 EFAs

Omega 3 EFAs are best known as brain food! Omega 3 EFAs make up the membranes of brain cells that allow for vital nutrients to flow in and waste products to flow out. Essential omega 3s allow for our neurotransmitters, the brain's chemical messengers, to be received. (2)

- Improve learning attention span and cognitive functions in children and the elderly
- Elevate mood, decrease depression
- Promote healthy skin
- Improve heart health, reduce heart disease
- Help manage stress
- Improve vision, especially night vision
- Improve metabolic (energy) rate
- Reduce inflammation
- Help control weight
- Lower triglycerides by up to 65%
- Necessary for brain development and proper function
- Produce hemoglobin in blood
- Help muscles recover from fatigue
- Convert to prostaglandins—PGE 3
- Soothe the body's defenses
- Keep blood thinner and healthier

Signs of Omega 3 Deficiencies

Symptoms can develop because of a deficiency of omega 3 essential fats over time. They may show up as:

- Learning issues
- Growth retardation
- Impaired brain function
- Impaired learning ability
- Muscle weakness
- Attention Deficit Hyperactivity Disorder
- Behavioral changes
- Irritability
- Mood swings
- Dry skin
- Low metabolic rate
- Tingling arms and legs
- High blood pressure
- Edema
- Poor vision
- Hormonal imbalances
- Inflammation
- Poor motor coordination

RECOMMENDATIONS FOR OMEGA 3 ESSENTIAL FATTY ACID

- Add more EFAs, especially omega 3 EFAs, to the diet.
- Eat a 3:1 ratio of omega 6 to omega 3 EFAs.
- Avoid Nutrition Vampire hydrogenated and partially hydrogenated oils
- Take a fish oil supplement if needed.

Omega 3 oils, like flax and walnuts, are fragile and can become damaged when exposed to light or heat. Damaged fats and oils could potentially become a source of inflammation and oxidative cellular damage.

It is best to store nuts and seeds, flax and fish oils in the fridge or a cool dark location. You can also freeze nuts and seeds for more extended use.

➤ Procedure: 1

Identify three different types of essential omega 3 and three types of essential omega 6 fats. Discuss their benefits.

➤ Procedure: 2

Demonstrate one's understanding of the vital role polyunsaturated omega 3 and omega 6 essential fats play in the body.

- Task students to highlight a particular omega 3 or 6 fat-containing food and do an in-depth study and present to the class on its fatty acid benefits. Have students write a report, do a skit, or make up a commercial, individually, pairs, or groups, focusing on the health functions essential fatty acids play in our bodies, issues with deficiencies and how to correct them.

EXAMPLE: ALMONDS

- What fatty acids ratios are found in almonds?
- What are the best ways to prepare and eat almonds?
- Where do almonds grow?
- What is the best way to store almonds?
- What are the health benefits of almonds?
- What is a portion size for almonds?
- What is the shelf-life of almonds?
- What different types of almonds are there?
- What are some interesting facts about almonds?

➤ Procedure 3

FATTY ACID FOODS POSTER, POWERPOINT, OR PRESENTATION

Make a pie chart using foods containing omega 3 and omega 6 essential fatty acids and the fatty acid ratios they provide. Use the Fatty Acid Chart found at the end of the Fats Chapter.

Assessment

Have a follow-up discussion with your class about the procedures they completed.

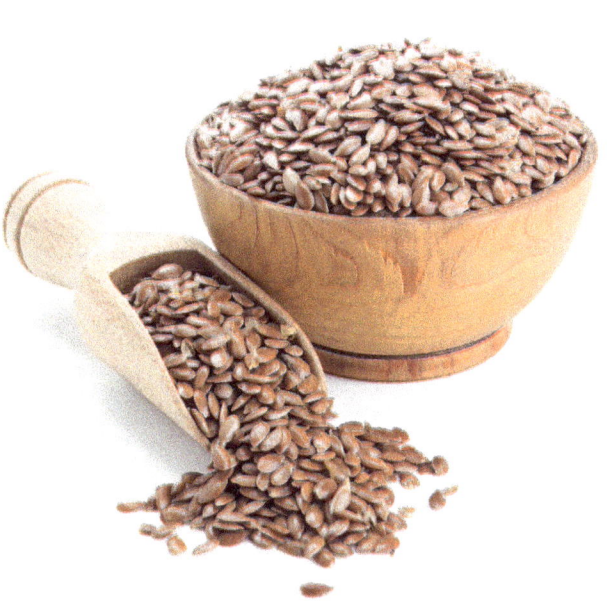

COMPREHENSIVE

Lesson: Problems Associated with Eating Damaged Fats and Hydrogenated Oils

➤ MATERIALS
- Samples of food products containing hydrogenated oils
- Samples of nuts or seeds

➤ GOALS
- Understand eating partially hydrogenated and hydrogenated oils, damaged or rancid oils and fats, including nuts and seeds, is unhealthy.
- Understand the importance of reading labels to avoid exposure to toxic hydrogenated oils and highly processed non-organic fats and oils.

➤ OBJECTIVES
- To learn to detect rancid fats and oils
- To make positive changes in the cooking fats and oils you use
- To create awareness in your home, school, and community about the dangers of consuming hydrogenated oils

➤ ACTIVATING PRIOR KNOWLEDGE
Ask students if they have ever experienced eating a nut or seed that had tasted bitter or sour. If that happened, suggest to them that they may have eaten a nut that was old or had become rancid. Also, ask if their parents ever cook and burn the butter or oil in a pan where it smokes. Again, this would be a case of fats or oils becoming damaged or spoiled. As well, ask students if they check food labels for partially hydrogenated oil before they eat any food from a package.

BACKGROUND DISCUSSION

It is important to teach your students about the different types of fats in foods that are not good for a person's health. Highlighted in this lesson are fats and oils that are considered unhealthy and, therefore, should be avoided.

Problems Associated with Fats
DAMAGED OR RANCID FATS
Avoid eating fats that are rancid, old, overheated, and overexposed to heat or sunlight. These types fats and oils may have become damaged, or rancid, and thus can cause oxidative cellular damage. Rancidity occurs when fats and oils are exposed to oxygen or when oils are overheated. (1) Heat, air, age, and sunlight can cause fats to become oxidized. Oxidation is the name of the chemical exchange that occurs. Eating these damaged fats may form free radicals in the body that cause a cascade of injury to tissues, cells, and potentially the DNA. Oxidation will change the color of the oil and may decrease the food's nutritional values. The same goes for nuts and seeds that taste bitter. They have spoiled so it is best to compost them. These fats can become toxic and are not suitable to consume! Sometimes the consumer may not be able to tell if they have spoiled because the oils have deodorizers or preservatives added to them.

Keep flax oil, sesame oil, and other light-sensitive oils in a dark cool place. Avoid exposure to heat or sun.

FAT STABILITY
The type of fat matters, as well. Saturated fats have a long shelf life and can withstand heat and light.

The more saturation (saturation refers to the number of water molecules on the fatty acid chain), the less damage may occur to the fat and making it less likely to become rancid. Butter and coconut oil are more shelf-stable than, for example, flax seeds or flax oil, which must be refrigerated and never heated.

SMOKE POINT

It is important to note that all fats and oils can become damaged and burn if heated past their smoke point. If oils reach their smoke point during cooking, toss them out and start fresh.

CONTAMINATED FISH, SEA FOOD, AND ENVIRONMENTAL POLLUTANTS

It is best to avoid eating fish contaminated with high mercury content. The burning of coal and global air pollution causes high levels of heavy metals to end up in the oceans where the fish become exposed. The food chain is such that the bigger fish eat the little fish. Guess what? We are at the top of the food chain and end up eating these toxins in fish. Check with the Environmental Working Group for the latest safety information.

EAT LOW MERCURY FISH WITH HIGH OMEGA 3 ESSENTIAL FATTY ACIDS

Anchovies, mussels, salmon, sardines, rainbow trout, Atlantic mackerel, oysters, pollock, and herring

We advise that children should avoid eating the fish listed below:

Halibut, lobster, mahi-mahi, sea bass, King mackerel, orange roughy, swordfish, tilefish, shark, marlin, tuna (canned, steaks) (2)

Hydrogenated and Partially Hydrogenated Oils

Avoid eating Nutrition Vampire hydrogenated and partially hydrogenated oils (PHOs). Hydrogenated oils are artificially manufactured fats made from vegetable oils like soybean or canola. Hydrogenated oils are also known as trans fats. (3) Hydrogenated and partially hydrogenated oils or PHOs are one of the top Food Tree Nutrition Vampires.

They are so terrible for you that hydrogenated oils have finally been banned from our food system by the Food and Drug Administration (FDA). The FDA removed hydrogenated and partially hydrogenated oils from the GRAS (Generally Recognized as Safe) list for food additives in June of 2018. However, they are still in circulation in the U.S. food system, so people still need to be vigilant and on the lookout for them in the foods they purchase. We suggest reading all package labels and asking your servers at restaurants for the ingredients in your meals when eating out.

WHAT ARE PARTIALLY HYDROGENATED AND HYDROGENATED OILS?

PHOs are factory-made oils that are chemically processed to act like saturated fat. Hydrogenated oils are added to foods to provide a longer shelf life and to increase flavor. What food manufacturers are striving for are food products that are shelf-stable and solid at room temperature, so they will last a long time. To alter the fat structure, companies artificially add hydrogen (water) molecules to vegetable oils, like soybean oil or canola oil. These types of fats are also known as trans fats. And they have been used ubiquitously since they are an inexpensive oil for restaurants and food producers.

One significant health concern to be aware of is that your body builds its cell walls out of fats and oils. Therefore, if you eat hydrogenated oils, your body will use those fats to build its cell walls. When eaten, these artificial fats harden the cells' outer membranes, which makes it difficult for nutrients to get in and waste to pass out. (4)

It is of utmost importance to avoid PHOs because of the link to serious health problems. Below is a partial list of adverse reactions that may occur from eating hydrogenated oils.

- Cause free radical damage
- Increase inflammation
- Damage to the immune system
- Increased risk of heart disease

- Links to ADHD and ADD
- Links to cancer
- Reduced cell membrane fluidity
- Impaired transport of nutrients
- Reduced water retention in cells
- Poor cellular communication
- Potential risk of malnutrition
- Diminished visual acuity
- Decreased testosterone
- Mood issues
- Skin problems
- Impaired hormone regulation

The Institute for Medicine concludes that "there is NO safe level for trans fats in the diet."

WATCH OUT FOR PARTIALLY HYDROGENATED OILS IN THESE COMMON FOODS.

You can find PHOs in hundreds of packaged, processed, and junk foods, including foods found in restaurants and even in hospitals. (5) Check labels carefully and be confident to ask servers when eating out.

- Bread
- Crackers
- Baked goods: pastries, cookies
- Tortillas
- Hamburger and hot dog buns
- Donuts
- Peanut butter
- Corn chips
- Potato chips
- Margarine spreads
- Microwave popcorn
- Ice cream and frozen yogurt
- Candy
- Fryer oil
- Fast foods
- Salad dressings
- Puddings
- Cake frosting
- Pie crust
- Vegetable shortening
- Non-dairy whipped dessert topping
- Beverages: Hot chocolate, sports drinks

▶ Procedure 1
NUT RANCIDITY TESTING

1. Divide students into small groups.
2. Provide each group with a small sample of oils, nuts, and seeds in separate jars.
3. Label the jars with the type of nut, seed, fat, or oil, and the starting date.
4. Put jars in an area of the room where you can expose them to air and sunlight so that they become rancid.
5. Beware of flammability factors. Do not place jars near any open flames.
6. After seven days, each group will observe what they see and smell.
7. Collect data on the scientific method sheet.
8. After one more week passes, have them look, taste, or smell the nut or seed and describe how the taste and smell of the nut or seed may have changed.
9. For more challenge, compare fats and oils with different fatty acid ratios to see which ones become rancid faster, if at all.
10. Flax will be the most fragile whereas coconut oil and butter are more resistant to light exposure and are more shelf-stable than other oils and fats.
11. Each group will present what they have discovered.

▶ Procedure 2
HISTORY OF HYDROGENATED OILS
Students write a paper or do a presentation explaining the history of hydrogenated oils and the adverse effects they have on the human body. The presentation can be a poem, PowerPoint, essay, commercial, illustration, cartoon strip, or student choice approved by the teacher.

▶ Procedure 3
BECOME A PHO FOE!
Students compose a persuasive letter to anyone, or anyplace, that may use hydrogenated oils: school administration, a restaurant, their parents, friends, or grandparents to suggest they remove all PHOs from the foods they offer or eat.

Students can become food activists by deciding "to help clean up" the food ingredients at one of the following places:

- School kitchen/cafeteria
- Foods served at parks, sports fields, and concession stands
- Candy fundraisers
- Vending machines
- Favorite restaurant or cafe
- Movie theatre
- Home

EXAMPLE ACTIVITY:
At school, set up a meeting with whomever is the decision-maker for purchasing school foods. Craft in a letter or presentation the information you have learned about the dangers of PHOs, especially for young growing kids. Respectfully request the removal of all hydrogenated oils from the foods served at the facility. Be sure to be positive and present viable alternatives to the current foods served. Be prepared to offer scientific studies to support your request.

Other ideas to create more engagement in healthy change:

- Involve the student council.
- Write about your PHO FOE campaign in the school paper.
- Blast about wanting healthy quality school foods on social media outlets.

AT HOME
Check your pantry, cupboard, refrigerator, and freezer for PHOs. Make sure to read small printed ingredient lists on your favorite items. Especially look at packaged bread, cookies, treats, dressings, corn chips, flour tortillas, and salad dressings.

AT RESTAURANTS
Ask food servers, cooks, chefs, the manager or owner about ingredients served in their establishment. Educate them on why you want to avoid eating hydrogenated or partially hydrogenated oils. Sometimes you may rather not know if your favorite foods have PHOs in them, but the truth is that these oils could be in anything!

Always check first with your wait staff. If the server comes back and says, the item is made with PHOs, you need to choose carefully whether you really want to eat it or not. Make your case to the staff, owner, or manager that you want to eat at their restaurant, but you also want to eat nutritious foods. Politely ask if they would be willing to make a switch to using a healthier oil.

Assessment
Discuss what your students learned about rancid oils, nuts or seeds, and hydrogenated oils. Talk about any behavior changes that they did or want to make.

DISCOVERY

Fat Calculations: Fat gram and calorie calculations for optimal daily nutrition

➤ MATERIALS
- Paper, pens, and pencils
- Calculators
- Sample fat-containing foods: empty cartons or packages from butter, coconut oil, yogurt, salad dressing

➤ GOAL
Understand that people need to eat a certain amount of fats to be healthy.

➤ OBJECTIVE
- To know how to calculate the amount of calories foods have in fat grams

➤ ACTIVATING PRIOR KNOWLEDGE
Discuss with your students if they know or are aware of how much fat to eat each day and that there is a calculation to help them figure out what that amount is.

BACKGROUND INFORMATION

A healthy balanced diet will include around 25%-30% of fats a day. Fats can be broken down into sub-groups called polyunsaturated, monounsaturated, and saturated fats. Calculations on the ratios of those specific fats needed can quickly be figured out.

Fat Calculation

1 gram of fat = 9 calories

2000 calorie diet = 500 calories/9 or 55 grams per day of fat

1500 calorie diet = 375 calories/9 g or 41-45 grams day or 15 grams per meal

Example:

3 oz. chicken = 19 grams

1 egg = 7 grams

⅛–¼ avocado = 18 grams

➤ Procedure 1
Find the fat content and calories found in different foods or oils. Break it down into the three fat subgroups for an extra challenge.

For instance, examine foods like avocado, nuts, yogurt, milk, eggs, walnuts, salmon, olives, sardines, snack bar, crackers, cookies, and candy bars, or oils like olive oil, butter, and coconut oil.

➤ Procedure 2
1. List one day's worth of food.
2. Determine the daily recommended intake of fat based on your daily diet.
3. Compare the daily intake of fat with the proper ratios of fats.

Assessment
Discuss the different amounts of fats found in various types of foods and oils. Discuss your students' reactions to learning about calculating calories in grams on the foods.

CLASSIFICATION OF FATS AND OILS

Saturated
- Butter
- Coconut oil
- Palm oil
- Cheese
- Beef tallow

Monounsaturated
- W9: Oleic
  - Avocado
  - Olive
  - Peanut
  - Poultry fat
  - Canola
  - Lard

Polyunsaturated
- W6: Linoleic
  - Corn
  - Soybean
  - Safflower
  - Sunflower
- GLA
  - Blackcurrant
  - Borage
  - Primrose

Polyunsaturated
- W3 a-linolenic
  - Flax
  - Hemp
  - Walnut
  - Dark leafy greens
- EPA-DHA
  - Seaweed
  - Fish
  - Grass-fed beef

FATTY ACID SPECTRUM IN FOODS AND OILS

		POLYUNSATURATED OMEGA N-3 %	POLYUNSATURATED OMEGA N-6 %	MONOUNSATURATED %	SATURATED %
VEGETABLE FATS	Olive Oil	1	9	76	14
	Avocado	0	14	74	12
	Cocoa Butter	0	2	38	60
	Canola Oil	11	21	61	7
	Coconut Oil	0	2	6	92
	Corn Oil	1	53	31	15
	Flaxseed Oil	57	18	16	9
	Grapeseed Oil	1	72	17	10
	Olive Oil	1	9	75	15
	Palm Oil -eco ban	0	11	39	50
	Peanut Oil	0	32	47	21
	Safflower Oil	1	14	77	8
	Sesame Oil	0	43	42	15
	Sunflower Oil	1	71	16	12
	Soybean Oil	8	54	22	16
	Walnut	12	61	17	10
ANIMAL FATS	Beef Tallow	2	3	40	50-55
	Butter	2	2	28	68
	Chicken Fat	0	22	48	30
	Egg	22 total PUFA		36	42
	Lard	1	9	45	45
	Salmon fat	46 total PUFA		37	17

From European Food Information Council, www.gbhealthwatch.com/Science-Omega3-Omega6.php, Oregon State University.

FREQUENCY OF EATING FATTY FOODS AND OILS

	DAILY	WEEKLY	MONTHLY	INFREQUENTLY	NEVER
Butter					
Almonds					
Avocado					
Avocado oil					
Flax oil					
Flax seeds					
Coconut milk					
Coconut oil					
Olive oil					
Salmon					
Corn oil					
Soybeans					
Peanut oil					
Safflower oil					
Lard					
Sesame seeds					
Pumpkin seeds					
Hemp seeds					
Hemp oil					
Walnuts					

Permission to reproduce. ©The Food Tree

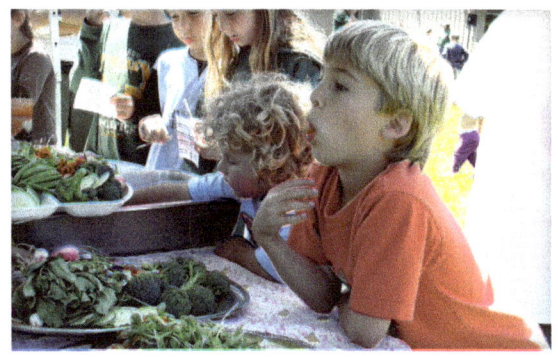

INTRODUCTION TO THE VEGETABLES FOOD GROUP

"No single fruit or vegetable provides all of the nutrients you need to be healthy. The key lies in the variety of different fruits and vegetables that you eat."

-Harvard School of Public Health (1)

THE FOOD TREE ANALOGY
The shiny, healthy leaves reflect a well-nourished tree and its vital life-giving energy like the health and vitality a person will receive when eating a diet rich in vegetables.

DAILY RECOMMENDED SERVING SUGGESTION: 5
20% of daily calories
Energy source, carbohydrate, four calories per gram

VEGETABLE FOOD SOURCES
Vegetables are rainbow colored plant foods that include edible roots like potato and carrot, stems like celery and rhubarb, and leaves like lettuce and collards.

WHAT ARE VEGETABLES?

Vegetables are the edible and nutritious parts of plants or trees that include stems, stalks leaves, flowers, tubers, and roots. Vegetables provide your body with vital vitamins, minerals, trace elements, phytonutrients, and fiber that are all necessary for your health and wellbeing. (1)

FOUNDATIONAL

Lesson: Getting to Know Vegetables

➤ MATERIALS

- The Food Tree Magnetic Board
- Examples and samples of different types and colors of vegetables: a jar of tomato sauce, an empty bag of frozen vegetables, sweet potato, onion, broccoli, and other fresh produce, photos, and pictures from magazines
- The Food Tree Nutrient Scroll, found in the appendix
- Activity—Plant Part Matching, found in the Activities Section
- The Food Tree Food Journal, found in the Activities Section
- See the Phytonutrient and Antioxidant lesson.

➤ GOALS

Learn about the wide variety of vegetable food sources to enjoy.

➤ OBJECTIVES

- To identify 5–10 different vegetables from each of the five rainbow colors (red, orange, yellow, green, blue/purple)
- To list and identify different types of vegetables
- To know what part of the plant a vegetable comes from
- To name one root, one leafy, and one cruciferous vegetable

➤ ACTIVATING PRIOR KNOWLEDGE

- Ask what the student's favorite vegetables are. Ask why and how they like to eat them.
- Do they think that vegetables are essential to eat? Why or why not? Discuss if your students eat or want to eat vegetables every day.
- Do they ever think about the fact that vegetables can be a leaf, a root, a stem, or a flower?

BACKGROUND INFORMATION

In this lesson, I encourage you to expand the vegetable horizon of your students. Get them excited about eating and cooking from a broader palate of food choices that can undoubtedly add to the pleasure, creativity, and nourishment in their diet.

Action Item!
Show your students The Food Tree Nutrient Scroll. This visual is a dramatic way to show the list of micronutrients necessary to eat daily or over three or four days. These are the nutrients a person needs to eat for optimal health.

What Are Vegetables?

Vegetables are plant foods that are part of the macronutrient group, carbohydrates, one of the three macronutrients. Vegetables provide four calories per gram as an energy source.

Eat a Variety of Vegetables

There are hundreds of types of vegetable varieties found from around the world, offering an equal amount of taste, texture, size, nutrients, and color. (2) Vegetables can come from many different edible parts of a plant or tree like the stem, leaves, flowers, fruit, seeds, tubers and roots.

Edible Plant Parts

Roots and tubers are the underground stems that carry water and nutrients to parts of the plant. Beet, carrot, ginger, potato, yam

Stems and stalks connect to the roots and transport water and nutrients to leaves, flowers, and fruit. Asparagus, celery, fennel, rhubarb

Leaves photosynthesize, release oxygen. Chard, kale, lettuce, spinach

EAT A VARIETY OF VEGETABLES

Eating and cooking from a broader palate of plants will undoubtedly add to the pleasure, creativity, and nourishment in your diet. Below are lists of vegetable categories to eat from.

CRUCIFEROUS VEGETABLES

- Arugula
- Bok choy
- Broccoli
- Brussels sprouts
- Cabbage
- Cauliflower
- Chinese broccoli
- Collard greens
- Daikon radish
- Horseradish
- Kale
- Maca
- Mizuna
- Mustard
- Napa cabbage
- Rapini
- Red radish
- Romanesco
- Rutabaga
- Savoy cabbage
- Spinach
- Swiss chard
- Turnip root
- Wasabi
- Watercress

LETTUCE

- Arugula
- Butterhead
- Frisee
- Green leaf lettuce
- Iceberg lettuce
- Lamb's lettuce
- Mizuna
- Nasturtium
- Oak leaf lettuce
- Purslane
- Radicchio
- Red leaf lettuce
- Romaine lettuce
- Round lettuce
- Watercress
- Dandelion
- Endive
- Escarole

LEAFY GREENS

- Arugula
- Beet greens
- Broccoli
- Collards
- Endive
- Escarole
- Kale
- Mustard greens
- Radicchio
- Spinach
- Swiss chard
- Turnip greens
- Watercress

ROOTS AND TUBERS

- Beet
- Carrot
- Cassava
- Celeriac
- Cumin
- Daikon, white radish
- Dandelion root
- Ginger
- Jerusalem artichoke
- Jicama
- Maca
- Parsnip
- Potato
- Radish
- Rutabaga
- Sweet potato
- Turnip
- Yam

ALLIUMS

- Chives
- Garlic
- Green onions
- Leeks
- Onion
- Shallot

NIGHTSHADES

- Tomato
- Eggplant
- Potato
- Peppers

> **VEGETABLE FOOD SOURCES**
>
> Arugula, artichoke, asparagus, beet, bok choy, broccoli, broccoli rabe, Belgian endive, Brussels sprouts, cabbage, carrot, cauliflower, celeriac, celery, chard, chili pepper, collards, corn, cucumber, dandelion greens, eggplant, fava beans, fennel, fermented vegetables, garlic, green beans, green onions, herbs, Jerusalem artichoke, horseradish, jicama, kale, kohlrabi, leek, lettuce, mushroom, nettles, onion, okra, parsley, parsnip, peas, pepper, potatoes, pumpkin, radish, rhubarb, rutabaga, salad greens, sea vegetables, spinach, squash, stinging nettle, string beans, sweet potato, Swiss chard, tomato, turnip, watercress, yam, zucchini

Flowers contain plant parts called pistils and stamens that make fruit. Broccoli, cauliflower, artichoke

Fruit produces seeds. Squash, tomato

Seeds contain the genetic material within a vessel to make a new plant. Beans, corn, sunflower seeds, sesame seeds

Eat Colorful Vegetables

The colors of vegetables expand over the whole rainbow of colors: reds, orange, yellow, green, blues, violet, and white. (3) Most American people eat a relatively limited range of vegetables and in limited quantities. (4) See the Phytonutrient and Antioxidant lesson.

➤ Procedure 1
PLANT PART MATCHING GAME

Play a matching game to learn about the different plant parts that we enjoy eating. See Plant Part Matching worksheet.

➤ Procedure 2
NAME THAT VEGETABLE

Play a guessing game with your students to see if they can name different types of vegetables. Bring in real examples of vegetables or gather images out of magazines, books, or the computer.

1. Show your students the vegetable.
2. Ask them to write down their answers as they go or have everyone say the names of vegetables out loud.
3. Divide the class into teams and have them play against each other to make it more competitive.

➤ Procedure 3

Have fun with your students finding places that have vegetables (and fruit) in their name. Below are some you may be familiar with. Ask students to research the locations they are named after and how they got their names.

- Belgium endive
- Jerusalem artichoke
- Swiss chard
- Thai eggplant
- Brussels sprouts
- Kalamata olive
- Bourbon vanilla
- Thai basil
- Anjou pear
- Key lime
- Rainier cherry
- Aleppo pepper

➤ Procedure 4
VEGETABLE LOVE

Talk with your class about their favorite vegetables. Discuss what vegetables are in season today. What are their favorite ways to enjoy eating vegetables? Talk about the many ways to prepare vegetables.

Assessment

Were the students surprised at the variety and types of vegetables they like and what a huge variety there is?

FOUNDATIONAL

Lesson: Serving Sizes and Daily Recommendations for Vegetables

➤ **MATERIALS**
- The Food Tree Magnetic Board
- Examples of different types of vegetables: real vegetables or other visual models. A jar of tomato sauce, an empty box of frozen vegetables, a sweet potato, an onion, broccoli, photos, pictures from magazines
- Measuring cups
- Vegetable Log Sheet
- The Food Tree Daily Food Journal, located in the Activities Section

➤ **GOALS**

Understand what the serving sizes and daily recommendations are for vegetables.

➤ **OBJECTIVES**
- To state the number of servings of vegetables needed to be eaten daily for the best health
- To illustrate serving sizes for raw and cooked vegetables
- To show an ability to choose appropriate portions of vegetables according to an individual's unique dietary needs

➤ **ACTIVATING PRIOR KNOWLEDGE**

Ask the class if they know how many servings of vegetables to eat every day and what a portion size looks like.

BACKGROUND INFORMATION

The Food Tree Vegetable Recommendations

The Food Tree suggests eating five servings of vegetables every day. Eating a range is valuable, too, as noted in the phytonutrient section. Strive to eat vegetables that are in season, locally grown, sustainable, fair trade, homegrown, and organic whenever possible.

- Eat a Rainbow. Eat a variety of nutrient-dense, colorful, antioxidant, and phytonutrient-rich produce. (2)

> **THERE ARE MANY WAYS TO PREPARE VEGETABLES.**
> *Explore them all!*
> Bake, Broil, Roast, Sauté, Blend, Dehydrate, Ferment, Fresh, Freeze, Juice, Puree, Steam, Stew

- Eat Fresh. Choose to eat fresh vegetables every day. Eat as close to the harvest time as possible. Fresh produce retains more nutrients than those that have been sitting around for a while. Exposure to air, heat, overcooking, water, processing, sun, and poor handling decreases a vegetable's nutrient value.
- Eat in season.
- Buy local. Check out your local farmer's market for the best produce.
- Frozen vegetables are a good choice. Vegetables are frozen immediately upon picking. They are quick to defrost, and you can easily add them to all kinds of dishes like soups, wraps, and salads.
- Jarred vegetables should be chosen over canned when possible. Buy and store vegetables in glass jars in water or their juices (i.e., olives, pickles,

sauerkraut, tomato sauce).

- Juiced vegetables are a great way to receive vitamins, minerals, electrolytes, and water quickly. Some juice may not contain vegetable fiber. Gulp vegetable juice down soon after you make it as it oxidizes when exposed to air and therefore, its nutrient value will be reduced.
- Shop, grow, and eat different varieties of vegetables. Avoid getting into a rut.
- Nutrient availability will vary according to each plant, how you prepare them, the time of harvest, type, length of storage, how you cook them, and the person's digestion and absorption capacity.
- Eat raw and cooked vegetables because they offer up different nutrients when cooked or eaten fresh. For instance, cooked carrots or tomatoes offer different nutrients than raw carrots and tomatoes. Some nutrients may get lost when cooked, whereas some vegetable nutrients are not affected when cooked, like onions.
- Eat a side of raw vegetables with every meal. Try sliced cucumbers, carrot sticks, or bell pepper slices.
- Grow vegetables at home and at school. You can eat them straight out of the garden and cook them instantly.
- Put them on your sandwich. Include vegetables like lettuce, cucumber, tomato, pepper, zucchini, and sprouts.
- Eat vegetables for breakfast. Have salsa or a veggie saute with your eggs or tofu scramble.
- Eat one cup of cooked vegetables and one fresh serving with dinner every night to equal three servings.

What other ideas do students have? Share your thoughts with your classmates and your community!

Serving Size Recommendations for Vegetables

ENERGY SOURCE FOUR CALORIES PER GRAM
20% OF DAILY CALORIES

However, like all things, it depends on the person and your unique requirements. Adjust the actual amount eaten to take into account a person's height, weight, age, caloric needs, and activity level. For serving size estimates for children, use the size of the palm as a serving.

- 1 carrot
- 1 cup chopped raw vegetables
- 1 cup of leafy vegetables or lettuce greens
- ½ cup of cooked vegetables
- 1 medium sweet potato
- ¾ cup of vegetable juice

➤ Procedure 1
SERVING SIZES

1. Discuss the list of the recommended serving sizes of vegetables.
2. Show examples of vegetable serving sizes. Use real food, models, or pictures.
   - For instance, show your students what a serving size of steamed broccoli looks like in a bowl.
   - Show a serving of salad greens.
   - Show a serving of salsa.
   - Show a serving of potatoes or baked yams.
3. How does this compare to the number of vegetables a student would typically eat?

➤ Procedure 2

MEAL PLANNING—VEGETABLES ARE NOT JUST A SIDE DISH

Have students create a day's worth or up to one week's worth of what eating five servings of vegetables looks like on a meal planning sheet. Students can also explain how each serving would be prepared, either raw or cooked. Have students include recipes and nutrition facts for an extra challenge.

Or, have students use an outline of The Food Tree. Students can write the foods in the canopy of a Food Tree image they draw or you provide. Students can also draw or cut and paste pictures from food magazines and glue onto The Food Tree.

RAW AND COOKED

Below is a sample meal plan to represent how to include five servings of vegetables a day in the diet.

Breakfast	½ cup tomato salsa = raw. Serve with beans, tofu, or eggs
Snack	1 carrot, peeled and cut into sticks = raw
Snack	1 stalk of celery = raw
Lunch	¾ cup steamed broccoli = cooked
Dinner	1 cup butternut squash soup, cooked = cooked
Dinner	½ cup kale = cooked
Dinner	1 cup fresh lettuce greens = raw

➤ Procedure 3

KEEP A VEGETABLE FOOD JOURNAL AND LOG

For young students, keep a simple food journal. For older students, have them journal and keep a Vegetable Log.

Create a Log

1. Across the top of the paper write: Date, Raw Vegetable, Cooked Vegetable, Serving Size, From Home, From School, From Restaurant.
2. Down the left side, write a list of vegetables.
3. Ask students to keep the log for one week.
4. Explore data findings. What were the most common sources of vegetables eaten?
5. Record the students' responses on a big wall chart. You can make this activity anonymous to protect the children's privacy.

Assessments

- What have students learned from looking at their diets compared to The Food Tree recommendations? Students can take this lesson a step further and calculate the number of vegetables that they are eating every day.

- Have students look at the list of vegetables they wrote down at the beginning of the lesson. Ask the following questions: Are you eating vegetables more often? Are you eating appropriate serving sizes? What changes have you or can you make to improve your diet?

- Ask students to write down the changes they could make. Challenge them to implement these changes, even if it's just one meal at a time.

FOUNDATIONAL

Lesson: Benefits and Functions of Vegetables

➤ MATERIALS
- The Food Tree Magnetic Board
- Food Props of vegetables. May use, for example, a jar of tomato sauce, an empty frozen vegetable bag, fresh produce, dried vegetables
- The Food Tree Nutrient Scroll, located in the appendix

➤ GOALS
Understand the health benefits of eating a diet rich in quality vegetables.

➤ OBJECTIVES
- Explain three health benefits obtained by eating vegetables

➤ ACTIVATING PRIOR KNOWLEDGE
Discuss students' favorite vegetables. Ask why and how they like to eat them. Ask your students if they think vegetables are important to include in their diets and why.

BACKGROUND INFORMATION

Benefits and Functions of Vegetables

Vegetables provide vital vitamins, minerals, trace elements, phytonutrients, and fiber that are all necessary for being a healthy person.

PROVIDE ENERGY SOURCE
Vegetables provide four calories per gram in the form of carbohydrates.

PROVIDE NUTRIENTS
Vegetables are rich in vitamins, minerals, and trace minerals. For instance, dark leafy greens have an abundance of vitamin A, vitamin B6, vitamin C, vitamin E, vitamin K, magnesium, calcium, potassium, manganese, choline, and folate. (1)

PROVIDE ANTIOXIDANT PHYTONUTRIENTS
Phytonutrients are the chemicals in foods that give plants their fabulous colors and are part of the plants' own defense system shielding them against damage caused by insects, sun, cold weather, wind, or other stressors.

Phytonutrients are the colors of fruits and vegetables that expand over the whole rainbow of colors: red, orange, yellow, green, blue, indigo, violet, and white. Phytonutrients like anthocyanins, flavonoids, and quercetin act as antioxidants. Antioxidants are known to help reduce damage from free radicals. A natural chemical reaction makes free radicals but when too many are created, they can cause illness and disease. Antioxidant chemicals from plants can, therefore, protect and decrease the risk of damage and disease. Phytonutrients are known to fortify the body against colds, flu, heart disease, cancer, diabetes, stroke, high blood pressure, hormone imbalance, and inflammation. (2)

PROVIDE FIBER
Vegetables are naturally high in fiber. Fiber is the tough part of plants, including the rind, skin, and seeds. Fiber is known to maintain gut health, keep the colon clean by ridding excess waste byproducts, aid in digestion and elimination, keep bowel movements

EAT A RAINBOW

Red fruit and vegetables like tomato, grapefruit, and cherry contain bioflavonoids and beta-carotene that are powerful detoxifier-compounds that help prevent cancer. (3)

Orange foods like carrots, sweet potato, and cantaloupe contain beta-carotene that studies show helps prevent colon cancer.

Yellow fruits and vegetables like pineapple contain bromelain that reduces inflammation found in people with allergies and rheumatoid arthritis. (4)

Green vegetables like broccoli and kale contain glucosinolates that are known to block cancer-causing substances. (5) They are rich in flavonoids known to be beneficial for healthy blood circulation and immune response.

Blue and Purple fruits and vegetables like blueberries, grapes, and purple potatoes contain anthocyanins that nourish heart health by improving circulation, strengthening blood capillaries, and circulating nutrients. They work to help detoxify the liver, skin, kidneys, and bowels. (5)

---

regular, and help maintain blood sugar, which is vital in the prevention of diabetes. (6)

Fiber helps feed beneficial bacteria in the gut that are necessary to reduce the possibility of intestinal problems like diverticulitis, indigestion, gas, and bloating. (7) Bacteria in the gut help to make vitamins, like the B vitamins.

BUILD IMMUNITY
The phytonutrients, vitamins, minerals, and fiber are all critical to maintain health and to help resist illnesses such as common colds and flu.

SUPPLY ENZYMES
Enzymes are elements that break down foods to assist in digestion. They are found naturally in fruits and vegetables, especially raw produce. The pancreas also produces enzymes. Amylase, found in beets, cauliflower, celery, and onions, is an example of an enzyme that breaks down carbohydrates.

ENGAGE THE SENSES
Vegetables supply a diverse variety of flavors, textures, and colors that all add joy in growing, shopping for, preparing, cooking, offering, sharing, and eating.

▶ Procedure 1
VEGETABLE HIGHLIGHT
Have students do a research project highlighting one vegetable and the potential health benefit it offers.

1. Present the information as a paper, PowerPoint, or poster board presentation.

2. Create a skit, commercial, or video selling the fantastic benefits of eating vegetables. Highlight the phytonutrients, minerals, vitamins, and unique attributes. Make sure to include ways to prepare and cook.

Assessment
Were the students surprised at how many health benefits vegetables provide? Were they motivated to eat more in their diet?

DISCOVERY

Lesson: Problems Related to Low Dietary Intake of Vegetables

➤ MATERIALS

- List of vegetables

➤ GOALS

Highlight the importance of including a variety of vegetables in the diet.

➤ OBJECTIVES

- To learn the importance of eating The Food Tree's recommended servings of five vegetables a day
- To show easy ways to add more servings of vegetables into a person's diet
- To evaluate common health problems people might experience when there is a lack of vegetables in the diet
- To illustrate how American children are deficient in servings of vegetables in their daily diet

➤ ACTIVATING PRIOR KNOWLEDGE

Ask the class if they have ever been nagged by their teachers, friends, parents, or grandparents to eat more vegetables. Ask them if they have discussed why it is so important to eat vegetables. Ask for a show of hands of kids in your class who think they eat one serving of vegetables a day. Then ask who eats two, then three, four, and then five or more servings a day.

BACKGROUND INFORMATION

The saying "eat your vegetables" may seem like an annoying thing a parent, teacher, and doctor would say. However, eating at least five servings of vegetables a day is one of the very best things a person can do for their overall short- and long-term health. Vegetables provide essential nutrients like vitamins, minerals, phytonutrients, and antioxidants. A diet deficient in these nutrients could potentially cause serious health issues. (1)

The United States government current CDC (Centers for Disease Control) statistics indicate that only ¼ of children eat the recommended amount of vegetables a day. Another way to say that is 75% of U.S. children are not eating enough vegetables. In particular, the intake of nutrient-rich dark green leafy vegetables and deep yellow varieties of vegetables are extremely low in the American child's diet. (2)

The systemic lack of eating vegetables in certain underprivileged neighborhoods, towns, and cities can be due to a fundamental lack of access to fresh fruits and vegetables, a lack of education on the importance of eating healthy foods, and limited time to shop for and grow vegetables.

Most Common Impacts of a Diet Deficient in Vegetables

We know vegetables provide nutrients that are vital to a person's health. Just as the list of positives is quite long, the list of harmful effects from a diet lacking in vegetables is just as lengthy. We encourage you and your students to explore this topic further.

- Digestive issues due to lack of fiber (3)
- Poor nutrient absorption

- Lowered immune system that may cause poor wound healing, frequent colds, infections
- Cognitive and attention span problems
- Skin, hair and nail problems
- Teeth, dental, gum, oral health issues (4)
- Obesity or overweight
- Metabolism problems
- Hormone imbalances
- Blood sugar issues
- Acidosis—Vegetables provide minerals that keep the pH (acid/alkaline) balanced.

Eating sweets, white flour foods, and meat requires minerals to digest and process them. But when eaten in high quantities, those foods may create an acidic ash in the body and cause a condition called acidosis. The Standard American Diet is typically high in sweet foods, processed grains, sugary drinks, and meat that can cause a mineral imbalance signaling a need for more vegetables (high in minerals) in the diet. (5)

There are many different reasons children do not eat enough vegetables:

- Lack of access to quality and variety of vegetables.
- Lack of parent and family education, awareness, interest, poor role-modeling, conflicted parenting styles.
- Lack of time, limited financial resources for shopping, and meal preparation.
- Lack of diversity/variety in vegetable choices. A person may get stuck on eating only carrots or iceberg lettuce, for instance.

What vegetables should you avoid eating?

- Overcooked vegetables will lose nutrients.
- Canned vegetables often lose significant amounts of their nutrients, specifically 50% of vitamin C (Evelyn Roehl, *Whole Food Facts*, 1996).
- The lining in cans may contain toxic chemicals, so beware.
- Dehydrated vegetables, however tasty and flavorful, have often been exposed to heat for long periods, potentially reducing their nutrient value.
- Microwaved vegetables lose enzymes and deplete nutrients that we need for proper digestion. (6,7)

▶ Procedure 1

Have students choose one health condition that may be improved by eating more vegetables and present that to the class or in a paper.

▶ Procedure 2
TAKE A POLL DOWN VEGETABLE STREET

1. Take a poll of people in your community on the amounts and the kinds of vegetables they eat daily. Brainstorm as a class, in groups, or individually questions to ask people. Your class can all ask the same set of questions, students can come up with their own set of questions, or students can do a mix of both. Questions will depend on what kinds of things you want to teach and students want to learn.
2. Then, decide as a class, in groups, or as individuals which communities to poll.
3. Ask students to carry out their poll either as a written or oral questionnaire.
4. Have students organize their results in a comprehensive written report or graphics display. Share results with the class or in the school newspaper.

Examples of Communities to Poll

- Classes at school
- An entire grade level
- School as a whole

- Faculty and staff
- School sports team
- Peer/friend groups
- Family
- School drama club, church group, etc.

Polling Questions Examples

- What kinds of vegetables do you typically eat? Would you eat them if they were in a different form? For instance, if they were cooked or fresh? Why or why not?
- Do you tend to eat the same vegetables daily or weekly? Do you think you eat a variety or lack variety in your diet? Or do you eat a wide range of vegetables? Do you change the types of vegetables for different meals? Or do you tend to eat the same thing for the same meal for days on end?
- On average, how many different veggies do you eat daily?
- What are your favorite kinds of vegetables?
- What are your favorite ways to make or eat them?
- Do you eat the same vegetables as your family, siblings, or friends? As your parents?
- What purpose do vegetables serve in a person's diet?
- What would you do differently regarding vegetables in your diet?
- Discuss having access to fresh vegetables. Do you live in a "food" dessert? Or is there an abundance of food in your home and your community.
- Ask questions about time or money constraints. (as appropriate)

➤ Procedure 3

Develop creative and practical ways to help your family, school, or community gain better access to fresh vegetables. Brainstorm ways to increase the number of vegetables your community eats and execute the plan.

Assessment

- What patterns did students notice from their survey? What surprised them? What was not surprising? Compare results. Did all students have similar results from their polls?
- Did people tend to eat differently depending on different factors like cultural background, age, gender, work hours, family life, etc.?
- Ask students to think about and contemplate why people's eating habits are the way they are. What are the most effective ways students can positively impact their diet and that of their communities?
- It is highly likely that each community will require different action steps to change the amount of vegetables they eat. Encourage students to put in the work and take those beneficial steps.

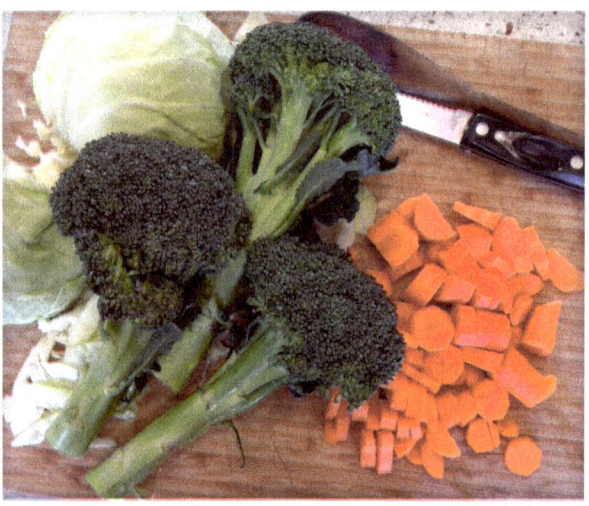

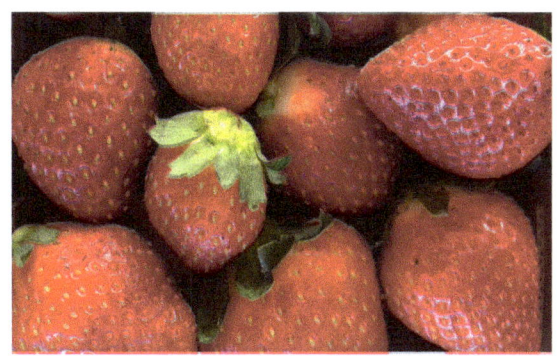

INTRODUCTION TO THE FRUITS FOOD GROUP

What fruit always travels in groups of two? Pears!

THE FOOD TREE ANALOGY
The Fruit represents the Fruits Food Group on The Food Tree. Metaphorically, fruit is symbolic of fertility. Fruit bear seeds that make new plants and trees. Like fruit, fully nourished people have enough to share with their families, communities, and the world. Fruits represent being creative, generous, and abundant.

DAILY RECOMMENDED SERVING SUGGESTION: 3
10% of daily calories
Energy source, carbohydrate, four calories per gram

SOURCES OF FRUIT
Apple, banana, blackberry, blueberry, cantaloupe, cherry, cranberries, dates, fig, grape, honeydew, kiwi, kumquat, lemon, lime, mango, nectarine, olallieberry, orange, passion fruit, pear, peach, persimmon, pineapple, plum, raisin, raspberry, strawberry, watermelon

WHAT ARE FRUITS?

Fruit are plant-based foods that are part of the macronutrient group, carbohydrates, one of the three macronutrients.

Fruits are the seed-producing part of a plant. They come in an enormous array of tastes, colors, sizes, shapes, and textures. The taste of fruit can be sweet, tangy, sour, bitter, or spicy. But they are typically sweet, juicy, and delicious. We have access to more fruits due to the ability to easily import and export crops from around the world.

FOUNDATIONAL

Lesson: Getting to Know Fruit

> **MATERIALS**
- Food Tree Magnetic Board
- Different examples of fresh fruit like apples, oranges, a bag of frozen berries, a jar of apple sauce,
- The Food Tree Nutrient Scroll, located in the appendix

> **GOALS**

Learn about the enormous variety of fruit.

> **OBJECTIVES**
- To list and identify a minimum of eight different kinds of fruit
- To name one fruit of each rainbow color

> **ACTIVATING PRIOR KNOWLEDGE**

Ask what your students' favorite kinds of fruit are to eat. Talk about the different types of fruit they enjoy. Ask why and how they like to eat them. Do they ever think about eating different types of fruit than they normally do? Do they wonder if the fruit they are eating is in season?

Do they think having fruit in their diet is essential, and why or why not?

BACKGROUND INFORMATION

What Is Fruit?

Fruits are plant-based foods and are the seed-producing part of a plant. They come in an enormous array of tastes, colors, sizes, shapes, and textures. The taste of fruit can be sweet, tangy, sour, bitter or spicy. But they are typically sweet, juicy, and delicious. Fruit grows in different regions around the world. Due to the ability to easily import and export crops, we now have access to more fruits that we would never have had a chance to try in the past unless a traveler.

Eat Colors

The colors of fruit expand over the whole rainbow of colors: reds, orange, yellow, green, blues, violet, and white. See the Phytonutrient and Antioxidant lesson.

Eat a Variety

There are hundreds of types of fruit varieties found from around the world and in your area, offering an equal amount of taste, texture, size, and color. Eating and cooking from a broader palate of food choice can undoubtedly add to the pleasure, creativity, and nourishment in your diet. Below is a list of common fruit categories.

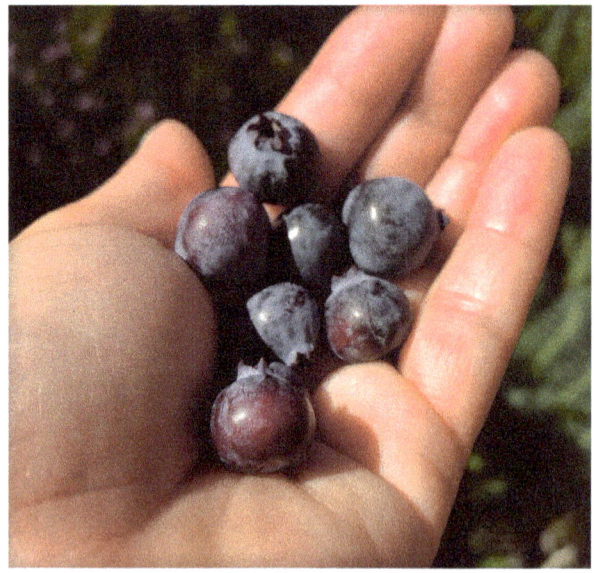

Types of Fruits

Berries
- Blackberry, blueberry, cranberry, kiwi, passion fruit, olallieberry, pomegranate, raspberry, strawberry

Melons
- Cantaloupe, honeydew, rock melon, Sharon melon, watermelon

Stone Fruits
- Apricot, cherry, peach, nectarine, plum

Tropical Fruits
- Banana, dragon fruit, mango, papaya, passionfruit, pineapple

Deciduous Fruits
- Apple, grape, fig, pear, kiwi, persimmon

Citrus Fruits
- Grapefruit, lemon, lime, mandarin, orange, tangerine

➤ Procedure 1
NAME THAT FRUIT

Play a guessing game with your students to see if they can name a variety of different types of fruit. Before you begin, bring in real fruit or gather images out of magazines, books, or the computer of examples of fruit.

1. Show your students the fruit. Have them write down their answers or have everyone say the names out loud.
2. To make it competitive, divide the class into teams and have them play against each other.

Assessment

Were the students surprised at the variety and types of fruit they like and what a huge variety there is?

FRUIT FOOD SOURCES

Apple, banana, blackberry, blueberry, cantaloupe, cherry, cranberry, date, fig, grape, honeydew, kiwi, kumquat, lemon, lime, mandarin, mango, nectarine, olallieberry, orange, passion fruit, pear, peach, persimmon, pineapple, plum, raisin, raspberry, strawberry, watermelon

FOUNDATIONAL

Lesson: Serving Sizes and Daily Recommendations of Fruit

Chinese proverb: "The best time to plant a tree was 20 years ago. The second-best time is now."

➤ MATERIALS
- The Food Tree Magnetic Board
- Examples of fruits: a jar of apple sauce, an empty bag of frozen berries, fresh produce, photos, and other illustrations
- Measuring cups
- Fruit Log Sheet
- The Food Tree Food Journal, located in the Activities section.

➤ ACTIVITY
Rainbow Foods

➤ GOAL
Understand what the serving sizes and daily recommendations are for fruit.

➤ OBJECTIVES
- To explain what the appropriate serving sizes and amounts are for fruit each day
- To demonstrate what a serving size of fruit looks like
- To identify six different types of fruit
- To make clear and educated decisions about the serving sizes and amounts of fruit needed in a daily diet

➤ ACTIVATING PRIOR KNOWLEDGE
Ask students what they think a portion size looks like and how many portions of fruit are recommended to eat in one day.

BACKGROUND INFORMATION

DAILY RECOMMENDED SERVING SUGGESTION: 3
10% of daily calories
Energy source, macronutrient carbohydrate, four calories per gram

Certain fruits do contain small amounts of proteins and fats, the other two macronutrients. Fruit is one of the five highly nutritious food groups on The Food Tree.

The Food Tree recommends an average healthy person eat at least three servings of fruit every day. However, like all things, it depends on the person and your unique requirements. Adjust the actual amount of fruit needed to take into account a person's height, weight, age, nutrient needs, caloric needs, and activity level. For serving size estimates for children, use the size of the palm as a serving.

The Food Tree suggests eating a variety of fresh fruits and to remembering to eat in season, locally, sustainably, fair trade, homegrown, and organic whenever possible.

1 medium apple
½ cantaloupe
1 small banana

Recommendations for Fruit
- Eat the whole fruit.
- Fresh is best.
- Frozen is good, too.
- Eat fruit alone or before a meal for better digestion and nutrient absorption.
- Add fruit to bread and muffins.

- Make a smoothie for a delicious snack.
- Pre-peel or slice oranges so it is easy to bring to school and eat.
- Add a banana, frozen berries, dates, raisins, or unsweetened cranberries to your bowl of hot cereal or oatmeal.
- Pack a side of fruit with your lunch every day.
- Eat frozen fruit. Try freezing grapes (wait till they are in season and then freeze and eat on hot days). Put frozen pineapple or mango on top of yogurt. Add frozen blueberries to whole grain pancakes and waffles.
- You can't go wrong with a snack of apples or bananas with nut butter.
- Celebrate special occasions, like birthdays, with fruit. Make fruit shish kebobs or melon balls for a fun presentation.
- Add fruit to salads.
- Get creative and save money by making your homemade fruit roll-ups.
- Eat fruit straight out of your home or school garden!

What other ideas do students have? Share your thoughts with your classmates and your community.

▶ Procedure 1
TALK ABOUT IT

Discuss the different types of fruit that may be in season where you live. What kind of fruit is in season in your area, and what are your favorite ways to eat them? Talk about why it is best, when possible, to eat seasonally and locally grown foods. For instance, seasonal fruit usually tastes better when picked ripe versus being picked unripe and then being shipped half way across the planet. Therefore, when eating in season, there is typically a much shorter shipping distance and often less or no packaging, to get it into your mouth.

> **Interesting Fact**
> It takes three to four oranges to produce just one cup of juice!

▶ Procedure 2
SERVING SIZES

1. Discuss the recommended serving sizes of fruit.
2. Show examples of fruit servings sizes. Use real food, models, or pictures. For instance, show your students a serving size of berries, melon, orange, or dried fruit.
3. How does this compare to the serving size they would usually eat?

▶ Procedure 3
MEAL PLANNING—FABULOUS FRUIT!

Have students create a day's worth of what

> **DELICIOUS WAYS TO ENJOY EATING FRUIT**
>
> There is a wide variety of fruit grown in our country and even more around the world to discover. Expand your horizon beyond the same two fruits you may be in the habit of eating every single day.
>
> - Fresh
> - Frozen
> - Shish kabobs
> - In Salads
> - In soup
> - On pizza
> - Roll-ups
> - Melon balls
> - Smoothies
> - Dried
> - Grilled
>
> Fruit is delicious, nutritious, and easily incorporated into recipes. It is perfect as a stand-alone snack. Each different kind of fruit you eat will offer a different nutrient profile. Therefore, eating a variety will be better for your health!

eating three servings of fruit looks like on a meal planning sheet.

1. Ask your students to write down how they would prepare each serving.
2. Have students include recipes and nutrition facts for an extra challenge.
3. Or have students use an outline of The Food Tree. Students can write the foods on the canopy of The Food Tree image. Students can also draw or cut and paste pictures from food magazines onto The Food Tree image.

Sample Meal Plan Ideas:
Three servings of fruit a day

Breakfast	Chopped apples, blueberries, banana on hot cereal
Snack	Frozen mango smoothie
Lunch	Two kiwis
Snack	Raisins (and walnuts)
Dinner	Half a grapefruit before dinner

➤ Procedure 4
KEEP A FRUIT FOOD JOURNAL

1. Provide students with a Fruit Log Sheet. Write across the top: "Date, Fresh, Frozen, Other, Serving Size, From Home, From School, From a Restaurant."
2. Down the left side, write a list of fruit.
3. Ask students to keep the journal for one week.

Explore data findings. What were the most common sources of fruit eaten? Record student responses on a big wall chart. You can tally up the data anonymously to protect the children's privacy.

Assessment

Discuss the students' changing views on the importance of eating fruit. Talk about all of the beautiful kinds of fruit they can eat and remind them to enjoy eating a variety.

1. Encourage students to pay attention to whether they are eating enough fruit every day.
2. What have students learned from looking at their diets compared to The Food Tree recommendations? Students can take this lesson a step further and calculate the number of fruit servings they are eating every day.
3. Have students look at the list of fruit they wrote down at the beginning of the lesson. Ask the following question: Are you eating fruit more often? Are you eating appropriate serving sizes? What about variety? What changes have you, or can you make to your diets? Ask students to write down the changes they could make. Challenge them to implement these changes, even if it's just one meal at a time.

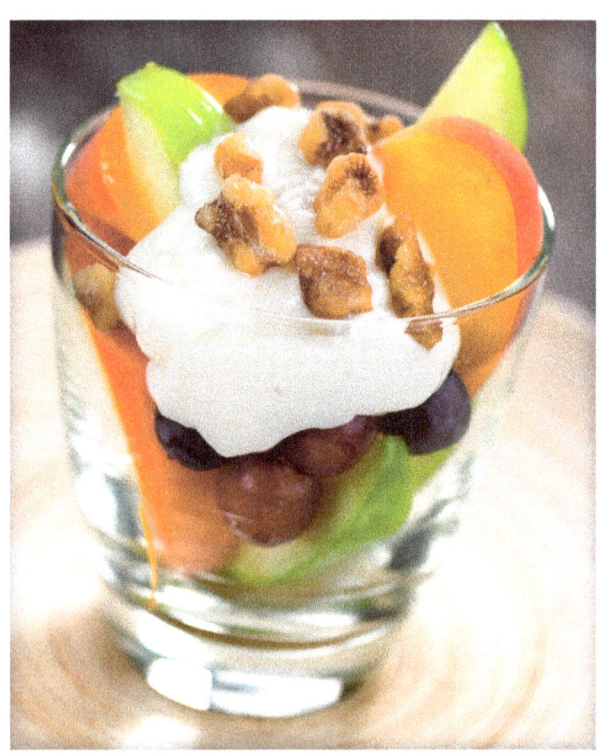

FOUNDATIONAL

Lesson: Benefits and Functions of Fruits

➤ MATERIALS
- Examples and samples of different types of fruit: a jar of apple sauce, an empty bag of frozen fruit, fresh fruit, dried fruit
- The Food Tree Magnetic Board
- The Food Tree Nutrient Scroll, located in the appendix
- The Food Tree Food Journal, located in the Activities Section

➤ GOAL
Understand the health benefits of eating a diet rich in quality fruits.

➤ OBJECTIVES
- To show the number of servings of fruit recommended daily
- To name six different kinds of fruit
- To explain the health benefits of eating fruit
- To explain why the different colors found in the fruit indicate different nutrients

***Action item**
Show The Food Tree Nutrient Scroll

BACKGROUND INFORMATION

Benefits and Functions of Fruit

Fruits are one of the Five Food Tree Food Groups that contribute to a healthy body. Fruits provide your body with vital vitamins, minerals, trace elements, phytonutrients, and fiber that are all necessary for your health and wellbeing. (1)

PROVIDE ENERGY SOURCE

Fruits provide four calories per gram in the form of a carbohydrate. Calories from fruit provide quick energy from the fruits' natural sugar, glucose.

EAT A RAINBOW

- **Red** fruit and vegetables like tomato, grapefruit, and cherry contain bioflavonoids and beta-carotene that are powerful detoxifier-compounds that help prevent illness.
- **Orange** foods like persimmon, sweet potato, and cantaloupe contain beta-carotene that studies show helps to promote healthy immunity.
- **Yellow** fruits and vegetables like pineapple contains bromelain that reduces inflammation found in people with allergies and auto-immune conditions like rheumatoid arthritis.
- **Green** fruits and vegetables like broccoli and kale contain glucosinolates that are known to block cancer-causing substances. Plus, they contain flavonoids beneficial for healthy circulation and immune response.
- **Blue and Purple** blueberries, grapes and purple potatoes contain anthocyanins that are good for heart health and to improve circulation, to strengthen blood capillaries, to circulate nutrients, and to help detoxify the liver, skin, kidneys, and bowels, which all help promote better health.
- **White** fruit and vegetables like banana contain vitamin B3, B5, B6, biotin, vitamin C, manganese, magnesium, and potassium. Potassium is a mineral that helps to balance salt in the cells.

PROVIDE NUTRIENTS
Fruits are rich in vitamins, minerals, and trace minerals. For instance, cantaloupe, blueberry, and lemon are all rich in vitamin C. (2)

PROVIDE PHYTONUTRIENTS
Phytonutrients are the chemicals in foods that give plants and their fruit their colors. They are the chemicals found in plants that provide antioxidants like anthocyanins, and the flavonoid, quercetin. Antioxidants are known to help to reduce damage from free radicals and protect against disease and illness like colds, flu, and cancer. Antioxidants decrease risk for heart disease, diabetes, and stroke by lowering blood pressure, helping with hormone balance, and reduction of inflammation. (3)

PROVIDE FIBER
Fruits are high in fiber. Fiber is the tough indigestible cellulose part of plants. Fiber is either soluble or insoluble. (See Lesson—Focus on Fiber). Fiber helps to maintain gut health, keeps the colon clean, aids in digestion and elimination by helping pass stools easily, and helps maintain balanced blood sugar. (4) Fiber helps feed beneficial bacteria in the gut that are necessary to reduce the possibility of intestinal problems.

SUPPLY ENZYMES
Fresh fruit, especially raw fruit, contain enzymes. Enzymes are elements that break down food and are necessary for digestion. Protease, found in pineapple and papaya, is an example of an enzyme that breaks down proteins.

ENGAGE THE SENSES
Eating a diet rich in colorful fruit engages the senses in taste and texture which adds to the joy of eating. Fruits supply an excellent variety of flavors, textures, and colors that provide a positive experience in growing, shopping for, preparing, cooking, offering, sharing, and eating them.

Problems associated with the lack of fruit in a person's diet

Current government statistics indicate that only twelve percent of Americans eat the recommended daily amount of fruit. A low intake of fruit may result in a lack of phytonutrients, antioxidants, and fiber.

What kinds of fruits should we avoid?

- Canned fruit packed in sugar water.
- Fruit juice. It is best to eat the whole fruit instead of drinking pure fruit juice. Even though fruit is healthy, drinking straight juice or juice with sugar added is one of the reasons for increased caloric intake among children. Fruit juice, without the pulp, lacks fiber and will increase glucose levels in the blood.

➤ Procedure 1
AN APPLE A DAY
Ask your class to highlight the health benefits of a certain type of fruit in a paper, posterboard, or presentation.

Assessment

Have a conversation with your class to see if they are motivated to include more fresh fruit in their diet knowing now how good they are for them.

COMPREHENSIVE

Lesson: Cost Analysis of Fruits

➤ MATERIALS
- Arrange to call or visit different stores that sell produce
- Data collection sheet

➤ GOAL
Understand the cost differentials of organic to non-organic fruit sold at different types of stores.

➤ OBJECTIVE
- To compare and contrast the cost of organic or non-organic fruit in your community

➤ ACTIVATING PRIOR KNOWLEDGE
No doubt eating organic food is better for us, our children, and the environment. Whether or not people have access to it, can afford it, or want it is another story. However, we wonder if sometimes there may be a misperception that buying organic produce is more costly. Is it? Does it have to be?

BACKGROUND INFORMATION

In this exercise, task students to compare different types of organically grown and conventionally grown produce sold at a variety of stores. To bring more nutritious, tasty organic foods to our communities, we first need to create a baseline of how people are currently eating and shopping so we can know the direction to pursue.

➤ Procedure 1

Compare and contrast the cost of organic or conventionally grown fruit in your community. Research the costs of organic or conventional to see if there are large, small, or no price differences. You may find that organic is more affordable than conventionally grown.

Choose at least three types of places that sell fruit. Here are suggestions to get you started.

- Big Chain Commercial Grocery Stores
  - Safeway, Stop & Shop, Giant Food Stores, Publix, Food Lion, Pathmark, Kroger, Nob Hill, WinCo Foods, H-E-B
- Big Chain Health Food Stores
  - Whole Foods, Sprouts, ALDI, Trader Joe's, Hy-Vee, Wegmans
- Box Stores
  - Walmart, Meijer, Sam's Club, Costco
- Independent Grocery Stores
- Local Shops
- Convenience Stores
- Farmer's Markets
- Farm Stands
- CSA's (Community Supported Agriculture)
- School Garden or Community Grown Vegetables
- Home Grown Vegetables

Ask the students to review their data collection and comment on what they found. Were their perceptions accurate? Did they debunk any myths? Have students prepare an analysis of their findings.

DATA COLLECTION SHEET

FOOD TYPE	STORE	PRICE	STORE	PRICE	STORE	PRICE

Permission to reproduce. ©The Food Tree

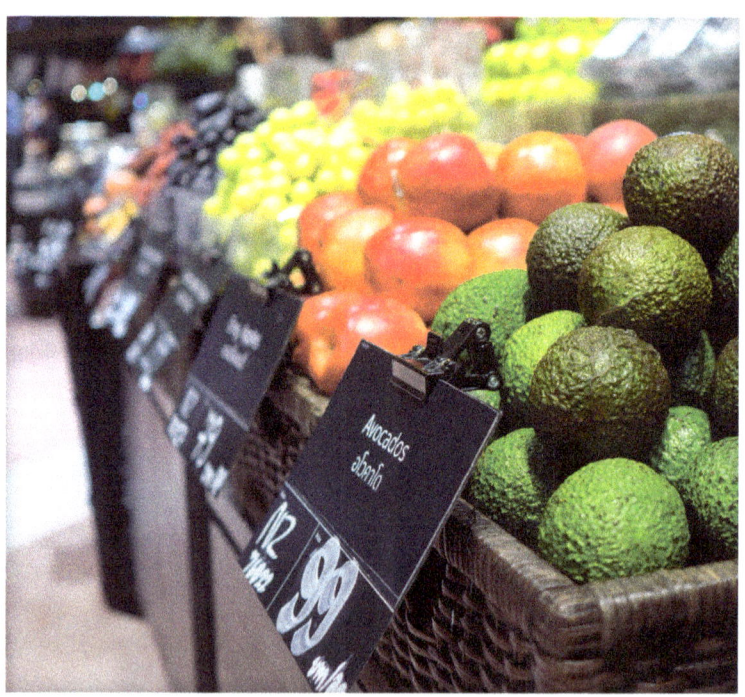

THE FOOD TREE

COMPREHENSIVE

Lesson: Eat Locally Grown and In-Season Fruit

➤ MATERIALS
- Fruit list
- Map of the United States

➤ GOALS
Understand that eating fruit in season and locally grown usually tastes better, is more nutritious, and is often more environmentally sustainable than fruit that travels far distances.

➤ OBJECTIVES
- To create awareness about the different growing seasons and climates of fruit
- To appreciate the concepts of Eat Locally Grown and Eat In-Season

➤ ACTIVATING PRIOR KNOWLEDGE
Rarely do you meet someone who doesn't like fruit. Ask the class to raise their hands if they eat at least one piece or serving of fruit every day. Ask if they think it is optimal to eat all types of fruit year-round. Why or why not?

BACKGROUND INFORMATION

In this lesson, we look at the model of "Eat Locally Grown and Eat In-Season". This concept supports the idea that fruit and vegetables are foods that are often best eaten fresh right after they are picked or harvested.

Discuss with your class the type of fruit that grows in your area. Discuss the fruits that are currently in season in your community or region. Discuss how the fruit is produced in different parts of the country and distributed.

The Food Tree encourages people to eat all foods and, especially, fruit grown locally, in season, organically, sustainably, and fair trade. It is important for students to understand that it is not natural to be eating grapes in December, whether you live in Vermont or California, for that matter! It's not just about the growing but what kinds of foods your body needs during different times of the year and what type of climate you live in. We encourage students to look carefully at their thoughts, beliefs, and behaviors around growing, accessing, providing, preparing, and eating fruit.

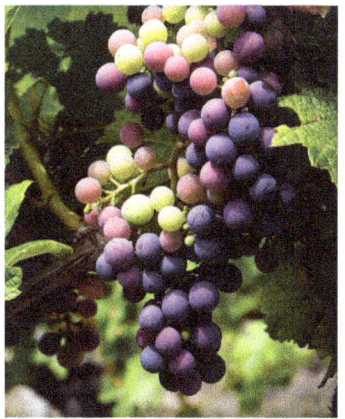
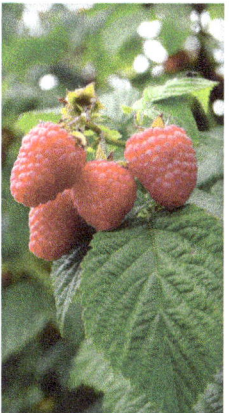
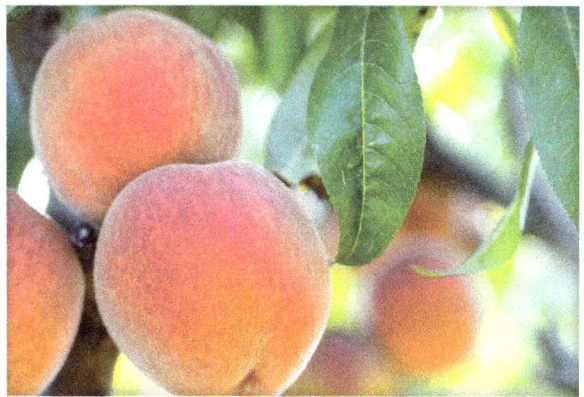

➤ Procedure 1
IMPORT/EXPORT

1. Divide your class into four sections. Each section will represent four parts of the U.S.
2. Research the different fruit grown in those regions. List common exports from the U.S.
3. Explore what fruit we enjoy in the U.S. such as bananas and mangoes that are imported.

➤ Procedure 2
GROW YOUR OWN!

Illustrate and create a year-round garden plan on how you would grow fruit at your school, home, or somewhere else in your community.

- What variety of fruit would grow?
- What types of fruit grows naturally in your area?
- Would you need a greenhouse to grow particular fruit?
- How is your access to water required to grow certain crops of fruit?
- What would be the harvest times of those fruits?
- What would be the costs? Seeds, time, maintenance, tools, storage unit, etc.?

Assessment

Do your students have a new appreciation for the growing season of fruit?

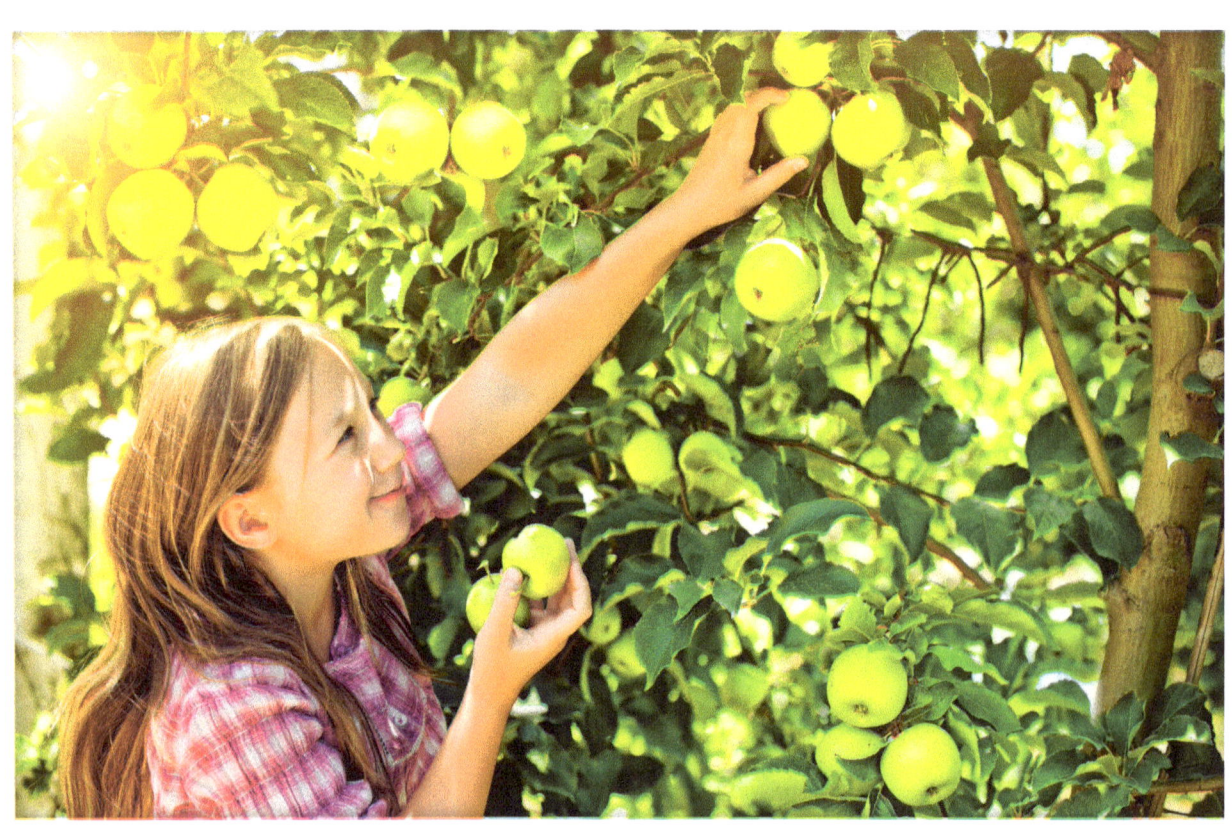

SUPPORT LESSONS

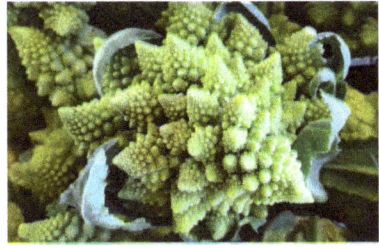 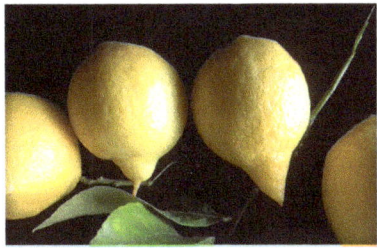 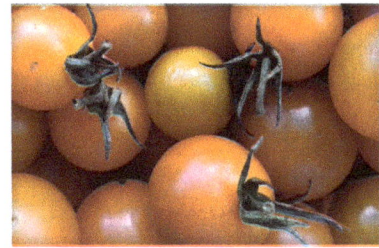

DISCOVERY

Lesson: Rainbow Food Phytonutrients and Antioxidants

➤ MATERIALS
- Rainbow Foods List
- Chalkboard and chalk or dry erase board and markers in all colors
- Variety of fruits and vegetables or vegetable food props: laminated pictures, felt cutouts, or model of fruits and vegetable foods
- Small cups
- Toothpicks
- Napkins
- Knife and cutting board

➤ ACTIVITIES
- Taste the Rainbow Game
- Plant Part Sorting Game

➤ GOAL
Understand the importance of eating the five primary food colors found in fruits and vegetables that are necessary to support growing a healthy body.

➤ OBJECTIVES
- To name at least three fruits and three vegetables from each of the five rainbow color food groups: red, orange, yellow, green and blue/purple
- To state how many servings of fruit and vegetables they need to eat every day
- To know the importance of "eating a rainbow" variety of fruits and vegetables
- To define and list two different phytonutrients found in one fruit and one vegetable

➤ ACTIVATING PRIOR KNOWLEDGE
Ask students if they have heard the phrase, "Eat A Rainbow." Ask them to name colorful fruits and vegetables. Discuss the foods they brainstorm. Help them add to the list by suggesting more foods they might be familiar with. Ask them why they think eating rainbow-colored fruits and vegetables are essential to their health. Ask students what their favorite colorful fruits and vegetables are. Guide them in noticing the rainbow of colors found in them. Do all vegetables and fruits have the same nutrients? What makes fruits and vegetables have different colors?

Discuss the health benefits. Talk about why variety is important and how different fruits and vegetables offer different nutrient profiles and phytochemicals. Fruits and vegetables provide vitamins, minerals, fiber, antioxidants, and phytonutrients. Demonstrate to the class what a serving size of fruits and vegetables looks like and how many servings of fruits and vegetables are recommended during the day.

BACKGROUND INFORMATION

It is essential for children to have an abundance of fresh and cooked fruits and vegetables in their lives. Yet, fruits and vegetables are lacking in the diets of Americans in general but, more alarmingly, they profoundly lacking in the diets of children.

One main reason to eat more fresh produce is for the phytonutrients. These phytonutrients are considered to be antioxidants. These powerful plant chemicals are fascinating as they can protect both the plant from mold and insects and, in people, from disease and illness.

Antioxidants help prevent, protect, and reduce damage to our cells from free radicals that cause oxidative damage. Free radicals are groups of atoms that are missing an electron-molecule, which causes the molecule to become unstable and reactive. Antioxidant molecules donate electrons to make the reactive atom stable. They are thereby reducing oxidative damage in the tissues of the body.

When oxidative damage does occur, it results in rapid aging, cell damage, disease, and ultimately cell death. Some people are more susceptible to oxidative damage. It may be due to eating a poor diet, having phytonutrient deficiencies, or just experiencing the natural aging process.

Fortunately, our bodies make a natural antioxidant from an enzyme called superoxide dismutase (SOD). This self-made antioxidant provides electrons that reduce free radical damage. SOD is in foods like broccoli and cabbage that are rich in minerals.

Eating antioxidant-rich colorful fruits and vegetables are vital for children, especially if they eat a SAD (Standard American Diet) of junk food, soda, and fast foods. People need to eat a variety of different types of fruits and vegetables to receive maximum health benefits.

Listed below are a few compelling reasons for eating a variety of colorful fruits and vegetables.

- Offer different amounts of nutrient-rich, antioxidant, free radical quenching phytonutrients and phytochemicals
- Prevent and reverse modern-day lifestyle diseases. (2)
- Provide the plant pigments that add amazing colors to fruits and vegetables
- Provide antioxidant benefits
- Improve the immune system that fights and prevents disease
- Reduce cellular damage
- Help prevent and decrease the risk of heart disease, diabetes, and stroke by lowering blood pressure (3)
- Reduce the occurrence and susceptibility to colds and flu
- Help prevent certain cancers
- Help with hormone balance
- Reduce inflammation

Eat Rainbow Colored Fruits and Vegetables

RED FRUITS AND VEGETABLES

Apple, beet, bell pepper, blood orange, cabbage, cherry, chili pepper, cranberry, papaya, pomegranate, radicchio, radish, raspberry, red bell pepper, red grapefruit, red grapes, red onion, rhubarb, strawberry, tomato, watermelon

Nutrients found in RED colored foods

- Beet—folate, iron, manganese, potassium, betanin, fiber
- Cranberry—vitamin C, iron, tannins
- Cherry—vitamin C, potassium, anthocyanins, ellagic acid
- Grape—vitamins B3, B6, biotin, potassium, selenium, zinc, anthocyanins
- Pomegranate—choline, folate, vitamin K, vitamin C, phosphorus, potassium, anthocyanins

- Red bell pepper—vitamin B6, vitamin C, beta-carotene
- Tomato—vitamin B3, vitamin C, beta carotene, potassium, lycopene
- Watermelon—vitamin A, potassium, vitamin C, phosphorus, lycopene

ORANGE FRUITS AND VEGETABLES

Apricot, butternut squash, cantaloupe, carrots, mango, melon, nectarine, orange, orange bell pepper, papaya, peach, pepper, persimmon, pumpkin, squash, sweet potato, tangerine, yam

Nutrients found in ORANGE colored foods

- Cantaloupe—beta-carotene, vitamin B3, vitamin C
- Carrot—beta-carotene, folate, vitamin K, calcium, chromium, iron, zinc
- Apricot—beta-carotene, vitamin C, calcium, iron, zinc, vitamin B5
- Pumpkin—beta-carotene, vitamin C
- Mango—beta-carotene, vitamin C, vitamin E
- Sweet potato—vitamin E, vitamin C

YELLOW FRUITS AND VEGETABLES

Apples, avocado, banana, carrots, corn, cucumber, leek, legumes, lemon, lime, grapefruit, pineapple, rutabagas, yellow beets, yellow bell pepper, yellow cauliflower, yellow tomato, yellow onion, yellow watermelon, zucchini

Nutrients found in YELLOW colored foods

- Pineapple—vitamin B1, vitamin B6, vitamin C, manganese, bromelain
- Lemon—vitamin C, folate, potassium, limonene
- Carrot—beta-carotene, folate, vitamin K, calcium, chromium, iron, zinc
- Squash—bromelain, vitamin C

GREEN FRUITS AND VEGETABLES

Artichoke, arugula, asparagus, avocado, bok choy, broccoli, Brussels sprouts, cabbage, celery, chard, collard greens, cucumber, escarole, green bean, green bell peppers, green grape, green olive, green onion, green pepper, green tomato, honeydew melon, kale, kiwi, leek, lettuce greens, lime, melon, okra, peas, snow pea, spinach, sea vegetables, sprouts, tomatillo, watercress, zucchini

Nutrients found in GREEN colored foods

- Arugula—beta-carotene, vitamin C, sulforaphane, volatile oils
- Avocado—vitamins B1, B2, B3, B5, biotin, vitamin E, vitamin K, carotenoids, folate, iron, magnesium, potassium, zinc, glutathione
- Broccoli, Kale—beta-carotene, vitamin B3, vitamin B5, vitamin C, vitamin E, folate, calcium, iron, zinc, glucosinolates, flavonoids, sulforaphane
- Kiwi—beta-carotene, vitamin B3, vitamin C

BLUE/PURPLE FRUITS AND VEGETABLES

Back beans, blackberry, black olive, blueberry, currant, eggplant, elderberry, fig, plum, prune, purple bell pepper, purple cabbage, carrot, purple grape, purple potato, raisins, sea vegetables

Nutrients found in PURPLE colored foods

- Blueberry—beta-carotene, folate, vitamin B2, vitamin C, vitamin E, anthocyanins, ellagic acid, tannins, fiber
- Purple grape—vitamin B3, vitamin B6, biotin, potassium, selenium, zinc, anthocyanins, ellagic acid

WHITE/BROWN FRUITS AND VEGETABLES

Apple, banana, beet, carrot, cauliflower, celeriac, daikon radish, date, garlic, ginger, jicama, kohlrabi, mushroom, onion, parsnip, pear, potato, turnip, white bean

Nutrients found in WHITE colored foods

- Banana—vitamins B3, B5, B6, biotin, vitamin C, manganese, magnesium, potassium
- Garlic—vitamin B6, iron, magnesium, phosphorus, selenium, zinc, sulfur, volatile oils
- Apple—vitamin C, flavonoids, malic acid, pectin

> ### DR. ANDREW WEIL'S TOP FOODS LIST
>
> Dr. Andrew Weil, the esteemed pioneer in the field of integrative medicine, shares his *Healthy Food List*, top choices for foods worthy of regularly including in the diet.
>
> Spinach, collards, kale, broccoli, cabbage, Brussels sprouts, cauliflower, turnips, sweet potatoes, carrots, mangoes, apricots, tomatoes, watermelon, papaya, pink grapefruit, blueberries, purple grapes, red cabbage, beets, plums, green tea, chocolate, and herbs

- Potatoes—vitamins B1, B3, B6, vitamin C, folate, copper, iron, potassium
- Onion—vitamin B1, vitamin B6, flavonoids, quercetin, sulfur

What are some ways to add more colorful fruits and vegetables into your diet?

FOR BREAKFAST

- Add berries to your whole-grain pancakes or hot cereal.
- Have sliced oranges or hot lemon water before you eat.
- Have sautéed or stir-fried vegetables like onions, broccoli, kale, and carrots.
- Add salsa to your eggs, beans, or tofu.

FOR LUNCH

- Pack one fruit and one to two vegetables every day.
- Add sprouts, lettuce, cucumber, tomato, green pepper, roasted red pepper, and zucchini to your sandwich.
- Have a serving of raw carrot sticks, celery, or pea pods.

FOR DINNER

- Eat three servings of vegetables with your dinner every night: two cooked, one raw, or two raw and one cooked.
- Add tomato sauce to pasta.
- Add fruit and vegetables to your salads like sliced red onions, sprouts, and chopped apples.

FOR SNACKS

- Enjoy grapes and blueberries as a snack between meals.
- Make and gobble up kale chips.
- Prepare raw vegetables like jicama, red bell pepper, celery, and green beans.
- Make a smoothie with frozen strawberries, banana, and frozen mango.

➤ Procedure 1

RAINBOW FOOD BRAINSTORM CHALLENGE

Brainstorm as many different fruit and vegetables you can think of in all the different color groups. Do this exercise individually, in pairs, in groups, or as a class. Use the ROYGBIV—red, orange, yellow, green, blue, indigo, violet acronym. Blue, indigo, and violet can all be grouped under blue.

1. List as many fruits and vegetables in each color group in a certain time frame.
2. Have your students write the names on paper or have the class call the rainbow foods out loud and then write on a board.
3. Be prepared with a list of lesser-known vegetables and fruit.
4. Ask what their favorite fruits and vegetables are and how they enjoy eating them.

➤ Procedure 2
SELL IT! KIDS LOVE VEGETABLES
Prepare a research paper, PowerPoint, computer meme, graphic art, or poster board highlighting and featuring the amazingness of one or more rainbow foods or color groups.

Showcase
- nutrients and phytonutrients that are abundant in it.
- optimal season to eat it in.
- how to grow and prepare.
- health and medicinal value.
- different types or varieties.

➤ Procedure 3
RAINBOW CHEF
Have your class participate in cooking demonstrations featuring vegetables and fruits. You can do an *Iron Chef*-style competition or an informational traditional cooking demo. Do this activity as an individual or in pairs.

➤ Procedure 4
RAINBOW RECIPES
Have everyone in the class share a favorite rainbow food recipe. Make copies so that all of the students go home with a collection of recipes from their classmates. You can create a fruit and vegetable cookbook for fun. For more impact, choose one recipe a week and make the dish as a class.

➤ Procedure 5
RAINBOW FOOD JOURNAL
Ask students to keep a journal of their fruit and vegetable consumption. Keep it for one week and up to an entire month.
- Draw pictures of vegetables and fruits eaten for each day in their journals.
- Draw a rainbow or apply a rainbow sticker to the calendar day for those days when you had a rainbow of vegetables and fruits.

Write something about the food in the calendar: Brainstorm suggestions of topics they might want to journal about.
- Did they like the new fruits and vegetables they tried?
- Did they explore new flavors and try new produce?
- Describe if it was easy or not to be consistent with eating enough vegetables every day.
- Explore if there were any challenges with getting the family to buy and prepare vegetables.
- Describe what the fruit or vegetable tasted like.
- How was it experimenting in the kitchen with recipes and cooking?
- Talk about how it felt ordering vegetables in restaurants and the difficulty or ease of it.
- What is it like talking to their friends about their new interest in making sure they eat enough fruits and vegetables?

➤ Procedure 6
Explore the nutritional content of common fruits and vegetables either as an individual or group project.
1. Read an article related to the health benefits of fruits and vegetables. Research the types and amounts of phytonutrient chemicals that are in them.
2. Use magazines, newspapers, online, or in medical journals.
3. Write a paper based on the article and then discuss it as a class or as a presentation.

▶ Procedure 7

Create a flyer or graphic poster featuring the health benefits of a specific fruit or vegetable. Include the vitamins, minerals, and phytonutrients found in them. Hang them around the school.

▶ Procedure 8

PLANT A SCHOOL GARDEN

Discuss the kinds of plants students would like to grow. Create a planting schedule based on the season, location, and specific growing requirements for various crops. Prepare the soil and start planting.

Assessment

- Discuss the health importance of eating a variety of colorful fruits and vegetables during the day.
- Talk about ways to add more colorful fruits and vegetables into the diet.
- Go to the Farmers Market.
- Shop and cook with your parents.
- Ask what new rainbow foods they want to try.
- Challenge the class to find ways to grow fruits and vegetables.

RAINBOW FRUITS AND VEGETABLES LIST

RED

Apple, beet, blood orange, cabbage, cherry, chili pepper, cranberry, grape, guava, papaya, pomegranate, radicchio, radish, raspberry, red bell pepper, red grapefruit, red onion, rhubarb, strawberry, tomato, watermelon

ORANGE

Apricot, butternut squash, cantaloupe, carrots, mango, melon, nectarine, orange, orange bell pepper, peach, pepper, persimmon, pumpkin, squash, sweet potato, tangerine, yam

YELLOW

Apples, avocado, banana, carrot, corn, cucumber, leek, legumes, lemon, lime, grapefruit, pineapple, rutabaga, yellow beet, yellow bell pepper, yellow cauliflower, yellow tomato, yellow onion, yellow watermelon, zucchini

GREEN

Artichoke, arugula, asparagus, avocado, bok choy, broccoli, Brussels sprout, celery, chard, collard, cucumber, escarole, green bean, green cabbage, green bell pepper, green cabbage, green grape, green olive, green onion, green pepper, honeydew melon, kale, kiwi fruit, leek, lettuce greens, lime, melon, okra, peas, snow pea, spinach, sea vegetables, sprouts, tomatillo, watercress, zucchini

PURPLE AND BLUE

Black bean, blackberry, black olive, blueberry, currant, eggplant, elderberry, fig, plum, prune, purple bell pepper, purple cabbage, purple carrot, purple grape, purple potato, raisin, sea vegetable

WHITE

Apple, banana, cauliflower, celeriac, daikon radish, date, garlic, ginger, jicama, kohlrabi, mushroom, onion, parsnip, pear, potato, turnip, white bean

DISCOVERY

Lesson: Focus on Fiber

> **MATERIALS**

Examples of foods containing fiber. Bring in various versions of the same food.
- A jar of white rice and a jar of brown rice
- Oat groats, steel cut oats, and instant packaged oats
- Whole grain wheat bread and refined white wheat bread
- Digestive tract hoses

> **ACTIVITY**

Digestive Tract Exercise

> **GOALS**

Learn about the different types of fiber that exist in foods and the roles they play in your body.

> **OBJECTIVES**
- To describe at least three health benefits of fiber.
- To name and identify different types of foods that contain soluble and insoluble fiber.

> **ACTIVATING PRIOR KNOWLEDGE**

Ask students what they know about fiber. Where does it come from? Is it good for you?

BACKGROUND INFORMATION

Fiber is made up of cellulose, the main component of plant cell walls. It is abundant in vegetables, fruits, legumes, and grains. (1) Fiber is not absorbed as a nutrient in the bloodstream. Instead, the role of fiber is to pass through the digestive tract. (2) There are two specific types of fiber found in food, soluble fiber and insoluble fiber.

Soluble Fiber

Soluble fiber breaks down during digestion and turns into a gel matter. It aids in the retention of water and helps to form the stool and ease the passage.

Sources of soluble fiber are found in:
- berries, nuts, seeds, apples, pears, citrus fruits, lentils, oats, rice, and beans.

Insoluble Fiber

Insoluble fiber acts like a broom inside the digestive tract by brushing away waste in the colon. Insoluble fiber does not break down in water.

Sources of insoluble fiber are found in:
- The bran or husks of whole grains, like whole wheat or brown rice.
- The skin of vegetables, like green beans, green peas, cauliflower, carrots, and beets.
- Nuts and seeds, like almonds, peanuts, and amaranth.
- The skin of fruits like prunes, apple or kiwi.

Benefits of Dietary Fiber

Eating a diet abundant in fiber-rich foods like beans, fruit, vegetables, and whole grains contributes to many positive health benefits in the body. (3) Fiber's primary role is to support digestion and gastrointestinal health. Here are a few facts about why fiber-rich foods are so essential to eat.

Fiber helps to:
- Keep the intestinal tract healthy by aiding in the elimination of waste. Fiber removes

carcinogens, toxins, and excess hormones.
- Help prevent the recirculation of those wastes when they are removed from the body. (4)
- Slow the transit time during the digestion of foods.
- Make the body more efficient in the absorption of vital nutrients. This reduces the risk of malabsorption (poor nutrient absorption).
- Regulate blood sugar. Too much sugar in the bloodstream causes illnesses that may include diabetes, hormone imbalance, obesity, and digestive problems. Fiber slows down digestion by allowing your foods' natural sugars to be released slowly and steadily.
- Promote the growth and colonization of beneficial bacteria living in the intestinal tract that help to keep you healthy.
- Make vitamins, like the B vitamin family.
- Create conditions to manufacture serotonin in the digestive tract. Serotonin is your brain's happy mood neurotransmitter.
- Maintain a healthy weight.

Health Recommendation

- Eat at least five servings of vegetables a day.
- Eat whole grains instead of processed grains.
- Eat three servings of in-season fruit a day.
- Enjoy one serving of beans a day.
- Include one serving of nuts and seeds daily. (5)

Experts in the field of holistic nutrition suggest a range of fiber intake. Dr. Bob Sears, a well-respected pediatrician from the United States, suggests we eat up to 25-35 grams of fiber a day (6), and Dr. Andrew Weil, another prominent MD, suggests we eat up to 40 grams of fiber a day. (7)

➤ Procedure 1
COMPARE AND CONTRAST

1. Compare the different types of fiber in various kinds of vegetables, fruits, and grain-based foods.
2. Compare examples provided by the instructor and nutrition information found online (www.nutrition.gov/whats-food or https://ndb.nal.usda.gov/ndb/search/list).
3. Use online data to research whole foods that are sold without packaging labels.

➤ Procedure 2

Discover and discuss the foods that have the most fiber in them. Investigate and compare the fiber content found in fruits, vegetables, beans, and grains.

1. What is the difference between the amounts of fiber in processed versus whole grains?

HIGH FIBER FOODS

Almonds	Brussels Sprouts	Kale	Spinach
Apples	Cabbage	Lentils	String Beans
Asparagus	Cauliflower	Lettuce	Turnips
Beans	Collard Greens	Oats	Watercress
Berries	Cucumbers	Peas	Whole Grains
Bok Choy	Eggplant	Peppers	Zucchini
Broccoli	Fermented Vegetables	Popcorn	
Broccoli Rabe	Flax seeds	Radishes	

THE FOOD TREE

2. Show your students the difference between white rice and brown rice, oat groats, steel cut oats, and instant packaged oats, and whole-grain wheat bread and refined white wheat bread. Compare nutrient panels for the fiber content.

3. Compare the difference in fiber between fruit juice and whole fruit. As a fun point of interest, talk about how many oranges it takes to make one cup of juice. It takes three to four oranges to produce just one cup of juice! Can students imagine eating three or four oranges at one sitting?

➤ Procedure 3

Keep a 3-day Food Journal to track and count fiber in their diets.

Assessment

- Are students eating enough fiber daily?
- Discuss what students discovered about the amount and type of fiber found in different types of foods. What information was new to them? What did they already know?
- Are the students more or less motivated to eat foods with higher fiber counts? Are they more motivated to choose brown rice over white rice? Whole grain wheat bread over white bread? Challenge students to pay attention to the amount of fiber on food labels and to choose whole foods whenever possible.

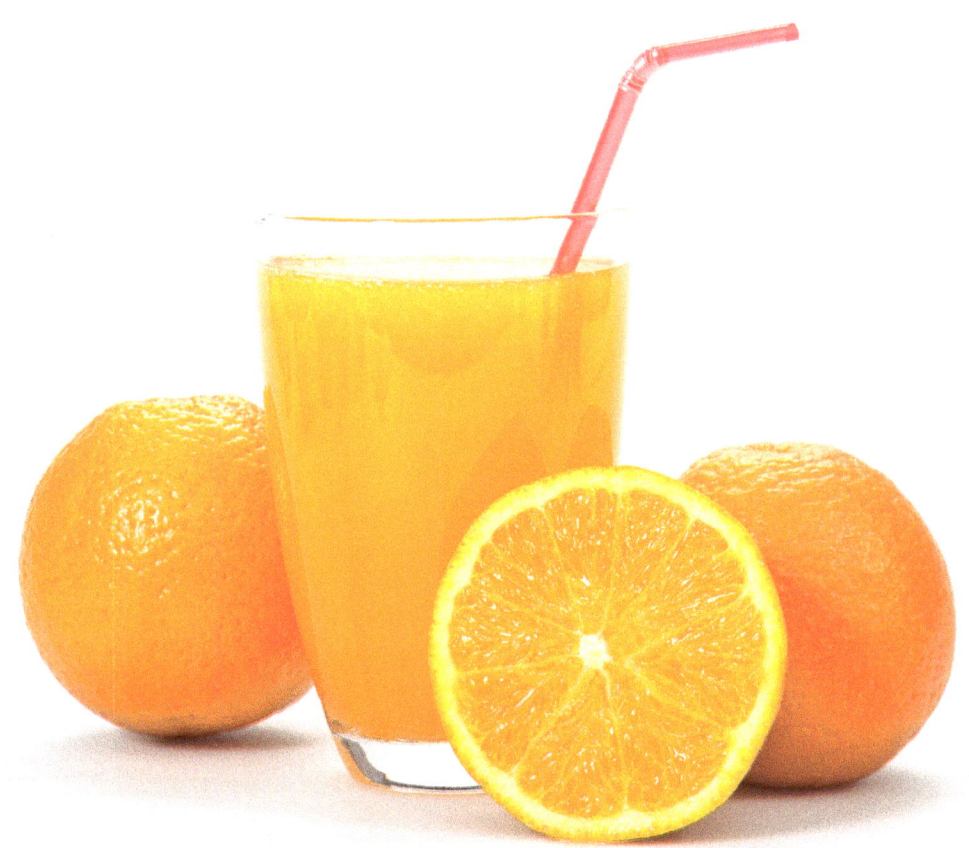

DISCOVERY

Lesson: The Delicate Dynamic Digestive Tract

➤ MATERIALS
- Digestive tract hose examples (make out of garden irrigation tubes or use string)
- Images of the digestive tract

➤ GOAL
Learn the essential functions of the gastrointestinal tract.

➤ OBJECTIVE
- To describe the importance and function of the digestive tract
- To demonstrate the layout of the physical structure of the gastrointestinal (GI) tract
- To explain the role the GI tract plays in nutrient absorption

➤ ACTIVATING PRIOR KNOWLEDGE
Ask students how closely they pay attention to their digestion. This particular topic may feel embarrassing to talk about; however, it is vital to discuss.

BACKGROUND INFORMATION

Take your students on a fascinating journey on learning all about the digestive tract. This lesson presents the physical representation of the gastrointestinal tract.

The digestive tract is the path, or tube, to health. The digestive tract consists of the:

- Mouth
- Esophagus
- Stomach
- Small intestine
- Large intestine or colon
- Rectum

There are eight different phases of digestion:

1. Thinking: The brain starts thinking about eating food.
2. Salivation: Saliva releases into the mouth.
3. Ingestion: Food enters the mouth.
4. Mechanical digestion: Chewing begins, food turns into a bolus.
5. Propulsion or peristalsis: An action causing the movement via rhythmic muscle contraction to move food, called chyme, through the digestive tract.
6. Chemical digestion from the secretion of digestive juices: The stomach secretes HCL, and the pancreas secretes digestive enzymes (pepsin) into the stomach and into the small intestine.
7. Absorption: The action of digested food in the new form of nutrients absorbing into the bloodstream and lymphatic system in the small intestine.
8. Defecation: The passing and release of undigested food, waste, and fiber through the colon or large intestine via the rectum and anus.

The Small Intestine

The small intestine of an average adult is 20 feet long. The small intestine absorbs many nutrients and most water. The majority of the food a person eats is broken down or digested and then absorbed through the walls of the small intestines. Nutrients and calories pass into the bloodstream through the small intestine or into lymphatic tissue. The small intestine is made up of three distinct parts: the duodenum, the jejunum, and the ileum. These three sections are responsible for the absorption of different nutrients and the absorption of ninety percent of the water you drink.

The lining of the intestines includes millions of villi, little rollercoaster-like bumps that make up the lining of the digestive tract. Villi extend into the lumen, or the intestinal cavity, about 1 mm. It does so to maximize the surface area for nutrient absorption of food molecules. Villi regrow every few days.

A diet high in refined grains and poor quality foods and drinks, plus having exposure to pesticides like glyphosate found in Roundup, may cause digestive issues and damage to your delicate gut lining and the villi. This pesticide may cause leaky gut and instigate other potentially adverse health conditions. (1)

Leaky Gut Explained

Because the intestinal tract lining is as thin as an eyelid, it is easily damaged. Injury to the gut lining can cause leaky gut and serious health conditions. Leaky gut, also known as gut permeability, is a situation in which little tears happen in the lining of the small intestine. These tiny holes allow undigested food particles to pass through into the bloodstream. The body perceives undigested food molecules as a foreign invader and its natural response is to activate the immune system.

Leaky gut may cause or worsen sensitivity or intolerance to foods, including the gluten protein molecule found in wheat. Possibly 5% of the population suffer from gluten intolerance. (2) A person may then be at a higher risk for allergies, food reactions, autoimmune diseases, and nutrient malabsorption. Symptoms of leaky gut may include gas, bloating, allergies, inflammation, bad breath, dental issues, and frequent illness. (3)

The Large Intestine

The large intestine, also called the colon, is 5 feet long in an average man or woman. It is where stool forms from the chyme and undigestible foods, like fiber. The colon takes any remaining water and re-circulates and reabsorbs it back into the body. The colon also absorbs electrolytes, produces vitamins, and absorbs any remaining nutrients. (4,5)

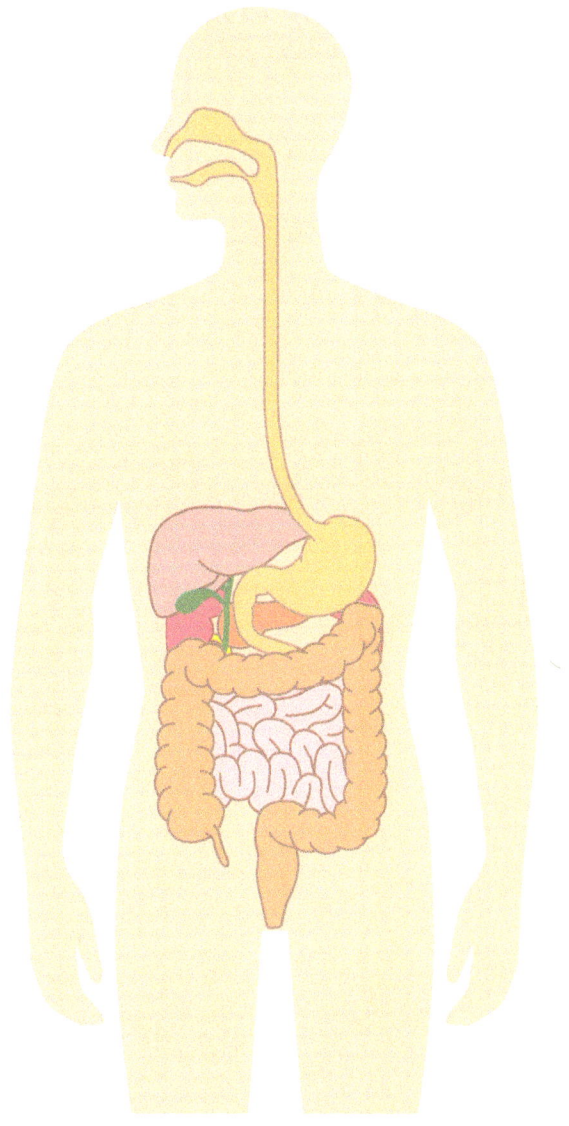

➤ Procedure 1

HOW LONG IS THE DIGESTIVE TRACT?

Show an example of how long the digestive tract is using irrigation hoses, tubes, rope, or string as a model. Explain that the digestive tract is made up of the small and large intestines. The small intestines in an adult measure up to 20 feet long. It is made up of three sections: the duodenum, the jejunum, and the ileum. The large intestine is also called the colon. It measures 5 feet long in an adult.

1. Cut two pieces of string or irrigation hoses in the length of the small and large intestine, 20 feet and 5 feet long, respectively.
2. Ask for student participation. Have students unravel the twenty-foot long hose. And then have another set of students unravel the 5-foot section of hose.
3. Enjoy the reactions you get from your students.

➤ Procedure 2

Have students create models of the digestive tract with recycled or found items. What everyday objects could represent the other parts of the digestive system? This exercise requires some creativity. For example, you can play around with:

Mouth = bottle caps

Esophagus = small plastic bottle or plastic piping

Stomach = inflated balloon

Intestines = socks, rope, string

➤ Procedure 3

Students do breakout investigations on the different sections and components of the digestive tract. They can write a research paper, create a PowerPoint, or create a poster board and present it to the class.

Assessment

- Use a graphic or illustration of the digestive tract to prompt further discussion of the wonders of digestion.
- Discuss how their perception, understanding, and appreciation of the digestive tract has changed or developed after this demonstration.

INTERESTING DIGESTIVE FACTS!

The entire intestinal tract is as thin as an eyelid.

An average full-grown person will have a small intestine measuring 20 feet long and a large intestine measuring 5 feet long.

The intestinal tract measures 2700 square feet or the size of a tennis court.

DISCOVERY

Lesson: Developing Critical Thinking Skills—Food, Diet, Eating, and the Media

➤ MATERIALS
- Access to the internet
- Magazines

➤ GOALS
Learn how to become a critical thinker in the digital age.

➤ OBJECTIVES
- To analyze how the media influences our dietary choices
- To become educated eaters through learning about holistic nutrition
- To learn to rely on your mind! Knowledge is power!

➤ ACTIVATING PRIOR KNOWLEDGE
Have your students explore how they and most people get their health and nutrition information. Discuss roles that parents, TV, social media, government, teachers, school, coaches, doctors, friends, even The Food Tree, play in their food choices and food preferences.

Strive to teach your students to become critical thinkers about the foods they choose to eat, why they made those choices, and the role of nutrition in their lives. Empower your students to navigate the unhealthy food messages they receive regularly. Strive to have them become educated on food issues, food politics, the food industry, and the science of human nutrition/human physiology. Using critical thinking skills is a trusted way for a person to have more success in creating life-long health while fostering a healthy society.

BACKGROUND INFORMATION

Have a candid discussion with your students about the role food plays in their lives. Have them contemplate the commercials they see on TV and online. Are junk foods cheaper than healthy foods? Do your peer groups influence your food choices? Have them reflect on the foods offered at school and in town while discussing the following points:

- Children exercise less and watch TV more than ever before in our society. The average American child watches at least 29 hours of TV or screen time each week.
- They will watch 11,000 junk food commercials a year.
- The Nielsen Company reports that Americans in 2018 spent on average TEN HOURS A DAY on their devices and looking at screens. (1)
- The junk food industry spends over two billion dollars a year on advertising to kids. Junk foods introduced to children as early as age 3 have a lasting negative impact on their health. These commercials reinforce false and misleading information with confusing messages. An astounding 98% of junk food commercials are for foods designed to be highly addictive. That means they are high in salt, bad trans fats/hydrogenated oils, sugar, and chemicals.

- American kids eat poorly. Only 1 in 5, or 20%, of children, eat the recommended amount of fruits and vegetables daily. According to the CDC, from 2007-2010, "93 percent of children didn't eat enough vegetables." (2)
- Forty percent of American children, from toddlers to teens, have diets from fast food restaurants. Shockingly, children in the U.S. get almost half of their daily caloric energy from fast foods. (3)

➤ Procedure 1
FOOD LITERACY: THE WHO, WHAT, WHERE, WHEN, WHY, AND HOW OF FOODS IN SOCIETY

Explore with your students their awareness of the "who, what, where, when, why, and how" of food and eating. Have students bring in junk food marketing ads and articles from the paper or online news sources relating to food, health, and nutrition and discuss in class the concepts of:

- Who grows your food? Who are the farmers who picked the food? Who prepared or made the food? Who owns the food companies from which you make purchases?
- What are the ingredients in the foods you eat? Investigate the ingredients found in packaged foods, in restaurants, in schools or hospitals, and identify them.
- Where was the food grown? How close or far to the consumer was this food grown? Was it produced in one country, then flown to another for processing and packaging, then shipped back to the original country?
- When was the food made or grown? How long does produce or packaged foods sit on shelves? Does this impact nutrition? Does this impact consumer choice? How does it affect quality, taste, or waste?
- Why do you make the food choices you do? What do you consider when deciding what to eat? Do you choose by flavor, convenience, cost, accessibility, peer or family pressure, or nutrient value?

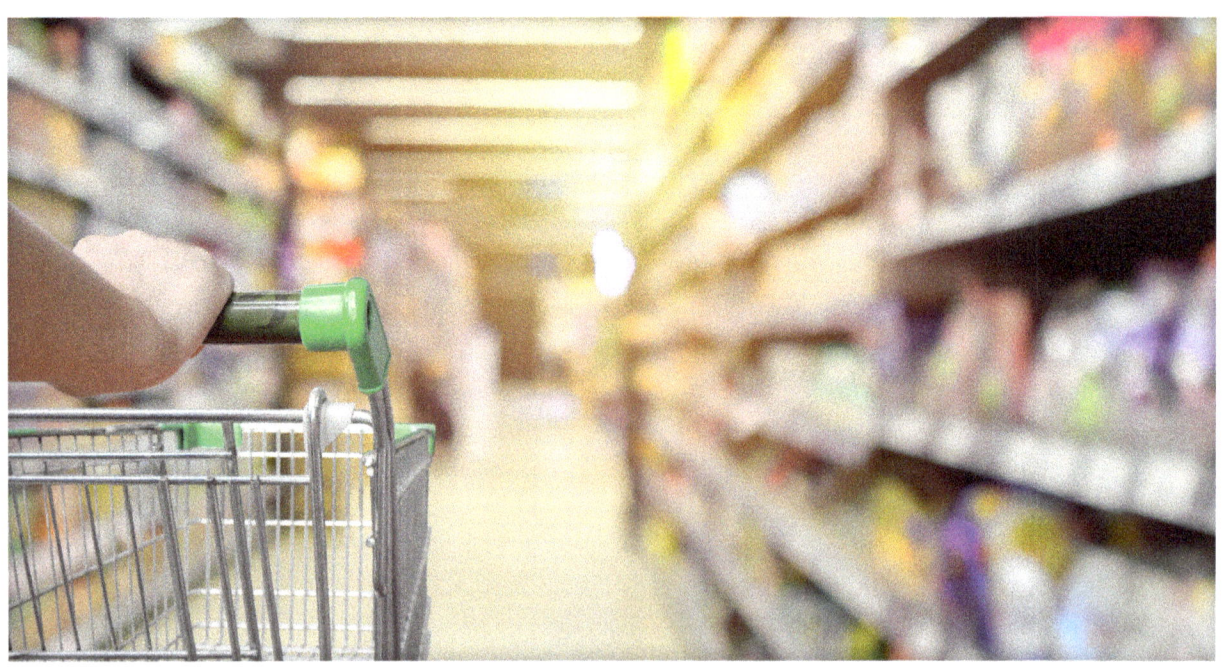

- How do your choices impact others? In your home, community, or globally? How are you influenced by your peers or marketing pressures from big food and beverage corporations?

➤ Procedure 2

Describe in a research paper, PowerPoint, meme, or skit how your peer group influences you regarding the kinds of food you choose to eat.

1. Distinguish if you receive positive, neutral, or negative messages from your friends or if there are certain pressures you face when making food choices.
2. Write a script and act out your observations.
3. Show your point of view on how friends and family may tempt and influence you in social situations. Then, act out a more positive and encouraging approach.

➤ Procedure 3
FOODS IN THE NEWS

Talk with your students about current health and nutrition trends, recent stories about food topics in the media, or news about the latest health food craze.

➤ Procedure 4
NUTRITION VAMPIRES

Have students compare and contrast, analyze, or use persuasive arguments regarding unhealthy food or something that is bad for your health but is not so apparent to the consumer.

1. Set up a debate between two people or create a panel to discuss the pros and cons of allowing Nutrition Vampires into the food system.
2. Identify all the covert, random, and subtle places we get bad food advertising.
3. Take photos in your town, of menus, or from another medium showcasing unhealthy foods.
4. Have students cut out magazine ads featuring unhealthy foods and analyze them.
5. Have the class vote on the most corrupt, convincing messages.

➤ Procedure 5
KNOW THY BODY, KNOW THYSELF

Examine how knowledgeable your students (and their community) are about basic human physiology and basic holistic nutrition. Do people today know more about how to fix bikes, program computers, or what the latest fashion trends are than they know about how the digestive system works? How much do you think our society knows about human nutrition and human physiology?

1. Have students conduct interviews with fellow students, teachers, parents, friends, and people in their local community about their knowledge of basic human physiology, food, and nutrition.

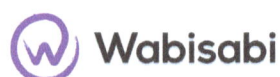

The Ultimate Cheatsheet for Critical Thinking

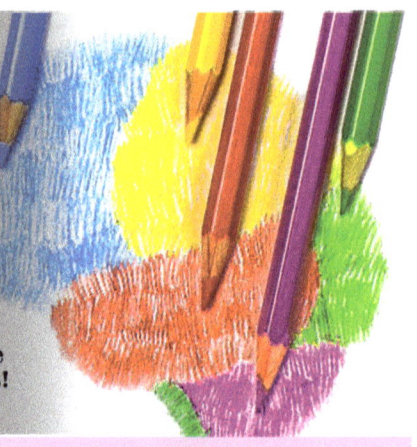

Want to exercise critical thinking skills? Ask these questions whenever you discover or discuss new information. These are broad and versatile questions that have limitless applications!

Who
- ... benefits from this?
- ... is this harmful to?
- ... makes decisions about this?
- ... is most directly affected?
- ... have you also heard discuss this?
- ... would be the best person to consult?
- ... will be the key people in this?
- ... deserves recognition for this?

What
- ... are the strengths/weaknesses?
- ... is another perspective?
- ... is another alternative?
- ... would be a counter-argument?
- ... is the best/worst case scenario?
- ... is most/least important?
- ... can we do to make a positive change?
- ... is getting in the way of our action?

Where
- ... would we see this in the real world?
- ... are there similar concepts/situations?
- ... is there the most need for this?
- ... in the world would this be a problem?
- ... can we get more information?
- ... do we go for help with this?
- ... will this idea take us?
- ... are the areas for improvement?

When
- ... is this acceptable/unacceptable?
- ... would this benefit our society?
- ... would this cause a problem?
- ... is the best time to take action?
- ... will we know we've succeeded?
- ... has this played a part in our history?
- ... can we expect this to change?
- ... should we ask for help with this?

Why
- ... is this a problem/challenge?
- ... is it relevant to me/others?
- ... is this the best/worst scenario?
- ... are people influenced by this?
- ... should people know about this?
- ... has it been this way for so long?
- ... have we allowed this to happen?
- ... is there a need for this today?

How
- ... is this similar to _____?
- ... does this disrupt things?
- ... do we know the truth about this?
- ... will we approach this safely?
- ... does this benefit us/others?
- ... does this harm us/others?
- ... do we see this in the future?
- ... can we change this for our good?

WABISABI LEARNING wabisabilearning.com

COMPREHENSIVE

Lesson: How to Read Nutrition Facts Panel and Package Labeling

➤ **MATERIALS**
- Empty food packages such as snack bars, yogurt containers, milk cartons, dry cereal, cracker boxes

BACKGROUND INFORMATION

Ninety percent of all foods eaten in America come from packages! Therefore, it is important to be able to read a packaging label or at a minimum, read the ingredient list. A nutrition label will be printed somewhere on the package or drink and list information required by the FDA. It will list the ingredients, calories per serving size, and nutrition facts such as what percentage of the food contains proteins, fats, carbohydrates, vitamins, and minerals.

➤ Procedure 1

It is important to know how to read a food packaging label to know how to find out the nutrients and ingredients found in the packaged foods you eat. Provide each student with several empty food packages. Students will also analyze false advertising found on food packaging. Look primarily for Nutrition Vampires like MSG derivatives and hydrogenated oils (trans fats).

1. Form small groups and have students brainstorm two to three food items they want to analyze.
2. Ask students to title a page called Nutrition Package Labeling.
3. Next to each item, as a group write F (fresh) or P (packaged).
4. Compare different brands and products.
5. Evaluate the macronutrient profiles: Proteins, Carbohydrates, Fats.
6. Compare vitamins and minerals across different brands to those found in fresh produce.
7. Calculate, compare, and contrast different nutrients from the Nutrition Fact labels of different food products.
8. Ask students to look at the different variables on the label.
   - Calculate and compare the vitamins, minerals, and fiber found in whole-grain bread vs. white bread or 100% pure fresh-squeezed orange juice vs. orange drink.

Refer to the Appendix for macronutrient calculations. Use the following calorie counting equation.

Fat (g) x 9 + carb (g) x 4 + protein (g) x 4 = ____

FAT FREE STRAWBERRY FLAVORED MILK

Notice the serving size is for 1 yet the values are for a 2,000 calorie a day diet.

Ingredients: Fat Free Milk, Sugar, Natural and Artificial Flavor and Color, (Red #40, Blue#1, and Beet Juice Color), Vitamin A Palmitate, and Vitamin D3.

Servings Per Container: 1

Percent Daily Values are based on a 2,000-calorie diet. Your daily values may be higher or lower depending on your calorie needs.

Amount Per Serving

	% Daily Value*
Total Fat 0g	
Saturated Fat 0g	0%
Trans Fat 0g	0%
Cholesterol 0mg	0%
Sodium 120mg	5%
Total Potassium 0mg	0%
Total Carbohydrate 22g	7%
Dietary Fiber 0g	0%
Sugars 22g	0%
Protein 8g	16%
Calories 120	Calories from Fat 0

Vitamin A	10%	Vitamin C	2%
Calcium	30%	Iron	0%
Vitamin D	25%	Phosphorus	0%
Magnesium	0%	Thiamin	0%
Folate	0%		

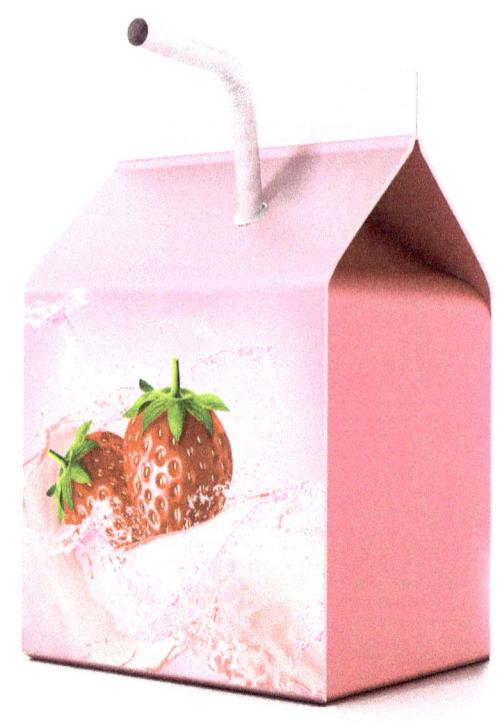

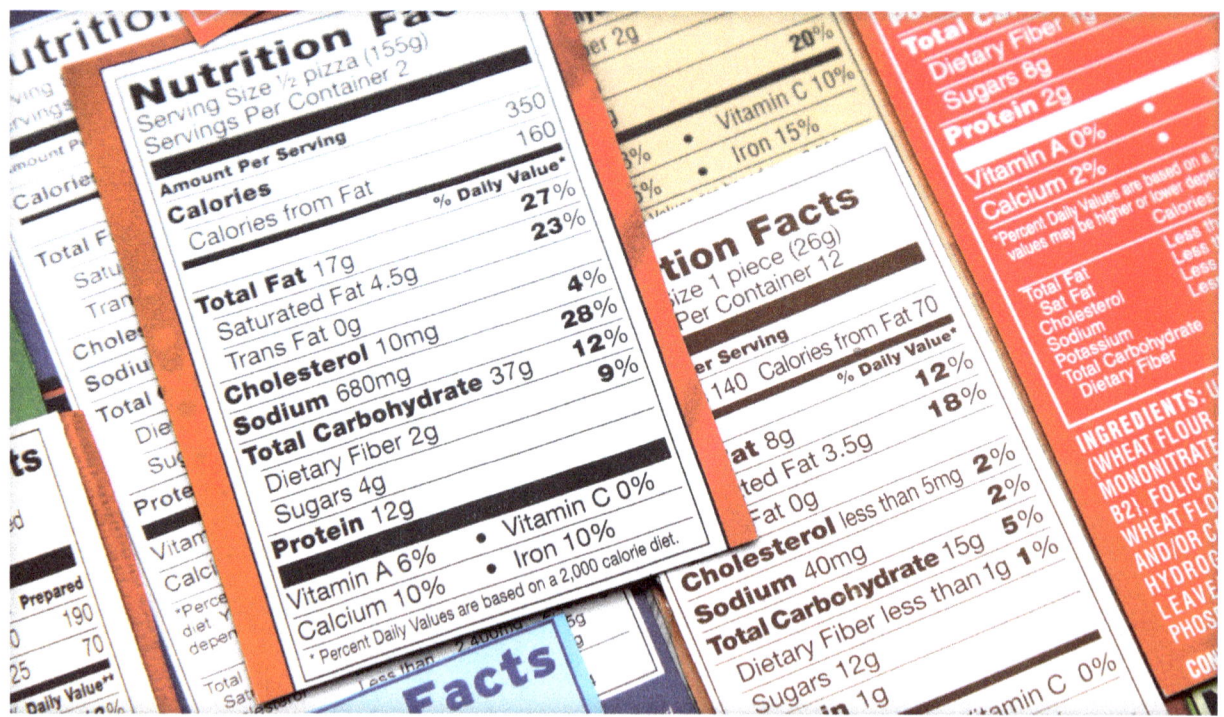

NUTRITION VAMPIRES

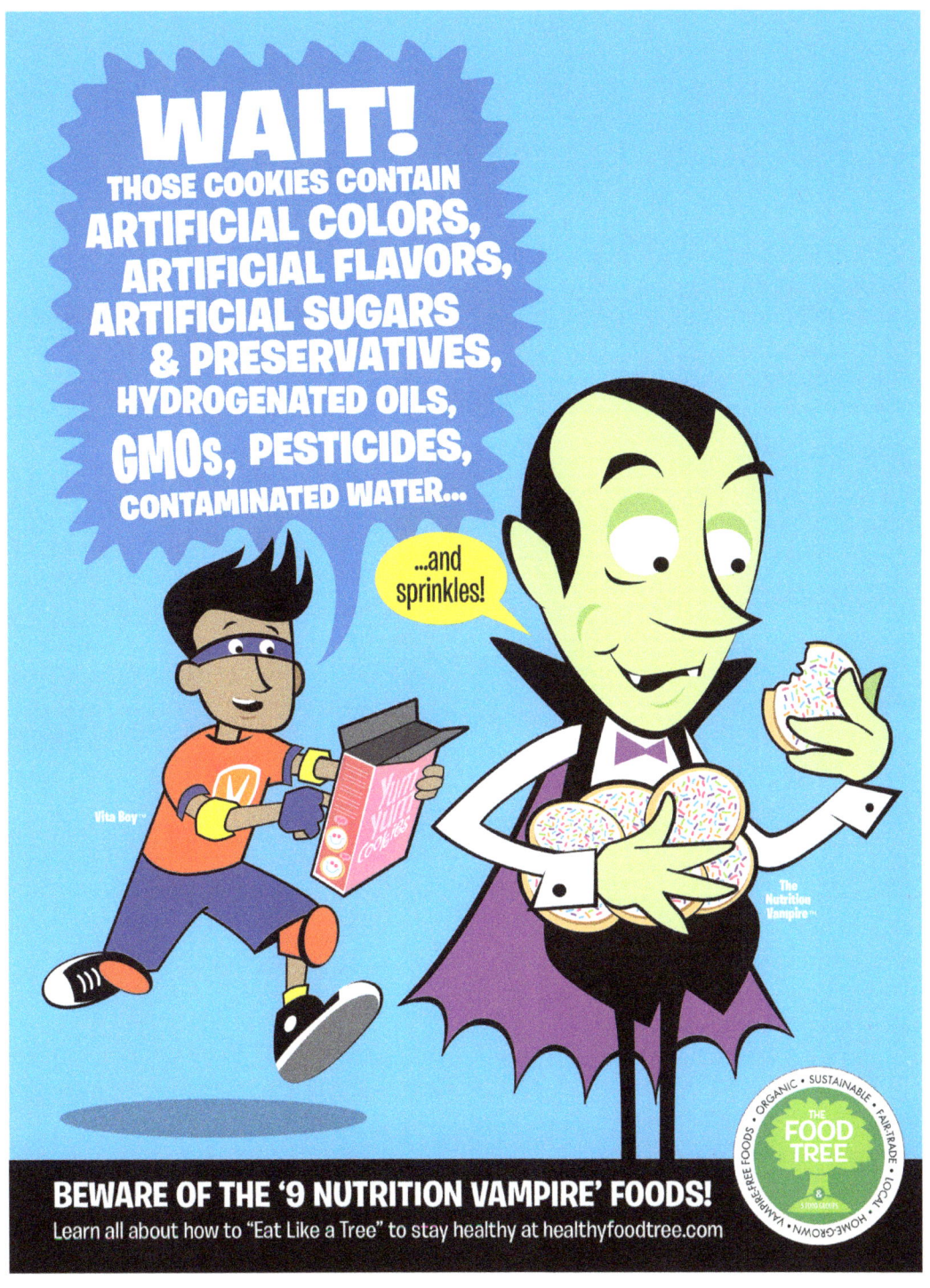

DISCOVERY

Lesson: The Nine Nutrition Vampires

"You never change things by fighting the existing reality. To change something, build a new model that makes the existing model obsolete."
BUCKMINSTER FULLER

➤ MATERIALS

- Examples of the Nine Nutrition Vampire Foods. Use actual food products or cut images out of magazines.
- Lesson: Problems Associated with Eating Damaged Fats and Hydrogenated Oils, in the Fats Chapter.

➤ GOALS

Learn about the Nine Nutrition Vampires found in our foods and the link in decline in human health.

➤ OBJECTIVES

- To list the Nine Nutrition Vampires
- To describe any issues or health concerns with eating processed packaged food containing Nutrition Vampires
- To explain how the FDA approves Nutrition Vampires into the American food system
- To share three ideas on how to create a Nutrition Vampire free diet

➤ ACTIVATING PRIOR KNOWLEDGE

How often do you question what is in your food or if, indeed, it is safe for you to eat? For instance, if someone gives you some cake at school, a friend's house, or at a restaurant, do you ask what the ingredients are? Do you think about food ingredients even though you believe food companies and our government say the food is safe? Do you get mad at yourself because you feel you are not eating right but, instead, you are hurting yourself with your negative thoughts or actions?

Discuss The Nine Nutrition Vampires as age-appropriate.

BACKGROUND INFORMATION

Nutrition Vampires are foods or ingredients added to foods that are considered by us, and many other health experts and scientists, to be unhealthy for people to eat. It is not my intention to incite fear, worry, and concern but to bring the Nutrition Vampires to you to create empowerment and awareness of these topics.

Processed and Packaged Foods

Nutrition Vampires can be lurking in pretty much any food or drink, especially ones that come from a package, bag, box, or bottle. These foods and ingredients are just not good or healthy for growing kids, or anyone for that matter. They are best to avoid as much and as often as possible. (1)

How do you know which packaged and processed foods may contain vampires? First of all, know what they are.

The Food and Drug Administration defines processed foods by seven food engineering criteria:

1. Is mass-produced.
2. Is consistent batch to batch.
3. Is consistent country to country.
4. Uses specialized ingredients from specialized companies.

> **THE FOOD TREE'S NINE NUTRITION VAMPIRES**
>
> 1. Artificial Colors
> 2. Artificial Flavors
> 3. Preservatives
> 4. Processed, Refined, and Artificial Sugars
> 5. Hydrogenated Oils and Damaged Fats
> 6. Genetically Modified Organisms (GMOs)
> 7. Herbicides, Fungicides, and Pesticides
> 8. Impure, Chlorinated, and Fluoridated Water
> 9. Your Vampire (particular food, thoughts, action, behavior)

5. Consists of pre-frozen macronutrients.
6. Stays emulsified.
7. Has a long shelf life or freezer life.

Nutrition Vampire Foods and Vampire Ingredients are found in thousands and thousands of processed, packaged, non-organic foods and beverages such as:

Potato chips	Tortillas
Corn chips	Fried food
Cookies	Donuts
Cakes	Diet foods
Candy	Fast foods
Gum	Pizza
Pastries	Salad dressing
Sports drinks	Canned foods
Energy drinks	Frozen food
Soda	Cheese
Bread	Animal-based foods
Crackers	Dairy with rBGH

HEALTH CONCERNS

Commercially grown foods, often filled with artificial and chemical ingredients, are staples in The Standard American Diet. Unfortunately, eating these kinds of foods daily can have a massive role in developing some severe health issues. We teach our children about wearing helmets and seat belts, stranger danger, and how to cross the road safely. As well, we need to teach children about current health concerns and the decline in Americans health related to foods that may contain harmful ingredients. No, not a fun job, but it is better to inform kids now than have to deal with sicker kids later.

- 60-90% of all food bought in America is packaged and processed. (2)
- 75% of all packaged foods are made with genetically engineered methods.
- 65% of teen boys drink soda and diet soda every day. (3)
- According to the CDC, the Autism Spectrum Disorder rates are currently 1 in 59.
- 1 in 13 children have asthma.
- 1 in 400 children will develop diabetes.
- 1 in 6 children aged 2-8 years have a mental, behavioral, or developmental disorder. (4)
- 30% of young adults have a mental disorder.
- Only 1 in 5 kids eat enough fruits and veggies every day.
- Obesity and preventable diseases are escalating in Americans and 75% of adults are obese.
- Approximately 30% of children are obese and 57% of children are on the path to becoming obese adults. (5)

TOXIC OVERLOAD

Children in the United States are sicker than ever. For the first time in history, children of this generation will not outlive their parents. We are facing a national crisis. The biggest health concern regarding vampires is not that infrequent eating will harm you but that regularly eating vampire foods over a lifetime just might.

Poor eating habits may contribute to a condition called Toxic Overload. Our detoxification pathways can only handle so much input of bad stuff. The liver,

> ### NUTRITION VAMPIRES
>
> **V** Void of Nutritional Value—nutrient-poor foods
>
> **A** Adulterated—foods altered from their natural DNA form
>
> **M** Manufactured—foods packaged, canned, or frozen using unhealthy ingredients
>
> **P** Processed—foods made with chemical ingredients or altered by chemical processing
>
> **I** Impulsive—foods and ingredients that trigger cravings like sugar and salt
>
> **R** Robs Health—foods that steal, deplete, and take nutrients away from the body
>
> **E** Empty—foods that leave you feeling dissatisfied, guilty, and regretful

kidneys, lymph and digestive system can't handle the onslaught of fast food and diet drinks. It is possible these chemicals and pesticides can alter a person's DNA.

Choose your food consciously. Make it a habit to always read the ingredient list on the back of all packaged foods. Check labels carefully and ask your servers at restaurants for the ingredients in the foods they serve. Eating all-natural treats crafted with quality ingredients are encouraged to be eaten and enjoyed.

➤ Procedure 1
KNOW YOUR VAMPIRES
Identify five vampire ingredients to watch out for in foods and describe their potential for harming human or environmental health.

➤ Procedure 2
READ LABELS
Watching out for Nutrition Vampires is about making conscious choices on the quality and quantity of food you eat. Write a top ten list of ways students can make good healthy Nutrition Vampire Free food choices wherever they are.

➤ Procedure 3
MAKE A HEALTH COMMERCIAL
Children and teens see over 11,000 junk food commercials every year. Instead of supporting those types of foods and food corporations that sell those products, have students brainstorm a junk food and ask them to create a commercial for healthier versions and alternatives.

➤ Procedure 4
TAKE A POLL!
Ask your friends and family to answer the following questions to get an idea about how other people regard food additives and their safety.

Sample Poll Questions

1. How often do you read the labels on the packaged foods you purchase?
2. Do you ever question the ingredients that are listed in the food?
3. Are you able to identify all of the ingredients in the foods you buy?
4. Do you know if they are safe for you?
5. When someone offers you cake at a restaurant, school, or the office, do you ever ask where it came from, who made it, and what are the ingredients it is made with?

Assessment
- List the top Nine Nutrition Vampires that can suck the life right out of you.
- Has this lesson created awareness that led you to develop better eating habits? If so, what are they?

DISCOVERY

Lesson: Too Much Sugar!

➤ MATERIALS
- Two pint-sized glass mason or clear glass jars
- One cup plus two teaspoons of white cane sugar
- Two bags or containers to hold sugar
- Examples of packaged foods with added sugar like yogurt, ice cream, chocolate milk, pastries, cookies, frozen foods, sauces

➤ GOAL
Understand that refined white sugar and its derivatives have permeated our food supply and can cause severe and adverse health effects in people who consume too much.

➤ OBJECTIVES
- To identify the sources and quantity of added sugar in foods students are eating
- To know how to read food package labels
- To list five names of sugar or other names of sweeteners
- To motivate students to reduce the amount of added sugar in their diets

➤ ACTIVATING PRIOR KNOWLEDGE
Talk to your class about sugar. Ask them who likes the taste of sugar. Do they eat added sugar every day? Ask students if they are aware of the amount of added sugar that they may be eating every day. Do they think there is a lot of sugar in their sports drinks, energy drinks, soda, or juice? Do they add extra sugar to foods like breakfast cereal? Discuss the way people used to eat hundreds, or thousands, of years ago compared to the way people eat today regarding added sugar.

BACKGROUND INFORMATION

There are many hidden sources of sugar in foods we eat every day. Sugar has completely infiltrated our packaged food and drink supply. The amount of added sugar in the average individual's diet is increasing rapidly and causing a host of unwanted health issues. Therefore, it is imperative for a person to be able to identify and reduce the sources of added sugar in their diet. (1)

Many people look forward to eating sweet foods or even have cravings for them. However, no matter how delicious sugary foods may taste, most, except for naturally derived sweeteners like honey, offer little to no nutritional benefit.

Overeating sugar is contributing to a decline in our nations' overall health and vitality (2) and is one of the major health problems facing American children today. Chronic illnesses are increasing dramatically among children who consume a diet high in processed sugars from junk food, soda, and processed grains (and its byproduct, sugar). People who eat a diet high in white flour products (such as bread, bagels, pasta, tortillas), white rice, soda, diet soda, table sugar, candy, cookies, baked goods, and other desserts, may be at a higher risk for illness. Eating too much sugar is not healthy. It is that simple. (3)

- Approximately 16% of American children's total caloric intakes come from added sugars, according to the CDC in 2012. (4)
- Processed sugar accounts for 20% of the average teenager's calories! (5)
- One teaspoon of white sugar has 15 calories.
- Consuming one soft drink a day, including diet drinks and beverages like Gatorade, gives children a 60% greater chance of becoming obese.

Annual Worldwide Deaths

The annual worldwide death from tobacco is 6 million people, whereas the annual worldwide death from sugar is 35 million people, six times as many! (6)(7)

Gut and Digestive Problems

Overeating added sugar and other sweeteners can cause a wide variety of health issues. Imagine those sugary foods turning into gooey white glue-like substance traveling through your system. Those types of foods can impair and cause damage to the fragile gut lining and may lead to a condition called leaky gut. (8) Another issue is that sugar kills off the beneficial bacteria that live in your intestinal tract and feed the "bad" bacteria that crave more sugar. (9)

Hormone Imbalance

Sugar can cause disruptions in the endocrine system that manages our hormones. Hormones are our body's chemical messengers that control different critical bodily functions. For instance, poor gut health caused by eating a sugary diet may translate into inadequate serotonin production because up to 90% of serotonin, your feel-good neurotransmitter, is made in the digestive tract.

Hormone imbalances can cause someone who is usually happy and focused to become disturbed and confused. Hormone fluctuations can lead to depression, mood issues, eating disorders, and other physical and mental health issues. (10) Studies show neurotransmitter and hormone imbalances can trigger ADD and ADHD, and hinder learning, especially in students. (11)

Addictive Quality

Eating sugar creates more sugar cravings and addictions. Sugar stimulates the opioid receptors found in the brain that feel pleasure. The brain likes feeling pleasure, so the more it gets that quick sugar hit, the more the brain wants it. (12)

Lifestyle Diseases

Sugar increases the risk of developing severe lifestyle diseases like heart disease, diabetes, overweight and obesity, arthritis, gastric issues, skin, and dental problems. (13) Sugar is stored in fat cells when the calories ingested are not burned up for energy. The fat eventually crowds out muscles and clogs veins.

The Food Tree Added Sugar Recommendations

The World Health Organization and the FDA suggest an adult should consume no more than 10% added sugar from honey, fruit juice, or syrup. For an adult with a 2,000 calorie a day diet, that is equal to 200–250

SOUR TRUTHS ABOUT OVEREATING SUGAR AND PROCESSED GRAINS

- Processed flour converts rapidly into sugar in the digestive tract. The sugar immediately gets absorbed into the bloodstream and causes a spike in blood sugar levels.
- The body responds to massive amounts of sugar by releasing insulin. Constant spiking may lead to metabolic diseases like insulin resistance or diabetes.
- An estimated 75% of the public will become insulin resistant. (14)
- By the year 2050, one in three people will be diagnosed with diabetes.
- High sugar diets are a cause of overweight and obesity, diabetes, ADHD, and other health conditions.
- Obese children are at an increased risk for these and other severe health conditions like cardiovascular disease, hypertension, cancer, and emotional and self-esteem issues.
- Eating sugar can cause sugar cravings and even create an addiction. Sugar can change your brain. It stimulates dopamine receptor sites on your mind. It is the part that feels pleasure.

calories from sugar or 12 teaspoons.

The Food Tree advises children to eat not more than 5% of calories from added sugars or fruit juice or not to exceed more than one to three teaspoons in their daily diet.

The American Heart Association recommends that adult males not exceed nine added teaspoons (or 36 grams and 150 calories) of sugar a day. Women are not to exceed more than six teaspoons (or 24 grams and 100 calories) per day. (15)

Ask your class to do the math to figure out what a healthy amount of added sugar would be for the average person in your class population.

Categorizing Sugars

Monosaccharides are made of one sugar molecule and can be absorbed directly in the bloodstream.

Fructose, Galactose, and Glucose

Disaccharides contain two sugar molecules.

Table sugar = Sucrose = glucose + fructose
Milk sugar = Lactose = glucose + galactose
Malt sugar = Maltose = glucose + glucose

▶ Procedure 1

SUGAR CONSUMPTION 200 YEARS AGO COMPARED TO TODAY

This activity demonstrates the drastic increase in sugar consumption from the 1800s compared to sugar consumption in the 21st century.

PREPARATION

1. Label one glass quart mason jar TODAY and label the other mason jar THE 1800s.
2. Have ready one cup plus two teaspoons of white sugar.
3. Fill one bag or container with one cup of pure cane sugar and the other with just two teaspoons of refined cane sugar.

DEMONSTRATION

At the beginning of the 1800s, consumption of added sugar was two pounds per person per year or the equivalent of 2.3 teaspoons of added sugar a day. By the early part of the 2000s, 200 years later, the average American

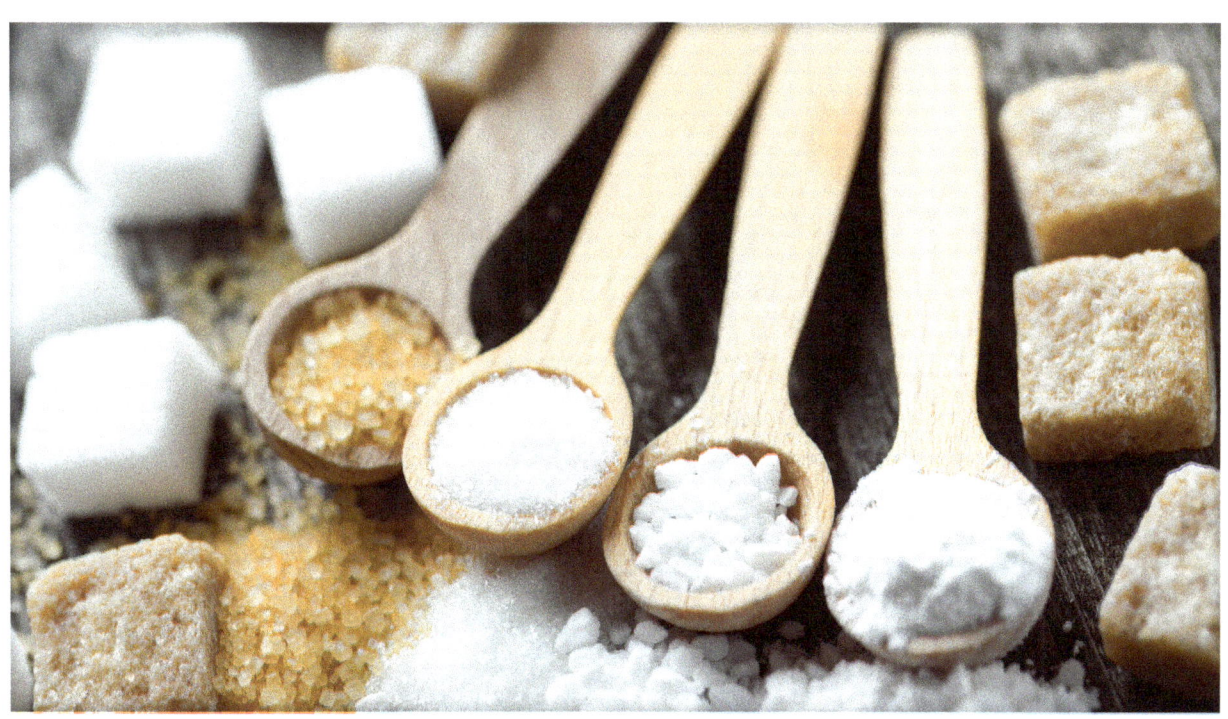

COMMON NAMES FOR SUGAR, ITS DERIVATIVES, AND OTHER SWEETENERS

Agave nectar	Crystalline fructose	Honey	Powdered sugar
Barley malt	Demerara	Icing sugar	Raw sugar
Beet sugar	Demerara syrup	Invert sugar	Refiner's sugar
Blackstrap molasses	Dextrin	Jaggery	Simple syrup
Brown rice syrup	Dextrose	Lactose	Sorghum syrup
Brown sugar	Ethyl maltol	Liquid invert sugar	Starch
Cane crystals	Evaporated cane juice	Liquid sugar	Stevia
Cane sugar	Evaporated cane juice crystals	Maltodextrin	Sucanat
Caramel		Maltose	Sucrose
Carob	Fructose	Malt syrup	Sugar
Carob syrup	Fruit juice concentrates	Maple syrup	Sugar cubes
Coarse sugar	Glucose	Molasses	Superfine sugar
Coconut nectar	Glucose syrup	Monk fruit	Syrup
Coconut sugar	Golden sugar	Muscovado sugar	Tapioca syrup
Corn sugar	Golden syrup	Oat syrup	Treacle
Corn syrup	Granulated sugar	Organic sugar	Turbinado sugar
Corn syrup solids	Gum syrup	Palm sugar	White sugar
Corn sweetener	High fructose corn syrup	Pearl sugar	Yellow sugar

** Monk fruit and stevia are natural plant-based foods that are wonderfully sweet and do not impact blood sugar or have any harmful impact on health.

---

eats 152-170 pounds of added sugar each year or the equivalent of one cup of added sugar a day, which is 42.5 teaspoons of added sugar a day or three pounds of added sugar a week.

1. Show the students the jar labeled THE 1800s. Show the students the jar labeled TODAY. Pour two teaspoons of sugar from the bag into THE 1800 jar. Then pour one cup of sugar into the TODAY jar.

2. You can measure out 42 teaspoons of sugar by using sugar cubes of one teaspoon or four grams each.

➤ Procedure 2
ANALYZING PACKAGED FOOD CONTAINERS FOR SUGAR CONTENT

1. Put students into small groups. Provide each group with at least two food containers that contain added sugars. (Ex: yogurt, ice cream, cookies)

2. Ask the students to look at the container and find the food label. Tell the students to read the food label and locate the sugars that are in that particular food. Call on the groups to share what they discovered.

3. Challenge students to spot sugar listed in one (or several!) of its many forms on the ingredient list.

4. How much sugar do the foods contain? How many teaspoons of sugar are in each serving? (4 grams = 1 teaspoon of sugar)

5. Record findings and have a class discussion on the types and amounts of sugar or sugar derivatives the students discovered in the packaged foods.

➤ Procedure 3
EXPLORE THE GLYCEMIC INDEX

The Glycemic Index is a scale used to indicate how fast and how particular foods raise blood sugar (glucose) levels in the body.

Assessment

- Discuss with your students if they were surprised about how little sugar people used to eat a hundred years ago compared to today.

- See if they were aware of all of the potential health problems that could arise from eating too many sweets, sugar, or refined grains.

- Were students surprised by the amount of sugar in packaged foods they eat regularly?

- Ask the following questions:
  - What can students do to limit the extra intake of sugar individually? As a class? At school? At home?
  - What are your weaknesses when it comes to being tempted by sweet foods?
  - What are some healthier alternatives you can choose?

- Further the sugar discussion by applying the gram/teaspoon conversion to math lessons, or researching the amount of natural sugar found in whole foods, like brown rice or berries. Have students examine why eating sugar from whole foods, like fruits and vegetables, are better for the body. Hint… It's the FIBER! See lessons on fiber for more information.

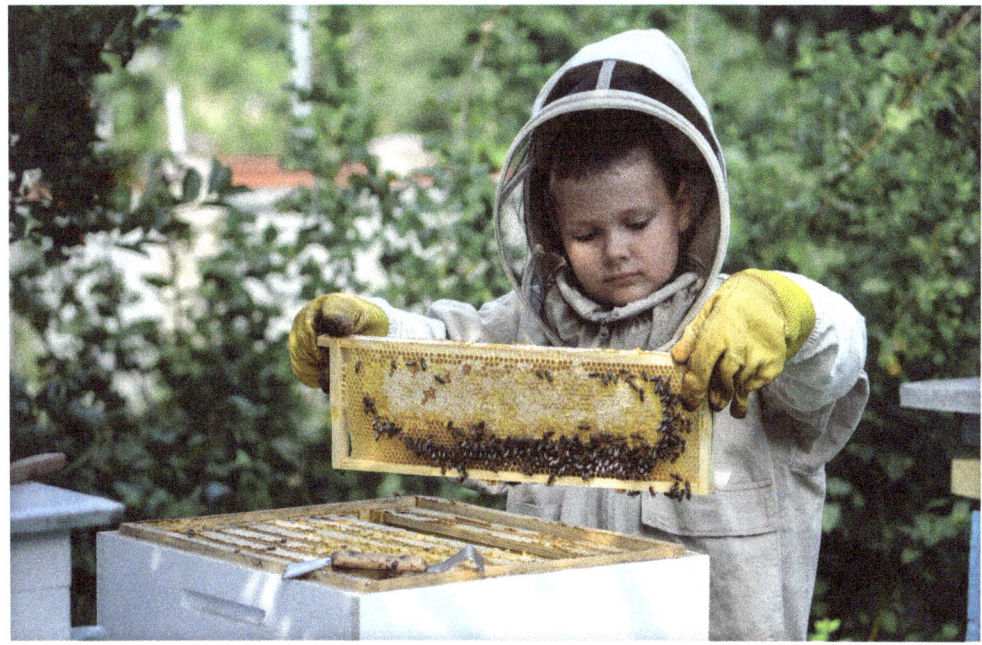

COMPREHENSIVE

Lesson: Nutrition Vampires and FDA Approval

➤ MATERIALS
- Nutrition Vampire List
- Examples of vampire foods
- FDA GRAS Chart located at the end of this lesson

➤ GOALS
Students learn how the Food and Drug Administration approves foods and chemicals.

➤ OBJECTIVES
- To create empowerment and awareness about how chemicals, additives, and pesticides are regulated and given approval for use in our food system

➤ ACTIVATING PRIOR KNOWLEDGE
Engage in a conversation to see if your students have ever thought about how food ingredients like preservatives, artificial colors, flavors, or additives are allowed into thousands of food products. Or, see if they have ever wondered if the government has everyone's best interest at heart regarding pesticides, herbicides, or insecticides used on crops and in animal feed. Are chemicals tested for human safety?

BACKGROUND INFORMATION

The food system in the United States has been taken over by corporations that are filling our foodstuff and ecosystem with all kinds of Nutrition Vampires. There has been a steady and drastic unhealthy change in the way we grow, distribute, and produce food over the last hundred years. We are witnessing the sordid effects these ingredients and industrial farming practices are having on the health and wellness of kids and adults.

The Food and Drug Administration (FDA) allows over three thousand food additives, colors, flavors, and preservatives into our food system. However, three thousand food ingredients still have not all been tested, nor have they been tested in all combinations of possible ingestion.

Nonetheless, the FDA believes in their safety and stands by every single one of them. (1)

While it is true that many ingredients are safe, natural, and relatively benign, many are suspect and the majority are guilty of causing harm and yet to be charged. It is worth contemplating why dozens of countries around the world ban ingredients and chemicals that are allowed for use, commercially and in households, in the United States.

How Are Food Ingredients Regulated for Approval?

Let's pretend that you have a fantastic new food chemical that you believe can make packaged foods last longer on the shelf. All you would need to do to attain approval is to pitch this new ingredient to the FDA and to follow one of these two ways to get your food additive in the marketplace.

OPTION 1.

You submit your item, the FDA evaluates whether your new product or substance is safe or not, and then decides whether it should be approved. The FDA must determine, based on the best science available, if there is a *reasonable certainty of no harm* to consumers when an additive is used as proposed.

OPTION 2.

You perform your safety studies, provide proof of safety to the FDA, and then the FDA approves your product. It is that simple. See the infographic provided by the Center for Science in the Public Interest.

Under the Food Additives Amendment, two groups of ingredients were *exempt* from the regulation process.

GROUP I—Prior-sanctioned substances that FDA or USDA had been determined safe for use in food before the 1958 amendment. Examples are sodium nitrite, and potassium nitrite used to preserve luncheon meats. Both of these additives are linked to cancer manifested after eating it thirty years later.

GROUP II—GRAS (Generally Recognized as Safe) GRAS approved ingredients that are generally recognized by scientific experts as safe, based on their extensive history of use in food before 1958 or based on published scientific evidence. The hundreds of GRAS substances include salt, sugar, spices, vitamins, and monosodium glutamate (MSG). Manufacturers may also request that FDA review the industry's determination of GRAS.

➤Procedure

Write letters to your local, state, and federal government and demand that harmful with a high probability to case harm be banned and removed from the U.S. food system.

Assessment

Have a follow-up discussion on how this lesson impacted their views on foods ingredients and Food safety.

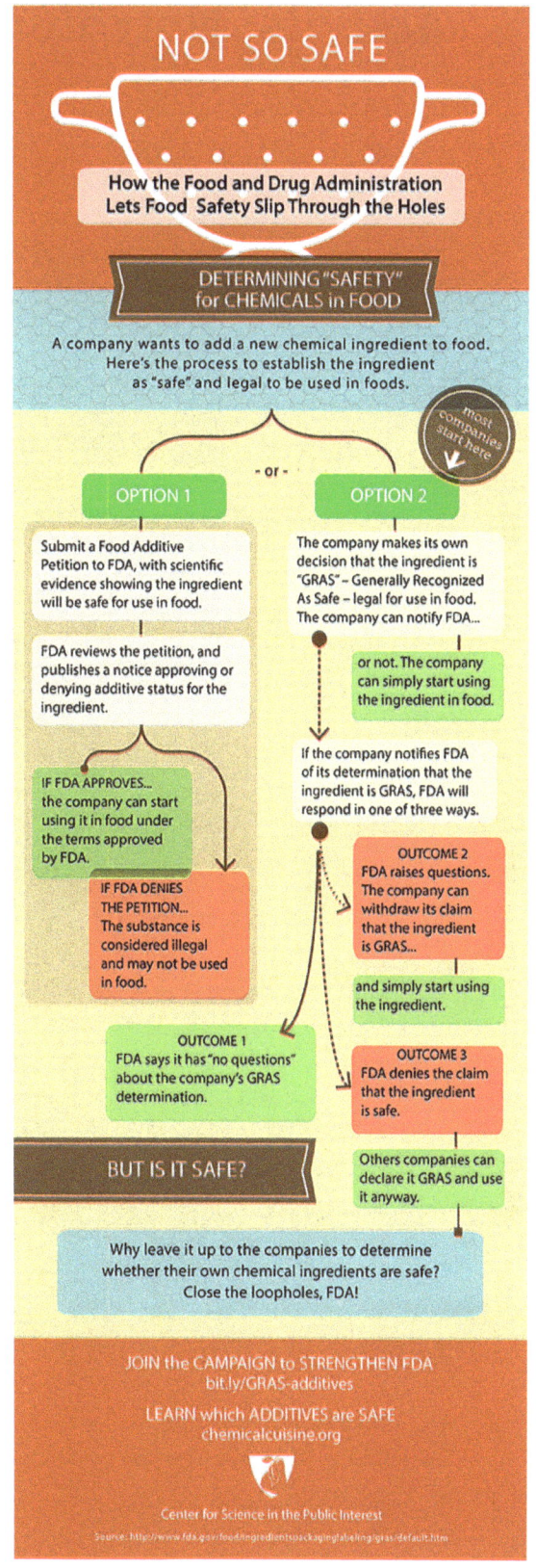

Activity: Nutrition Vampire Snack Attack

You can find packaged junk snack foods everywhere. Let's face it, they tempt us almost anywhere we go. So, if you choose to eat foods that come from a package, it is best to know and understand what the label means so you can make an informed decision for yourself.

➤ MATERIALS
- An assortment of Nutrition Vampire filled packaged foods, box labels, or photos of them including pop tarts, soda, Gatorade, gum, canned fruit in corn syrup, etc.
- An assortment of healthy snacks: fresh fruit, carrot sticks, whole grain crackers, and nut butter
- Snack Attack Reporting Sheets

➤ GOAL
Students learn to recognize Nutrition Vampires found in common foods.

➤ OBJECTIVES
- To understand how to read labels and be able and empowered to ask about nutrition vampires in restaurant foods
- To research the ingredients found in processed and packaged foods
- To evaluate and critique the FDA and the agency's additive approval process
- To illustrate how to make healthier food choices
- To identify five ways to create a Nutrition Vampire free diet

➤ ACTIVATING PRIOR KNOWLEDGE
Is it typical for you to eat packaged foods and, if so, do you read the labels so you know exactly what ingredients are in the product?

BACKGROUND INFORMATION

Nutrition Vampires can and may rob nutrients from the body and sabotage health. They are not suitable for growing kids, or anyone else for that matter.

Nutrition Vampires lurk in foods like chips, cookies, candy, pastries, packaged foods, gum, sports drinks, energy drinks, and sodas. It is best to avoid these foods as much as possible. Make it a habit to always read the ingredient list on the back of all packaged foods so you are fully aware of what is going in your body.

➤ Snack Attack Activity
DIRECTIONS
1. Set up five to ten Snack Stations. At each station, place two types of snacks. One should be a Nutrition Vampire filled snack and one The Food Tree Friendly healthy snack.
2. Split students into pairs or have them do the activity solo.
3. Ask the students to visit each station and list on a sheet of paper the 20 different snacks.
4. They can compare cookies, nuts, drinks, kinds of milk, chips, snack bars, bread, and muffins.
5. They will have to determine if the food would be considered a healthy snack or a vampire snack. Remember, even one Nutrition Vampire can make it a vampire snack.

SNACK ATTACK REPORTING SHEET

SNACK STATION	FOOD TREE FRIENDLY SNACK	VAMPIRE SNACK
1.		
2.		
3.		
4.		
5.		
6.		
7.		
8.		
9.		
10.		

Permission to reproduce. ©The Food Tree

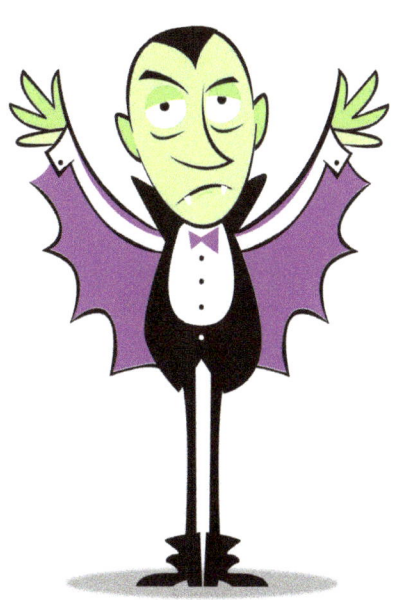

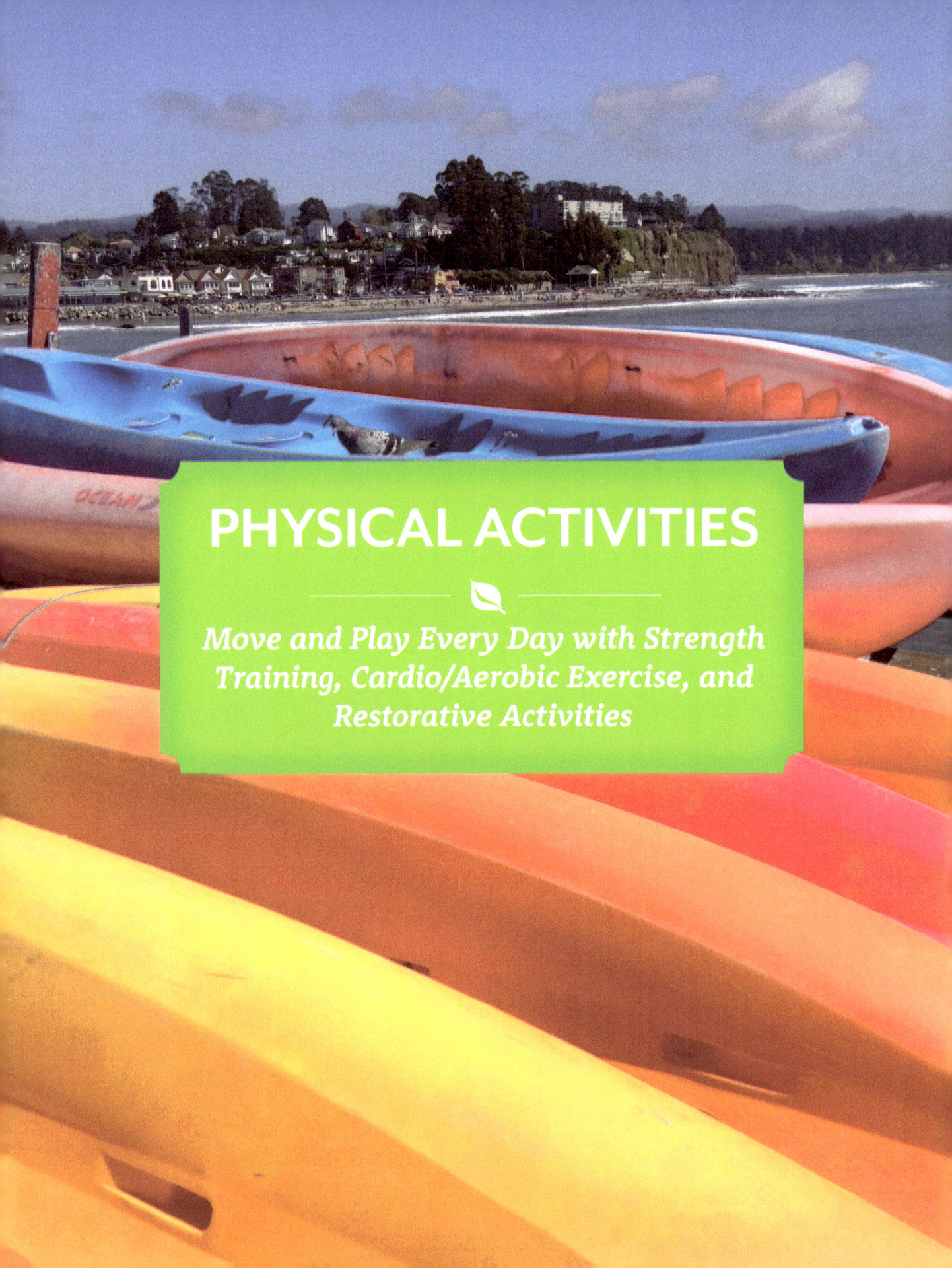

THE FOOD TREE

FOUNDATIONAL

Lesson: Introduction to Physical Activities

➤ MATERIALS
- Sports and Activities List—found at the end of this chapter
- The Food Tree Monthly Physical Activity Chart located at the end of this section
- Popsicle sticks, cardstock
- Markers in red, green, and blue or three colors of your choice

➤ GOAL
Learn the importance of regular daily physical activity and fitness and the impact on a person's long-term wellness and vitality.

➤ OBJECTIVES
- To demonstrate a knowledge of the difference between strength training, cardio training, and restorative activities
- To compare the reasons why all of the three main types of physical activities are important to engage in for overall health

➤ ACTIVATING PRIOR KNOWLEDGE
Ask students what their favorite physical activities are. Ask them how often they are exercising, playing sports, or doing a physical activity.

BACKGROUND INFORMATION

The Food Tree Curriculum focuses on the importance of including three different but important types of exercise and physical movement; Strength Training, Cardio/Aerobic Exercise, and Restorative Activities.

Whether you are a fitness buff or not, make sure you bring joy and fun into teaching your students about physical activities. Your positive and encouraging energy will instill into their lives a passion for movement. So, guide your students to develop a healthy attitude towards sports and exercise and not something to finish and get over with quickly. Reinforce that exercise and engaging in physical activities can be a positive experience and a time to look forward to.

It is a fundamental lesson to impart when children are young because taking care of their physical body is how they can show themselves that they love themselves and are worth taking good care of. The great thing is, the more people are active, the more they want to be active. One of the unsung benefits is that when people feel better, they tend to have a more positive outlook on life. And we all know that exercise makes us feel better.

The take-home message is to Take Care of Yourself. Nobody else can do as good of a job knowing what you need for your health than you.

Strength Training
Strength training is the act of building muscle in both small and large muscle groups. Building lean muscle mass is especially beneficial for developing core strength, developing strong bones and burning energy more quickly.

Cardio/Aerobic Exercises
Cardio/Aerobic exercises get the heart and blood pumping! These types of activities include running, swimming, climbing, and biking. Any activity that elevates the heart rate is considered a cardiovascular or aerobic exercise.

Restorative Activities
Restorative activities are known to help a person achieve a more calm and relaxed state of being. Restorative activities include activities like yoga,

stretching, tai chi, chi gong, and walking.

Many excellent restorative activities can help to achieve a peaceful nature. I have highlighted a few of my favorites in this chapter. Explore them all and see which ones become your favorites. Refer to the Mindfulness section for activities that are complementary and support the restorative activities.

➤ Procedure 1
KEEP AN ACTIVITIES JOURNAL

Ask your students to challenge themselves to do a physical activity every day for the next month. Have them keep track in a journal which physical activity they plan on doing and then have them journal about their experience. Suggest to your students that they write specific times in their calendar to help reinforce a successful outcome.

- Bike ride with Katie, Thursday @ 4 pm, meet outside the town library
- Hike with Dan, Santi, and Gabriel, 10 am Saturday. Meet at Dan's house
- Karate training, Monday 6 pm, Dad will drive me over and take me home
- 10 minutes of stretching in the living room before dinner
- 5 minutes of plank, sit-ups, push-ups and pull-ups Monday, Wednesday and Friday before breakfast

Below are a few sample exercise discussion topics and journaling ideas to support your students' reflections.

- How did you feel before, during, and after the exercise?
- Was the activity easier or harder than you thought?
- Did you try new activities you thought you never would?
- Did you follow through on what you said you were going to do? Why or why not? If you didn't do the physical activity, did you notice what got in the way? What could you do differently next time?
- Can I allow myself to move on, not feel bad, and be able to be gentle on myself if I didn't get to my goal?
- Did I pat myself on the back for doing the sport and sticking to it?
- Can I consider participating in that activity as something good I did for myself?

➤ Procedure 2
U-PICK ACTIVITY! READY, SET, GO!

Write each category of exercise in a different color with the names of the exercise on popsicle sticks or card stock. Once a day, have a student pick an exercise and have the whole class do three sets, five poses, or five minutes of that physical activity.

Strength Training – Red

- Plank
- Sit-ups
- Push-ups
- Squats
- Leg raises
- Lunges—forward, backward, lateral
- Chin-ups

Cardio/Aerobic – Green

- Jumping jacks
- Running in place
- Running up steps
- Jumping rope
- Dancing
- Hula hooping

Restorative – Blue

- Yoga poses
- Stretching
- Tai chi
- Walking
- Balancing poses

CARDIO/AEROBIC EXERCISES
The meaning of aerobic is "with oxygen".

It is of vital importance to include aerobic, heart pumping, blood circulating, oxygenating activities in a child's daily life to promote optimal health. We achieve an aerobic state when we get our heart rate pumping to 60%–80% of our maximum heart rate.

Playing and having fun is an important part of doing cardio/aerobic activities. Many cardio exercises involve team sports or competition. However, it is not always practical to play a team sport, and some don't want to have to compete. Therefore, foster a love of participating in diverse activities in your students so that they will always know how to be active, either solo or when free for a pick-up ultimate frisbee game.

Benefits of Cardio/Aerobic Exercise:

- Improve blood flow
- Promote waste removal
- Strengthen heart
- Increase oxygenation to muscles
- Transport immune cells
- Remove carbon dioxide
- Move lymphatic fluid (dead cells, toxic debris, waste, heavy metals)
- Improve digestion
- Increase energy
- Improve stamina
- Decrease fatigue
- Deliver nutrition
- Elevate mood, reduce depression
- Build bone density
- Lower blood pressure
- Maintain healthy blood sugar levels

Target Heart Rate Zone

The formula for a target heart rate during the peak of aerobic exercise is 60%-80% of a person's maximum heart rate. The maximum heart rate is the limit the heart can take before health problems occur from exercise stress. Don't push it too hard. Watch for signs of dizziness, muscle cramps, nausea, and vomiting.

The Target Heart Rate measurement used for adults *is not* the same for children.

TARGET HEART RATE FOR ADULTS:
Subtract your age from 220.

TARGET HEART RATE FOR CHILDREN:
Adjust the target heart rate for children under the age of 18 to fit the needs of the individual child. Consult a physician to find out what this is. There is little difference in heart rates between girls and boys at a young age. *Here is a shortlist of some of the various ways to get the heart rate up. Strive for 30-60 minutes of aerobic activity a day.*

- Hiking
- Climbing
- Running
- Jogging
- Jumping rope
- Soccer
- Ultimate Frisbee
- Trampolining
- Bicycling
- Swimming
- Jumping Jacks
- Dancing
- Hula Hooping

INTERESTING FACTS ABOUT THE HEART

- Made of muscle.
- Beats, on average, 100,000 times per day.
- Beats over 35 million times a year.
- Pumps over 2,000 gallons of blood daily.
- Contains over 60,000 miles of veins, blood vessels, and capillaries.
- May break. Heartbreak is a real syndrome caused by a stressful or emotional event.

STRENGTH TRAINING AND RESISTANCE EXERCISES

Muscles and bones. Building and maintaining muscles and building and maintaining bones is what strength training and resistance exercises are all about.

The reasons for being strong are straightforward. Muscles give you the power and strength to move your body. Muscles burn calories and are fat-burning machines. Muscles burn fat constantly, twenty-four hours a day, even while asleep. The more muscle you have, the more fat you burn, and the more fat you burn, the leaner and stronger you will be.

There are many ways, techniques, and disciplines that help a person create muscle mass. I have included a few common resistance and muscle building exercises that can be performed almost anywhere with anyone. One of the perks of doing these types of exercises is that they do not require any fancy gadgets, tools, or expensive fitness machines. You can use your own body for resistance, common household items, or gym weights.

BENEFITS OF BUILDING STRONG MUSCLES:

- Burn more calories
- Increase strength
- Improve balance
- Increase mobility and flexibility
- Cushion bones
- Increase muscle mass
- Build bone density

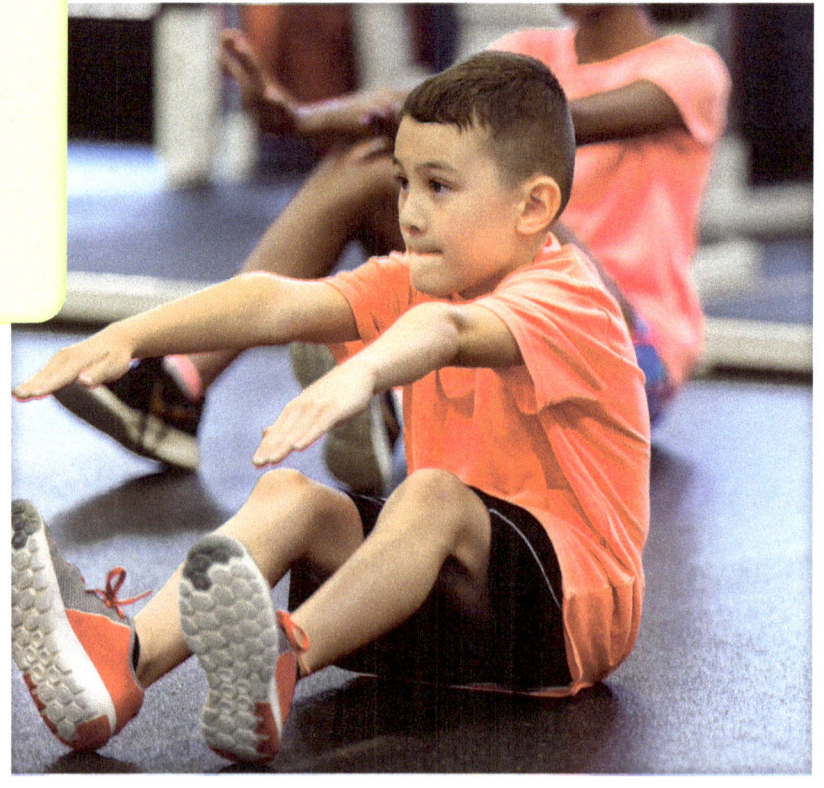

COMMON RESISTANCE AND MUSCLE BUILDING EXERCISES

Strive to engage in strength training resistance exercises 2 to 4 times a week. One of the goals when working out is to stress muscles to fatigue frequently. The fatigue creates a breakdown and actual injury and damage to the muscle. The body then repairs damaged muscle that builds up muscle mass. This action is called hypertrophy.

Plank

Begin on a firm, stable, flat, and comfortable surface like carpet or a yoga mat. Lie with your belly down flat on the floor.

1. Place your palms facing down directly underneath the shoulders, keeping your legs and feet together.
2. Curl the toes under and press your body up with your arms, pushing your hands into the floor as you extend your elbows.
3. Create a strong long line from the legs to the crown of the head.
4. Keep the belly, and the core engaged and pulled up toward the spine.
5. Keep the whole body aligned.
6. Breathe normally. Relax the jaw. Soften your gaze.
7. Hold the position for 30 seconds or longer. Repeat three times.
8. To release from the position, lower knees to the mat and bend your elbows as you return to a lying position. You can rest in Child's Pose (a yoga pose).

VARIATIONS:
Instead of #2, place hands in a fist and keep forearms down on the mat, tucked next to your side with elbows at a 45-degree angle. Continue with #3.

Walk Uphill or Run Up Stairs

1. Find any hill or stairwell and walk or run up them! You will feel resistance in your calves, thighs, hamstrings, and buttocks from the rise in the elevation.
2. Set a goal of how many times up and down you will go or for how long you will engage in the exercise.
3. Track your heart rate at certain time intervals. Make sure to stay in a healthy range.
4. Fun places to find stairwells to climb are in apartment buildings, malls, movie theatres, your school, stadium, stairs to the beach, in parks, or any building with at least two floors. Always take into consideration your and others' safety and noise (that you would make), of course. Ask permission where necessary and appropriate.

Sit-ups

1. Lie on your back with your knees bent.
2. Press your back flat against the floor.
3. Place your arms behind your head, so hands gently support and cradle the base of your head where it meets your neck.
4. Take a nice deep breath in, and on the exhale lift halfway with your elbows out to the sides, engage your core, and gaze slightly upwards.
5. Inhale on the way down.
6. Do three sets of twelve.

VARIATIONS

1. On the up, twist your body side to side, using your elbow of one arm to reach towards the opposite knee. Alternate with the other elbow and opposite knee, go back to center, and then release your body back down to the mat.
2. Place one foot on the opposite knee and sit up as noted above. Then alternate using the other foot.

Push-ups

1. Begin on a firm, stable, flat, and comfortable surface like a carpet or a yoga mat. Lie with your belly down on the floor.
2. Place your palms facing down directly underneath the shoulders, keeping your legs and feet together.
3. Curl the toes under and press your body up with your arms, pushing your hands into the floor as you extend your elbows.
4. Create a strong long line from the legs to the crown of the head.
5. Keep the belly, and the core engaged and pulled up toward the spine.
6. Keep the whole body aligned.
7. Breathe normally. Relax the jaw. Soften your gaze.
8. To modify the pose, rest knees on the mat. As well, you can lower the feet, and continue as with the basic pose.
9. Do as many push-ups as you can. Start with eight and build up to a hundred!

Squats

1. Stand with your feet shoulder-width apart, arms at your side, engage the core.
2. Raise arms straight out in front of you, parallel to the floor, fingertips pointing ahead as you lower yourself into a squatting position, forming a 90-degree angle with your thighs parallel to the floor.
3. Keep your back straight, knees in line with your toes, and feet anchored into the floor.
4. Alternatively, you can bring your arms and hands in a gentle fist close to your shoulder as you squat down. Or, clasp hands in front of you to form a 90-degree angle with your arms as you squat down.
5. To release from the position, push through your legs and drive the heels into the ground as you stand back up.
6. Perform three sets of twelve.

Lunges

FORWARD LUNGE

1. Stand with your feet shoulder-width apart, arms at your side, or hands on your hips. Engage the core. Keep the back straight and strong.
2. Take a big step forward with one leg as you dip down, forming a 90-degree angle at the knee with the opposite leg straight or gently bent.
3. To release, press down on your forward foot and lift up coming back to a standing position, core engaged, and breathing steadily.
4. Repeat with the other leg.
5. Perform three sets of twelve.

REVERSE LUNGE

1. Stand with your feet shoulder-width apart, arms at your side, engage the core.
2. Take one leg and reach behind as you dip down.
3. To release, press firmly with the ball of your foot and toes to come back to a standing upright position.
4. Repeat on the other side.
5. Perform three sets of twelve.

LATERAL LUNGE

6. Stand with your feet shoulder-width apart, arms at your side, engage the core.
7. Take a wide step to one side, arms out in front, or hands clasped together in front of the chest, as you squat down.
8. Keep the back straight and strong.
9. To release press into your foot and come back to a standing position.
10. Perform three sets of twelve.

STRETCHING MOVES

Stretching. Humans do it. Animals do it. And there are many good reasons why stretching is so popular. Studies show it relaxes muscles, lubricates joints, moves lymph fluid, is good for the back, eases mental tension and fatigue, and calms the mind.

Stretching is easy to do almost anywhere, anytime, with anyone. Make it part of your daily wake-up routine or wind-down time at the end of the day.

Upon waking is a satisfying time to stretch as you have just been sleeping for eight hours. Have you ever noticed how dogs do the downward dog yoga pose when they get up from sleep or a long rest? Follow suit.

The following exercises focus on stretching all of the major muscle groups. Those muscles include your neck, shoulders, quads, glutes, and hips.

GENERAL INSTRUCTIONS

Take a deep breath and move into your stretch. Breath calmly for a count of eight seconds. Push your body just enough to feel you are getting a good, nourishing stretch. After all, that is the point of this exercise. However, you want to make sure to gently breathe into the stretch and not push yourself to the point of strain, pain, or injury.

With each repetition, you will most likely be able to deepen the stretch as your body warms up, and you become naturally more limber and flexible. Hold all stretches for eight seconds. Release and repeat twice or as desired. Practice stretching once or twice a day and notice how good you feel.

▪ Full-Body Stretch– Standing Up

1. In a standing position, take a deep breath in and reach your hands up to the sky.
2. Move to standing on your tippy-toes.
3. Look up to the sky. Reach, reach, reach your arms up high in the air!
4. Alternate reaching upwards to the sky, with one hand, and then the other, while counting to twelve.

▪ Full-Body Stretch– Laying Down

1. Lie on your back.
2. Reach over your head and clasp hands together and turn palms outwards.
3. Point toes.
4. Take five full breaths in and out.
5. Relax feet and bring arms to the side.

Standing Twist

1. Stand with knees slightly bent and shoulders relaxed.
2. Make a soft fist and punch out in front of you, starting with the right arm and then the left.
3. Alternate your punches while counting out loud or silently, one, one, two, two, etc.
4. Punch out gently but firmly while looking forward with a soft gaze and relaxed jaw.
5. Keep the core engaged.
6. Do one set of twelve punches on each side.

Touch Toes

1. Stand up straight with knees slightly bent.
2. Bend at the waist, so you lean forward.
3. Allow the head to hang down.
4. Reach down, without straining, to touch your toes. Use a chair, block, or table to hold on to modify the movement.
5. Gently and easily turn head to the left and right.
6. Breath calmly for a count of eight.
7. Gently roll up, vertebrae by vertebrae, to a standing position.

Seated Forward Bend

1. While sitting in a chair, bend over at the waist, letting your head drop gently down.
2. Bring your arms forward over or next to your knees and allow your hands to touch the floor.
3. Take a few deep breaths.
4. When ready, roll up, vertebrae by vertebrae, with the neck and head last.

Neckroll

1. *Be gentle with this move.
2. Drop head and neck down in front with the chin reaching towards the chest. Keep jaw relaxed.
3. Gently roll the head up toward the right.
4. Then roll the head up to the left.
5. Do three repetitions, alternating each side.

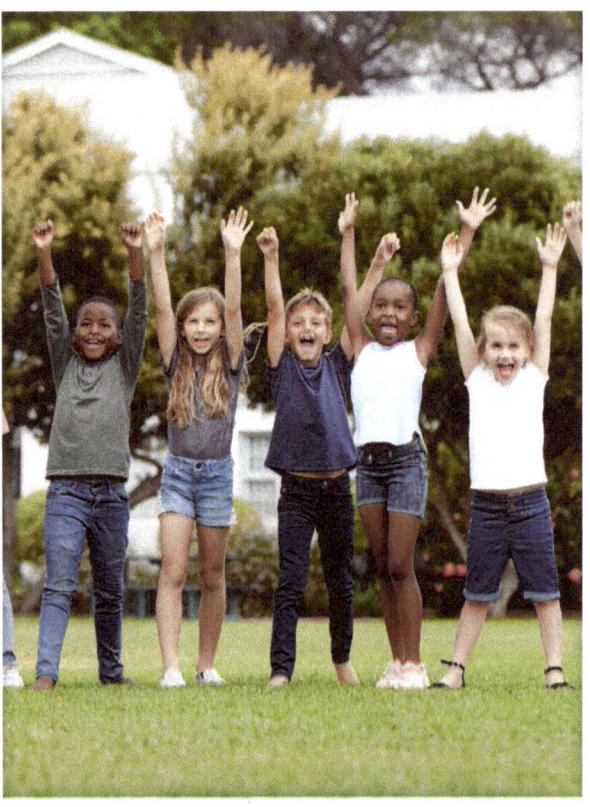

YOGA POSES

The Food Tree invites you to explore a range of simple yoga poses, also known as asanas. Yogas roots are from Hindu traditions stemming back to fifth and sixth BCE. Mental, physical, and spiritual components are at the heart of yoga. Practice care when performing yoga, just as you would in participating in any physical exercise.

■ Mountain Pose

Tadasana

Stand up tall, big toes touching, heels slightly apart, straight spine, eyes looking forward, core engaged, and shoulders relaxed. Stand with your weight evenly balanced, spreading toes comfortably apart. Press shoulders together, expanding the chest, while arms are at the side with palms facing forwards. Relax eyes and jaw. Allow the tongue to rest flat on the bottom of the mouth. Steady the breath. Stay in the position for 30 seconds to one minute.

BENEFITS:

The foundation of all poses. Teaches awareness of balance, alignment, breath, and posture.

■ Child's Pose

Balasana

Begin on your hands and knees. Lower your hips down towards your heels while you bring your big toes together, keeping your knees spread apart. Continue lowering yourself towards the floor so that your belly and chest rest on or between your legs. Stretch your arms out in front of you, with palms faced down. Allow your forehead to rest on your mat or folded blanket. For a deeper pose, lay your arms next to your side with your palms facing up. Close your eyes and stay in this position for one minute. Breathe.

Use this pose as a rest between more challenging poses.

BENEFITS:

Calms the mind, releases fatigue and stress. Opens up the hips, thighs, and stretches the back and torso.

■ Cat/Cow Pose

Marjaryasana/Bitilasana

Begin on your hands and knees. This position is also known as All Fours or Table Top. Point fingertips towards the front of your mat. On the inhale, relax the belly towards the floor while lifting the head slightly. Gaze softly upwards to stretch the eye muscles. Keep your wrists directly under shoulders and the knees under the hips, hip-width apart. On the exhale, round your back into an arch, pulling the belly to the spine. Gently release the neck. The head is heavy, and the chin moves slightly toward the chest. Repeat 10-20 times.

BENEFITS:

Loosens and stretches the back, induces relaxation, reduces stress, improves circulation, and stimulates the movement of spinal fluid. Facilitates digestion.

■ Downward Dog Pose

Adho Mukha Svanasana

Begin on your hands and knees. Press the hands into the ground, spread the fingers wide, tuck toes, and lift hips towards the ceiling so that you are forming an upside-down V with your body. Keep the legs hip-distance apart. Press chest to the thighs while lifting the hips, keeping arms straight but not locked. Engage abdominals. Hands are shoulder-width apart. Keep wrist creases parallel with the front of the mat. Keep legs straight or create a little bend in the knee. Hold the pose for five to ten breaths. Release. Repeat 2 more times.

BENEFITS:

Stretches the entire back, legs, arms, shoulders, and hands, and opens up the chest, improving breathing. Lengthens the spine. Increases blood flow to the brain. Benefits digestion. Relieves fatigue.

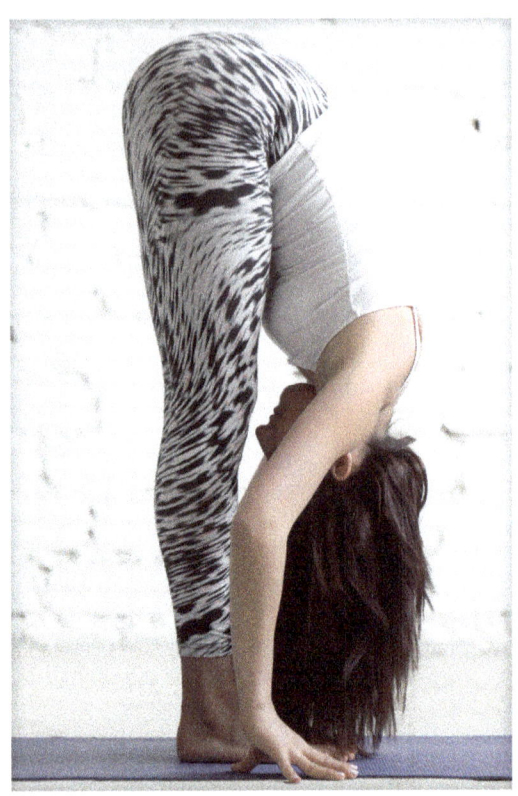

Standing Forward Bend (Rag Doll)

Uttanasana

Stand up tall with a straight spine, eyes looking forward, core engaged, and shoulders relaxed, as in Mountain Pose. Take a deep breath and bend at the waist folding forward, arms reaching toward the ground. Keep the knees slightly bent as you reach to touch the floor. For a more challenging stretch, slowly straighten legs while keeping the spine long. Do not strain! If you can't touch the ground with legs straightened, keeping knees bent will allow the lower back to extend safely.

A forward bend is a powerful pose that stretches the entire back. This pose impacts the feet, legs, lower back, neck, scalp, and the point between your eyebrows! Gently roll up one vertebra at a time. Stay in this pose for 5-10 seconds. Repeat once.

BENEFITS:

Relieves anxiety, alleviates headaches, quiets the mind.

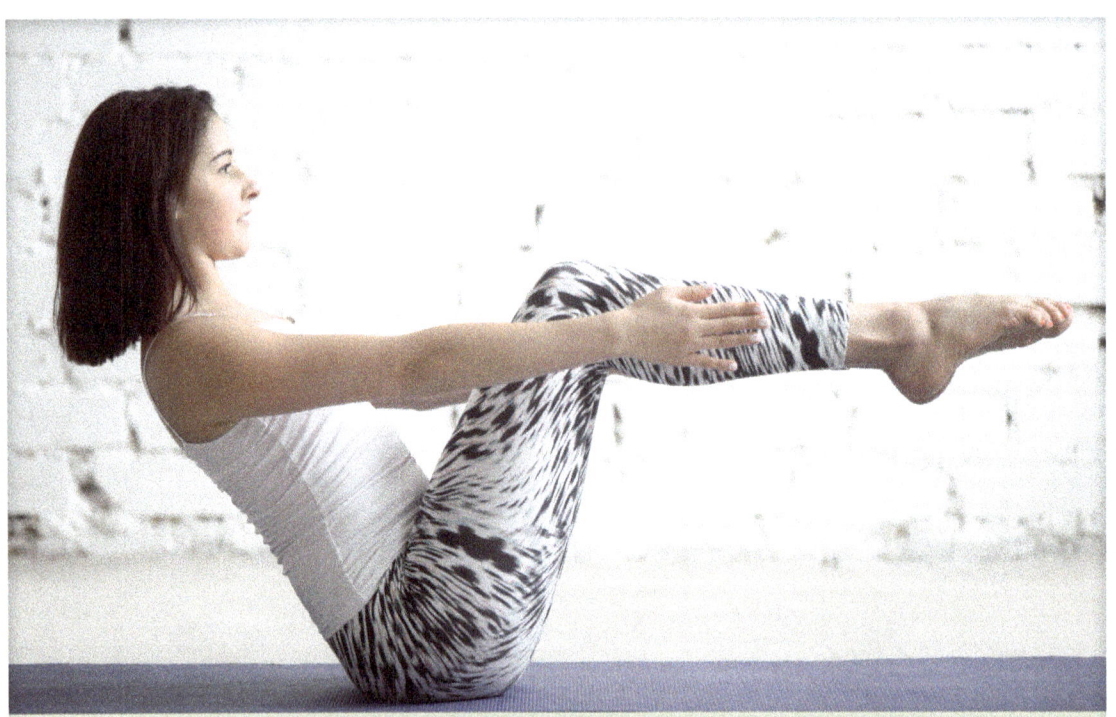

Boat Pose
Paripurna Navasana

Begin sitting down with your legs straight out in front of you. Place the hands on the floor behind your hips. Point your fingers towards the feet. Lean back while engaging your core, bend your legs and take hold of the back of your knees at a 45-degree angle to the floor. Lift your feet off the floor and balance on your tail and sits bones. You can hold underneath your knees or place your hands on the floor to add stability.

For a more difficult challenge, extend the legs and release and extend your arms out along the side of your thighs with your fingers spread wide open. Tilt chin slightly towards the sternum. Stay in the pose for 10-20 seconds and build up to one minute.

BENEFITS:

Good for balance. Opens hips. Strengthens abdominal and back muscles. Builds core strength.

Bridge Pose
Setu Bandha Sarvangasana

Begin by lying down on your back with your knees bent, feet on the floor, and your arms beside you with the palms pressing down. Keep your feet planted firmly on the ground facing forwards, hip-width apart, and knees over ankles. As you exhale, lift your hips and chest up off of the mat. Release inner thighs down towards the mat. You can support your lower back with your hands. Or, for more of a challenge, bring your hands together, roll shoulders towards each other, and interlace fingers underneath you, keeping arms on the mat.

To exit the pose, release hands and extend arms overhead. Then lower yourself down, one vertebra at a time, beginning closest to the shoulders and neck.

Pause and take a few breaths. Then, bring your knees to your chest, wrap your arms around, and give yourself a good hug and back massage. Hold the pose for 5-10 breaths.

BENEFITS:

This pose opens the chest and shoulders, creates a flexible spine, relaxes the mind, strengthens hamstrings, back, and glutes.

Legs Up the Wall
Viparita Karani

Sit with your shoulder next to a clear open wall. Put your legs out parallel to the wall. Lay back, pivot, and swing your legs up on the wall. Move your bottom and heels as close to the wall as comfortable. Place a smoothly folded towel under your hips for added support. Note that there will be a slight natural curve in the lower back. Rest arms by your side. Close eyes and relax in this pose for one to three minutes.

BENEFITS:

Improves blood flow, allows receptivity, boosts energy, alleviates lower back pain.

Corpse Pose
Savasana

Lie down on your back with legs slightly apart, close eyes, arms by the side with palms up. Remain awake and aware while calming and relaxing the mind and body. Get comfortable; use blankets, eye pillow, and bolsters under knees. Take a deep, cleansing breath to send a message to your parasympathetic nervous system to rest and relax. Practice for a few minutes and up to 20 minutes, especially at the end of your yoga session.

BENEFITS:

Works to relax and calm the body and mind. Relieves headache and stress. Overall, can rejuvenate energy.

GROUNDING, EARTHING, AND WALKING BAREFOOT

Getting in Touch with Nature Brings You Close to Your Nature

Earthing is probably one of the oldest activities for personal relaxation and restoration known to humankind. The act of Earthing consists of the most basic of all activities, walking barefoot on the earth. Or hugging trees, but we will get to that later.

The eye-opening truth is that most people rarely, if ever, go barefoot on the actual earth. And if people do go shoeless, they are often indoors. Why is allowing your feet to touch the ground, sand, grass, or forest floor so crucial to your wellness? What is going on underneath the surface of our soles?

We now understand our connection to the planetary magnetic field and how it directly impacts our health. The simple act of earthing, or grounding barefoot on the Earth, can raise your vibration, absorb antioxidants, and heal not only yourself but potentially others.

An electromagnetic grid surrounds the earth that emits electrical rhythms necessary for normal biological functioning. Not surprisingly, humans and animals are all-natural receptors to these energetic grids. When you connect to electromagnetic energy lines in the earth, your body absorbs free, negatively charged electrons that create grounding and balance.

Electrons donated to us from the earth are considered to be antioxidants. Antioxidants quench oxidative damage caused by free radicals. Oxidative damage occurs through normal human actions such as metabolism, breathing, exercise, digestion, elevated stress levels, exposure to environmental toxins, and nutrient-poor diets.

When molecules become oxidized, they lose an electron-molecule, creating unmatched electrons in cells. Unmatched electrons make them become a free radical atom. This free radical atom is unstable and can cause cellular oxidative damage. So, in response, the body craves antioxidants to protect its cells. The free radical searches for an electron to make it whole again. Sometimes it needs to steal electrons from other molecules if there are not many electrons available. This action causes other molecules to become unstable! And, so goes the chain reaction.

WHY ARE ANTIOXIDANTS SO IMPORTANT?

Many lifestyle diseases that stem from chronic inflammation, such as sleep issues, mood imbalances, and poor health, may be result of antioxidant deficiency. So, grounding, earthing, and walking barefoot are free and easy ways to add antioxidants to the body, offering the potential to feel better. (1)

All You Need is Half an Hour

Research studies conducted over the last decade show when people spend at least half an hour grounding into the earth, they experience a reduction in pain and inflammation, improved sleep, reduction in stress, balancing of cortisol levels, reduction in blood pressure, and improved overall health (2).

Additional scientifically proven benefits of grounding include:

- Keep you centered, balanced, clear, and aware

- Increase mental relaxation
- Promote a state of bliss and contentment
- Instill a sense of harmony with the natural world
- Calm the central nervous system
- Reduce jet lag
- Improve chronic pain
- Increase energy levels
- Regulate stress hormones
- Reduce headaches and mental fatigue
- Speed healing

Seriously. What could be more promising than that? If this is the case, why do most people never walk around without their shoes on?

WHAT ARE THE BEST MATERIALS TO USE TO CONDUCT ENERGY?

Barefoot is the best.

The soles of your feet absorb the electrons directly into your body. Wearing natural materials on the soles of your feet are excellent conductors of electron energy. (3) Natural fibers, moccasins, and leather-soled shoes work well because the foot perspires, which allows the earth's energy to transfer through the moistened material. Amazingly, all of this is happening on a molecular level. Water and concrete are also suitable transmitters. The human body is made up of 60% water and minerals. Both of these elements can transfer electrical currents. That is why the soles of the feet and the palms of the hands are wonderful conductors of the Earth's negatively charged electrons.

Materials that do not conduct free electrons are rubber, plastic, wood, pavement, asphalt, synthetic materials, and glass.

➤ Procedure 1
GROUNDING GARMENTS

Challenge your students to create fashionable grounding garments and footware that are able to absorb the earth's electrons.

➤ Procedure 2
GO BAREFOOT

Ask your students to see how often they go barefoot on natural materials. Have your students keep track of how long they ground for each day, how they do it, and if they notice beneficial results.

WHAT YOU CAN DO TO GROUND!
Take your shoes and socks off!!
Walk barefoot at the beach.
Walk barefoot on warm grass.
Walk barefoot through a forest.
Walk barefoot on warm concrete.

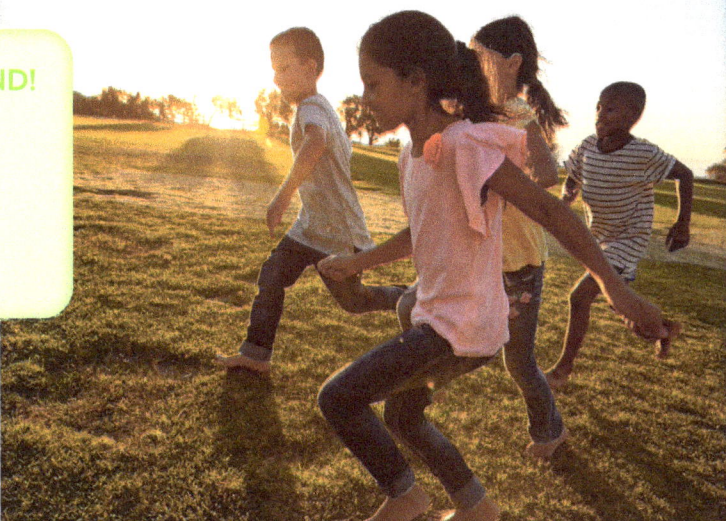

Mirror Reflection Exercises

This exercise is all about exactly copying another person's movements and facial expressions. It is fun to see and observe others deeply and with intention, and it is great to be seen. This exercise can build empathy, compassion, and awareness of others' feelings using nonverbal communication.

This exercise is great fun and exciting to do at any age. This is a useful classroom management tool for teachers to use when wanting to get every student's attention! Choose a symbol or gesture for the day or week, and when you flash that sign, the students will know to stop what they are doing, quiet down, and pay attention.

INSTRUCTIONS

Basic Mirror

Have two people face opposite each other. One person will be the person "looking in the mirror" and the other person will be acting as the "reflection in the mirror." The person looking in the mirror will begin making facial expressions and gestures. It will be the mirror's job to reflect the movements and expressions precisely as the person looking into the mirror.

TO BEGIN:
Match participants in pairs.

Start by having students in the "looking position" do only facial movements and expressions. As the group becomes comfortable and gets the hang of it, you can add in hands and arms. To amp it up, have the students do full-body motions and movements.

Remind the person always to keep eye contact with the "mirror" so that the reflection can easily and intuitively follow. Try to get your movements so close together that an observer wouldn't be able to tell who is the person and who is the mirror.

Basic Mirror Variations 1: Emotions

Have students act out emotions such as feelings of being:

Happy	Contemptuous
Courageous	Elated
Sad	Suspicious
Disappointed	Fearful
Angry	Pleased
Frustrated	Spooked
Excited	Contented
Scared	Joyful
Bored	Loving
Confused	Eager
Disgusted	Grateful
Surprised	Anxious

EMOTIONAL SCALING

Ask students to act out the emotion on three different levels of intensity with 1 being the mildest and 3 being the strongest. For instance, try a mad level 2, a surprised level 3, or a confused level 1. Ask students if they can figure out the emotion and at what level of intensity.

Variation 2: Common Behaviors

Have students act out common behaviors such as:

Brushing teeth	Cooking
Combing hair	Playing basketball
Opening a door	Playing the guitar
Reading a book	Tying shoe laces

Variation 3: Full-Length Mirror

Have students act out things like trying on a sweater, swishing hair back and forth, looking side to side, sitting down, eating, and posing in different positions with arms and legs.

Variation 4 Circle Mirror Exercise

The Circle Mirror Exercise is a group exercise designed to follow the movements of the person in front of them. This is a fun activity with the potential for lots of creative innovations.

DIRECTIONS:

1. Have everyone stand in a circle.
2. Ask participants to take a 90-degree turn to the right so that everyone is facing somebody else's back.
3. One person begins with a simple body movement.
4. Use the legs, the head, and the body.
5. Perform motions out to the sides so the person behind can see what the person in front is doing.
6. The person standing behind the person making the motion can take a one-second delay before making the motion.
7. When the motion comes back to the person who started the round, have them do the motion one more time to signal to the person behind that the round is complete.
8. Then, the next person behind performs their unique motion until everyone in the circle has had a chance to lead a move.
9. Try to create a unified flow as the motion goes around the circle.

VARIATIONS

1. Speed it up or go very slowly.
2. Add music.
3. Add a word, noise, or sound to each movement.
4. Add ribbons, materials, flags, or strips of fabric.

Have participants take turns going into the middle of the circle for extra fun and a unique vantage point. They can stand, lie down, or sit.

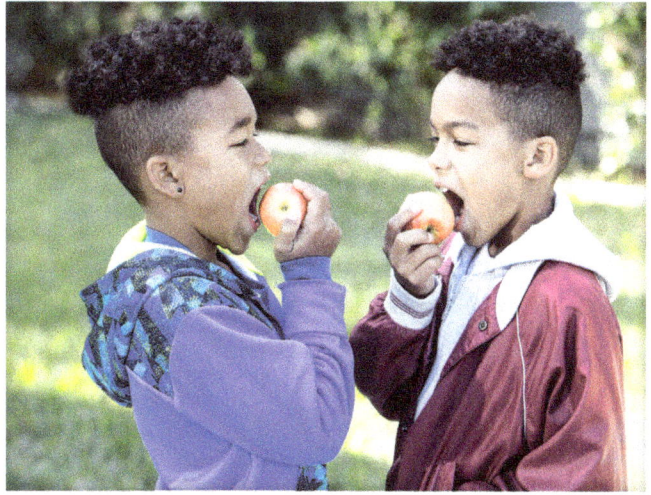

SPORTS AND ACTIVITIES LIST

Aerial Arts, Acrobatics, Aikido, Badminton, Baseball, Basketball, Beach Volleyball, Biking, Body Surfing, Bodyboarding, Capoeira, Chi Gong, Cycling, Dance, Disc Golf, Diving, Judo, Jump Rope, Hiking, Karate, Fencing, Golf, Gymnastics, Lacrosse, Hiking, Hockey, Horseback Riding, Hula Hooping, Handball, Ice Skating, Kayaking, Ping Pong, Polo, Racketball, Rock Climbing, Rollerblading, Roller Skating, Rowing, Rugby, Running, Sailing, Skateboarding, Snowboarding, Stand-up Paddle Boarding, Soccer, Surfing, Swimming, Tai Chi, Tennis, Trampolining, Ultimate Frisbee, Walking, Volleyball, Windsurfing, Yoga, Weight Lifting, Wrestling

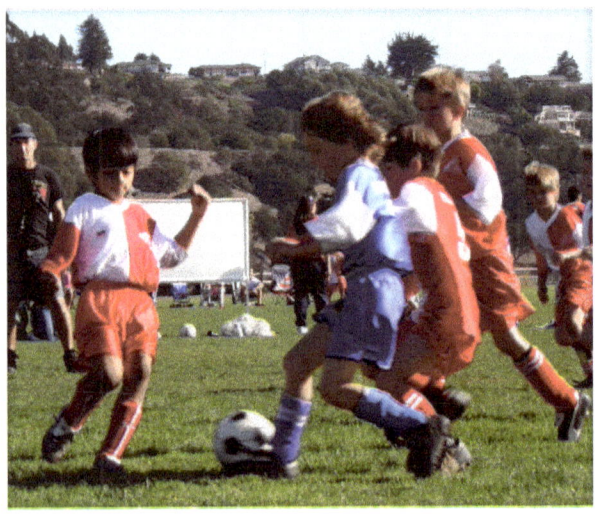
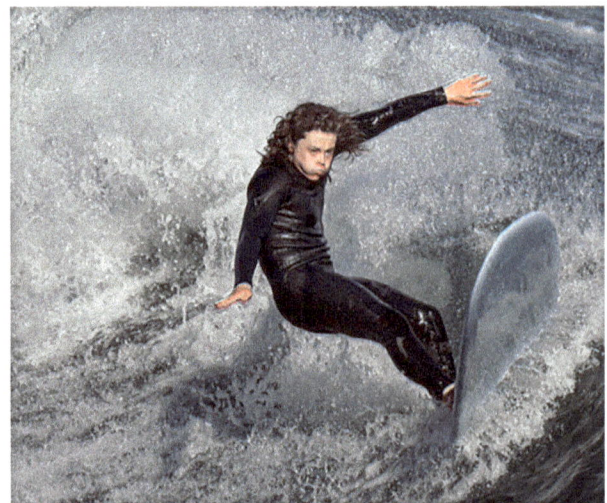

MONTHLY PHYSICAL ACTIVITY CHART

Plan out your monthly calendar with fun, exciting, calming, joyful, silly, fast, slow, challenging, relaxing, amazing, chill activities, exercises, and outings!

SUNDAY	MONDAY	TUESDAY	WEDNESDAY	THURSDAY	FRIDAY	SATURDAY

Permission to Reproduce. ©The Food Tree

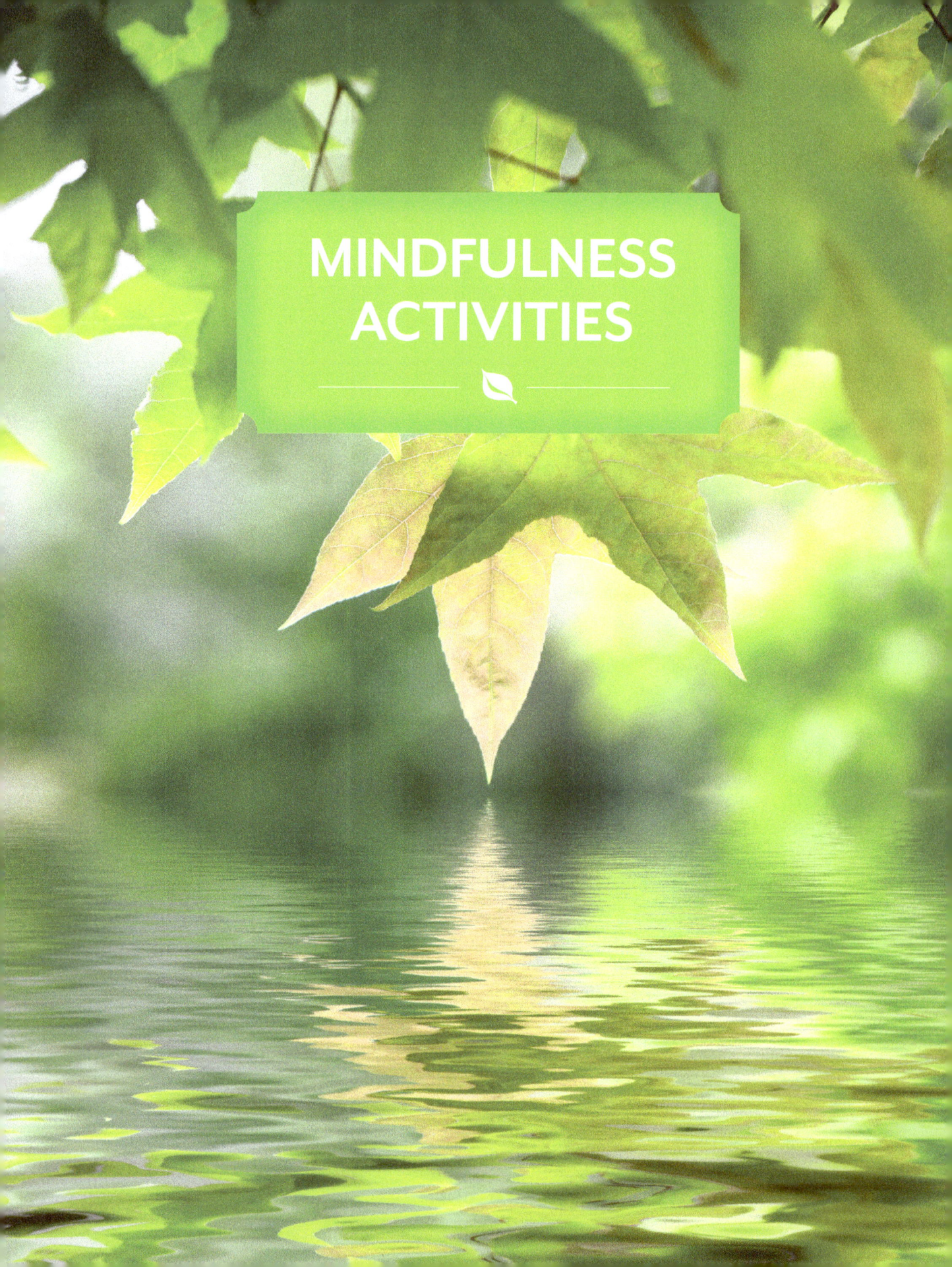

The mindfulness activities are designed to tap into the soulful side of a person. I highlight activities that will open oneself up to the reality that we all are connected energetically and share a common human bond to our inner self, each other, and the planet upon which we all live and depend.

Mindfulness activities, like the simple act of being grateful, offer a way to explore the emerging field of quantum physics, which is now able to measure the human energy field. Scientists, like those at Heart Math, measure these realities using breakthrough technology. In fact, they can measure energy emanating from the heart and how it impacts others, even your pet.

Empirical findings from a paper published in the Journal of Consulting and Clinical Psychology analyzing thirty-nine studies totaling 1,140 participants receiving mindfulness-based therapy for a range of conditions, including cancer, generalized anxiety disorder, depression, and other psychiatric or medical conditions suggest that mindfulness-based treatment is a promising intervention for treating anxiety and mood problems in clinical populations.

I will share these cutting-edge discoveries to catapult everyone's potential for healing and to thrive on an abundant planet. Dig in, enjoy, and feel the light!

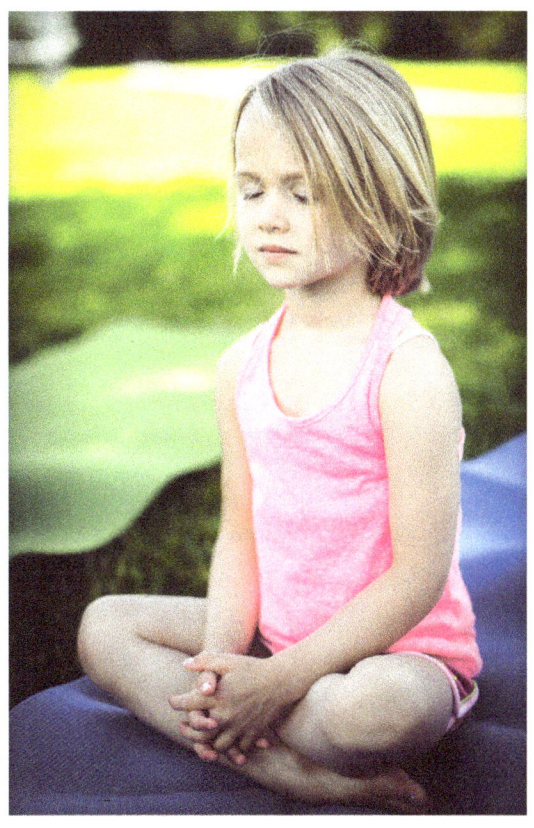

MINDFULNESS AFFIRMATIONS, MANTRAS, AND MEDITATIONS

Mindfulness practices, like meditation, saying affirmations, and using visualization techniques in schools has had a clear and positive impact on the wellbeing of the students.

Neuropsychological researchers over the last few decades have noticed improved school-wide GPAs, increased self-esteem, less stress and burnout, increased emotional intelligence, a reduction in anxiety, and a decrease in school violence in children engaged in mindfulness activities. (1)

Because of its relative newness in the western world, there is a significant need for more scientific studies. I encourage you to explore some of these exercises and while you do, keep rigorous records of your program results to capture evidence-based data on its potential benefits.

AFFIRMATIONS AND MANTRAS

Affirmations are not just lovely things you say to yourself. Affirmations are powerful words that your brain believes. (2) Yes, your mind believes what you tell it. In that case, it is best to fill it up with good thoughts and kind words.

To affirm something is to agree to the good and right intention that you want to bring into being. Repeating the affirmation is necessary as it reinforces the positive message you are declaring.

And when you say affirmations over and over, they are called a mantra.

There are endless mantras and affirmations. You can borrow them from any spiritual discipline or religion, explore the internet, find them in self-help books, or make up your own. Mantras and affirmations can be said aloud, quietly, silently in your mind, or you can write them down in a journal. You can use them in your meditation practice as a tool for stilling the mind and calming the body.

They can even be said while walking as in a walking meditation in a garden or along a path. Mantras and affirmations can be used as a quieting exercise to still restless bodies or refocus a classroom full of students or any bustling group.

To begin, start your affirmation or mantra with an "I" or "My" as in:

- I trust myself.
- I trust my inner wisdom.
- My heart is open to the creative energy of the universe.
- I honor the divine within.
- I am present in this moment.
- I am beautiful inside and out.
- My mind is calm and relaxed.
- I experience ease and flow in my life.
- I am content with all that is right here and now.
- I cultivate acceptance and gratitude daily.
- I allow abundance to flow into my life.
- I honor my worth and value.
- I trust all my needs will always be met.
- I am enough.
- I am awesome.
- I am perfect in the moment in every way.
- I say kind things to myself and about myself.

CREATE YOUR UNIQUE MANTRAS

Write three positive mantras or affirmations. These will be your mantras to say to yourself. You can also say selfless mantras that are in service to others or the world.

1. _____
   _____
2. _____
   _____
3. _____
   _____

An Exercise in Self-Healing

To practice self-healing, create a special place in your mind just for healing. Go there any time and visualize healing energy surrounding you.

Relax and repeat these self-healing affirmations any time that you want. Before you go to sleep is an excellent time for repeating healing affirmations because it helps prepare you for a rejuvenating and restful sleep.

- Excellent health is the natural state of my being.
- I awake rested, peaceful, and rejuvenated.
- I am filled up with positive and compassionate energy.
- Every cell in my body is regenerating with optimal health.
- My heart is healthy and pumps steadily.
- My lungs fill with cleansing oxygen.
- When I exhale, I release stress and negativity out of my body.
- I am relaxed.
- I take calm, deep breaths.
- I am a vibrant, radiant person.
- I am full of peace, love, and joy.

MEDITATIONS

"Meditation is a way of clearing away the mental clutter that surrounds the subconscious. And when our minds are clear, we can see and experience the joy of our own soul." Gurmukh

Meditation is a tool that can be used to quiet the mind and body and to bring you closer to yourself. The word meditation comes from the Latin root, *meditatum*, which means *to ponder*. There are endless different meditation techniques that have been used around the world for perhaps over 5000 years, with records illustrating the beginning roots in the Hindu and Buddhist religions. To be clear, meditation, as described here, is non-denominational and all-inclusive.

Schools across the country are engaging their students in all kinds of mindfulness techniques. They are having particularly great success with meditation. Visitacion Valley School in San Francisco rings a gong twice a day to alert the sixth, seventh, and eighth graders to engage in a fifteen-minute meditation session. The administrators noticed a 79% drop in suspensions and a dramatic increase in academic performance and school attendance. Meditation practiced in classrooms has proved to have great success in increasing happiness and reducing stress, anger, and depression. (1)

COMMIT TO MEDITATING

The most straightforward way to begin a new meditation practice is by setting aside a few minutes once or twice a day at the same time and in the same location.

Two Minute Quiet Time Meditation

To Calm, Relax, and Foster Joy in Children

Begin by having students settle down into a comfortable sitting position. Sound a gong, chimes, or bells.

Give the following directions:

1. Close your eyes.
2. Take three deep, slow, cleansing breaths.
3. Clear your mind of random thoughts. Allow any idea that comes in to pass on out.
4. Relax your forehead.
5. Relax your jaw.
6. Relax your shoulders.
7. You can repeat an affirmation or mantra.
8. Continue to breathe deeply and slowly.
9. Relax your belly.
10. Continue for at least two minutes or as desired.

Progressive Muscle Relaxation Meditation

Progressive Muscle Relaxation Meditation is a meditation that has some movement involved yet delivers deep relaxation. Dr. Edmund Jacobson developed this deep relaxation technique in the 1920s. It is known as progressive relaxation therapy. This process helps to alleviate tension and stress in the mind and body.

GUIDE YOUR STUDENTS WITH THE FOLLOWING FLOW.

To begin, tell your students that you are going to take them on a journey to relax the whole body. Have students:

1. Settle and lay down on their backs and get into a comfortable position.
2. Close your eyes.
3. Clear your mind.
4. Take a few cleansing breaths.
5. Relax your forehead.
6. Relax your jaw.
7. Allow any thought that comes in to pass on out.
8. Continue to breathe slowly, shoulders relaxed, belly relaxed.
9. Say out loud to your class:
    - Bring your awareness to your right foot.
    - Tighten up your right toes and foot. Squeeze them tightly, curl your toes in slightly, tighten, and release.
    - Now relax your foot completely, releasing all tension.
10. After the release, you may feel tingling or energy pulsing.
11. Use the same guided imagery for the rest of the body.
    - Right foot and toes, left foot and toes
    - Right calf, left calf
    - Right knee, left knee
    - Right thigh, left thigh
    - Both legs and feet altogether
    - Buttocks
    - Belly
    - Chest and shoulders
    - Neck
    - Face and scalp
    - The entire body all at once. Do it twice.
12. Do each hold for about two deep breaths while keeping the rest of the body relaxed.

With eyes closed, take steady slow breaths for a few minutes to continue the relaxation and calm that will come over you.

MINDFUL AND INTUITIVE EATING

There is much talk about the importance of incorporating mindfulness into one's daily life. In this exercise, you apply the art of being mindful in the act of eating.

I encourage you to take some time to explore your attitudes and daily practices when it comes to shopping for, preparing, cooking, eating, and even cleaning up after a meal. Discuss with your students their "negative" or self-sabotaging habits and rituals around food and eating. They can raise their hands as you read the list, or they can write down the behaviors that resonate with them and then create an opposite action as a replacement..

Often, we...

- Rush while eating
- Eat in the car
- Skip meals and don't eat at all
- Are emotionally upset when eating
- Aren't eating what you really want or need
- Eating what you want but NOT what you need
- Are concerned about food scarcity
- Are hungry but don't take the time for a healthy snack or meal
- Are thirsty and don't drink water
- Aren't hungry but eat anyway
- Overeat
- Feel peer pressure to eat junk food
- Are teased or mocked for wanting to eat "clean", vegan, organic, or healthy foods
- Are unaware of the ingredients in what you are eating
- Eat in front of a screen
- Eat standing up
- Don't question anything and eat whatever is in front of you
- Eat slouched over
- Complain about the food
- Engage in negative self-talk or food shaming
- Participate in dieting

MINDFULNESS MEAL IDEAS AND EXERCISES

Trust Yourself, Trust Your Body, Trust Your Intuition

The following passage can be read aloud to your class.

Do you trust and listen to your inner voice? Before you go for the next quick snack or have a mindless munching attack, close your eyes and breathe for a minute. Ask yourself, your body, what it needs. Slow down and trust the first ideas that come into the mind. Your intuition is something that will always guide you. The goal is to trust it. The more you do this practice, the more you will be able to access that intuitive part of yourself quickly.

Have you ever craved something? Cravings are a sign from yourself to yourself. So, listen up! Do you listen to your body when it needs food? Perhaps you get a sudden urge to eat an orange.

Maybe your body is asking for vitamin C, and a piece of citrus fruit will do the trick. Or you get a hankering for some nut butter. Perhaps you need a dose of healthy fats or protein.

Even craving "bad foods" like sugar can give you a lot of information about what your body needs. For instance, craving something sweet could mean you have low blood sugar, and you are running low on energy. You could also be tired and need to rest because sugar would give an energy boost. You could be experiencing stress and crave sugar to help calm you down because it stimulates the release of endorphins, a feel-good chemical.

The same goes for water. How often do you get that nudge to drink water but you just can't be bothered to get up off the couch, out of bed, off the computer, or off the field to take a break and hydrate? Yet when you finally do, you guzzle down the water and realize how thirsty you were. Perhaps if you didn't act on getting that water, you'd develop a headache, mental fatigue, a feeling of being faint, or eat food due to a false sense of hunger.

The body will always take what it needs from different parts of the body to keep your major systems functioning. It will take minerals from your bones if you don't get enough minerals from your diet. Yikes. But the beautiful message is that your body knows what it needs, so start listening! The next time you get a sweet tooth, take a breath, listen, and instead of eating a candy bar, have some nuts, seeds, and an apple. And trust yourself!

Banish Negative Self Talk

Identify your negative or self-sabotaging behaviors, thoughts, and self-talk about your relationship to food, your body, and eating. These negative or self-sabotaging behaviors can seriously impact a person's mental, spiritual, and physical wellbeing. The only way to change the behavior or thoughts is first to have an awareness that they exist and then identify what they are.

It is only then that you can begin to alter course and correct the behavior with alternative positive and self-loving behaviors, thoughts, and self-talk. Write down both the negative thoughts or behaviors on one side of a piece of paper or in your journal and on the other side, write down the positive antidote. Flip your negative self-message to a more positive message.

One of the world's leading therapists, Marissa Peer, shares a few tips to create a more confident and self-loving person. She encourages people to write 'I AM ENOUGH' on mirrors or to post it on paper so that you will be reminded often of this positive message.

- Always speak kindly about yourself.
- Stop criticizing yourself.
- You are enough.
- Stop beating yourself up.
- Sometimes other people can't or won't say what you want them to say.
- Be your own cheerleader, helpful coach, loving parent, or encouraging teacher.

Eat in Silence

Eating in silence is a common practice in spiritual communities. Being quiet offers time to slow down the mind and business of one's life. It allows space to focus on your breath, the beautiful and nutritious food in front of you, and the simple and pleasurable act of eating. You may be surprised at how good it feels.

Eat with Your Eyes Closed

Keeping your eyes closed while eating is a unique experience for those of us who are blessed to have sight. It is not often that we would elect to close our eyes during a snack or a meal, unless it's been a long day and you are falling asleep. Closing your eyes will allow you to fully concentrate on the taste, textures, and smell of the food you are eating.

You can feed someone else, too, who is blindfolded. Have the person taste a raisin, mango, pineapple, or blueberry. Have them really take the time to savor the taste, smell, and texture of the food.

Keep a Weekly Food and Mood Journal

Share in your journal the ways you feel about food, eating, your health, and your body. Write about your willingness to create more trust in yourself around food and eating. Write about all the times you received the internal message about hunger or thirst and either listened to them or didn't listen to them. What was the outcome? How did you feel afterward? Write about your feelings before, during and after a meal. Talk about how you feel physically before, during, and after eating a snack or meal. Journaling will connect your mind to your intuition and heart.

Creating Sacred Meals

Create sacred meal time wherever you eat: at home, the school cafeteria, or at work. Have fun and enjoy the good feelings you will bring to your next meal. Creating sacred meals is about the intention behind your action, not on how elaborate or simple your action is.

- Set the table.
- Use cloth napkins, placemats, and tablecloths.
- Use real plates and utensils instead of paper plates or plastic utensils.
- Place flowers or small plants on the table.
- Say a blessing, gratitude, wish, or prayer before you eat.
- Thank the chefs and cooks for preparing your meal for you.
- Create your own lovely rituals to add sacredness to your food growing, preparing, and eating.

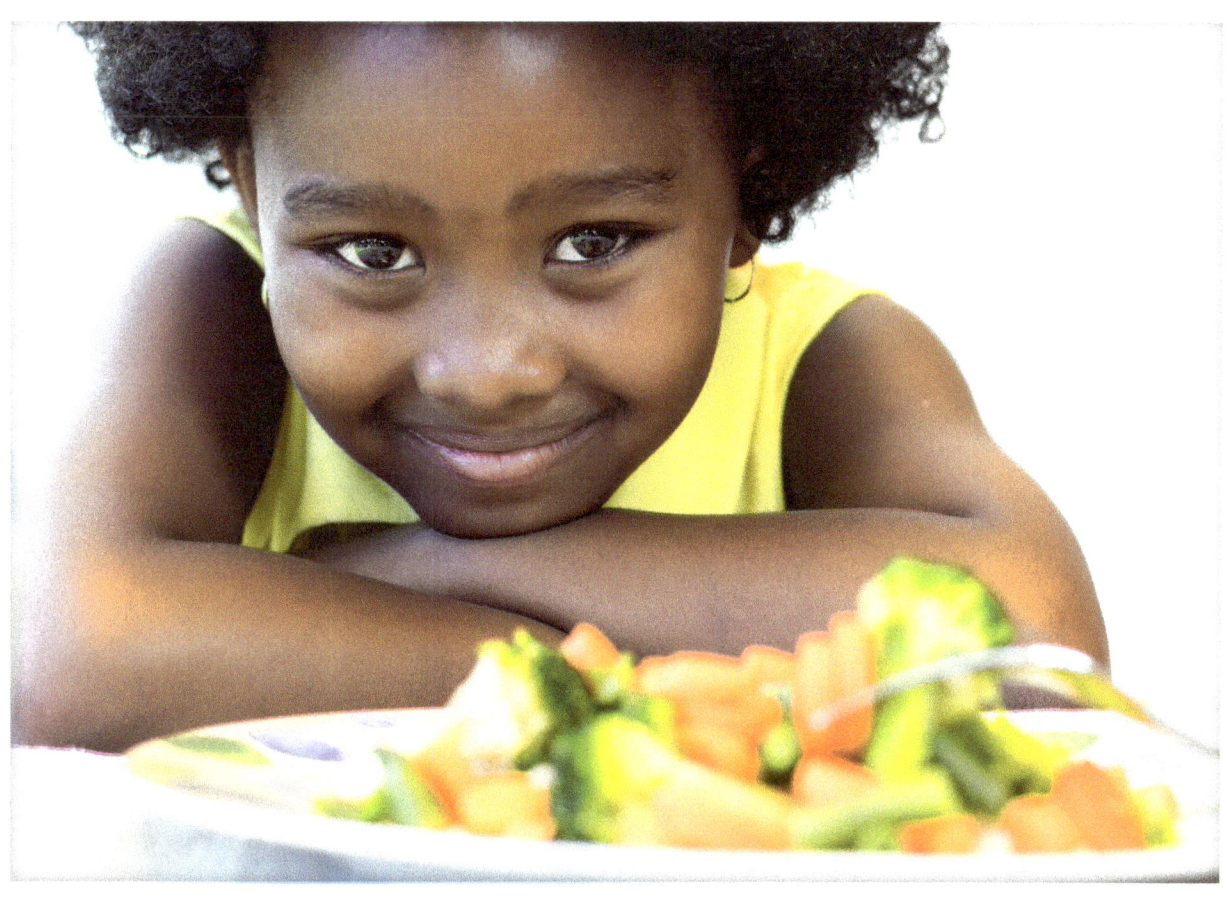

GRATITUDE JOURNALS AND IDEAS

Who knew that feeling more peaceful, grateful, and joyful in daily life is attainable with simply a piece of paper and pen? Being mindful of what you are grateful for regularly has many proven health and spiritual benefits. A study in the Journal of School Psychology led by Dr. Robert A. Emmons with early adolescents showed that counting blessings were associated with "enhanced self-reported gratitude, optimism, life satisfaction, and decreased negative affect." Noted in particular was an increase in satisfaction and gratitude with their school experience. We are sure most parents and teachers would welcome such attitudes.

Have fun exploring the five empowering and inspirational ideas to express what you are grateful for.

Gratitude Journals

Gratitude journaling is a straightforward, private, and insightful way to express the reasons you are grateful. Gratitude journaling has been shown to reduce stress, improve relationships, reduce blood pressure, and heal heartache. Every day, write down in a journal or any notebook three to ten things that you are grateful for. Thinking of using a tablet or computer? Keep that screen powered down. Mindfulness experts say putting pen or pencil to paper makes a more meaningful neurological link to the brain, which is a point worth noting.

So now that you are excited to share your blessings, the question is, where and when to journal? To create more success, do your gratitude journaling around the same time and the same location daily. You can journal at the bus stop, at your school desk, in your bedroom, in your office, or at your dining table. It is nice if you can create that familiar habit and ritual. Some people like to keep a journal on their nightstand so they can journal in the evening before going to bed to clear the mind. Some folks prefer to journal first thing upon waking so that they can start the day with a positive mind-frame.

Chalkboard Painted Gratitude Wall

Find a wall or space in your home to collect gratitudes. Ideally this is a section of wall in the classroom or on a door that is visible and easily accessible. You can paint this special spot with chalkboard paint. Chalkboard paint comes in a rainbow array of colors with just as many specialty chalkboard markers that will surely go with your décor. Or, if you don't want to overthink it, you can't go wrong using old-school black or green chalkboard paint.

Fill the space up with gratitudes every day, every week, or every month and keep adding for however long you like. When the area is all filled up, or you want to start fresh, wipe it clean to start the next collection of gratitude. It may be a fun project to take a picture of them and collect in a booklet to remind you of all your blessings. Whoop! Are you feeling the good vibes already?

Jar of Gratitudes

Use a mason jar or any wide-mouthed glass vessel to hold your thoughts and words of gratitude. Find colorful paper of your choice and write down three things you are grateful for. You can write your words on the same paper or three different pieces of papers. A special effect is to use metallic pens on black paper. Or use cardstock and cut the edges with crinkle or shape edged scissors for fun edging. The creative options are endless.

You can write down the date so you can go back and reread them over time. With little kids, use stickers, markers, stamps, and pictures you cut out and glue on paper. Everyone in the classroom or your family can choose their own style of paper. This activity is best to do every day. At school, before you

GRATITUDE JOURNAL

TODAY, I AM GRATEFUL FOR…

_____

_____

_____

_____

_____

_____

_____

_____

_____

_____

_____

_____

_____

_____

_____

_____

_____

_____

_____

_____

Permission to reproduce. ©The Food Tree

begin class, ask students to write down what they are grateful for. At home, do this before dinner and even when friends and guests come over.

Gratitude Tree

Find a tree branch and secure it in a spot in your classroom, home, office, or an accessible area at a special event. On a slip of paper with a small hole punch through it, ask people to write a gratitude or positive message and then tie it to the branch using string or yarn. The hanging branches filled with colorful notes are lovely to create for a special occasion, as in a going-away party or for a birthday celebration. Write the gratitude on interesting paper with colorful or metallic markers.

Photo Journaling

Take a picture every day, print it out, and paste in a journal with a short caption of why you took the picture and why you are grateful for the experience.

THE "I WONDER" EXERCISE

The "I Wonder" exercise is intended to foster imagination, creation, manifestation and to build JOY and CURIOSITY in your life. Rumor has it that Leonardo Da Vinci had his students do this every day! The "I Wonder" statements can be academic, spiritual, funny, or personal. There are no rules as that would defeat the purpose of this exercise.

Ask your students to say 10 to 100 "I Wonder" statements out loud or write them down on paper using a pencil or pen. It is most powerful for the brain when you say your words out loud, or when you write them down on a piece of paper. Therefore, do not type the list into a computer. Students can create their own I Wonder Journals, or begin the day saying them as they get ready in the morning or before going to bed at night.

"I WONDER" EXAMPLES

I wonder what I am going to have for a snack today.
I wonder what new idea will pop into my head.
I wonder what I will laugh about today.
I wonder what songs I will sing.
I wonder what music I will play on my guitar.
I wonder what I will learn today.
I wonder what the test will be like.
I wonder what kinds of animals I will see on my walk.
I wonder when my grandmother is coming over.
I wonder if it is going to rain today.
I wonder what weekends I am going to go skiing this year.
I wonder what baseball team I am going to get on this year.
I wonder how my puppy is doing today.
I wonder how my mom is doing today.
I wonder what book I will read tonight.
I wonder who I will play with today.
I wonder what kind of habits I can improve.
I wonder what song I am going to write today.
I wonder what music I will listen to later.

THE SCALE OF HUMAN CONSCIOUSNESS

The Scale of Consciousness is a guide, or map, to the human range of emotions that was created by psychiatrist Dr. David Hawkins. He discusses his philosophy in his acclaimed book, *Power vs. Force: The Anatomy of Consciousness* (Veritas Publishing, 1995). Researchers studied the impact one person's energy has on another person with thousands of test subjects from around the world ranging in age from young children to the elderly. They measured a person's energy frequency in response to stimuli using Applied Kinesiology (AK), also known as muscle testing. This scale uses logarithmic calibrations to measure the different levels of human consciousness. Each leap to the next level increases to the tenth power. The results were astounding.

The researchers found that most of humanity, seventy-eight percent, is functioning at a level of 200 or less. That means most of the world's population operates in the destructive negative zone. However, change and growth can happen and shift. Scientists have discovered that one person at level 300 counterbalances 90,000 individuals below level 200. One person at level 400 counterbalances 400,000 individuals below level 200. One person at level 600 counteracts the negativity of 10 million individuals below level 200.

This scale certainly brings to light the idea and importance of raising your vibration! The intention is to create and foster more self-awareness of the energy you emit and bring to a space.

Challenge yourself to see if you can increase your power to feel courageous, which is the beginning of the positive levels. See if you can muster up willingness and acceptance about your current life and circumstances. At these levels, you can lift and transmute someone else's energy that is feeling shame, guilt, apathy, and fear. Just by shifting your energy. Wow. Notice when you get to the level of willingness, acceptance, and reason, you will feel a more expanded energy while experiencing the emotions and energy below that level will be experienced as a more negative feeling of contracted energy.

Dr. Watkins suggests that we can move between levels but often stay within a certain range, called the Level of Consciousness or LOC. Nonetheless, it is entirely possible to move up levels and shift your energy to a more positive vibration.

THE SEVENTEEN LEVELS OF HUMAN CONSCIOUSNESS

SHAME 1-20
People experience feelings of humility, low self-esteem, contempt, and not trusting others in this state. They may exhibit harmful and destructive behavior and have thoughts of murder or suicide.

GUILT 30
In this state, a person feels remorse, blame, regret, or guilt. A person may experience a sense of worthlessness and have a difficulty forgiving theirself.

APATHY 50
The state of apathy includes indifference, lethargy, dependency on others, and feeling stuck, hopeless, and numb.

GRIEF 75
The dominant energies at this level are feelings of sadness, loss, regret, anguish, and heartbreak. It includes a belief that the opportunities in your life are gone, you feel like a failure.

FEAR 100
The primary emotion at this level is one of anxiety, panic, concern, and unease. Some feel suspicious and paranoid.

DESIRE 125
People at this level have feelings of wanting, ambition, and passion with the potential to lead to positive

change but the downside is that the person could also go the other direction towards greed, need, and addictive behavior.

ANGER 150
This level is the result of unmet desires which creates frustration leading to anger. In this state, people may feel resentment and outrage. They can get stuck here or be motivated to move out of it.

PRIDE 175
A person will feel satisfaction, pleasure, and honor. They have a positive outlook and feel optimistic. However, the ego may become inflated. A person at this level may have a false sense of feeling good because of dependence on external factors like wealth, popularity, fame or being in positions of power. In a sense, their happiness is out of their control and may disappear.

COURAGE 200
People at this level are empowered. They know that they can harness power to create the life they want. This person knows that they are in control of their success and growth. They know they are the source of making their dreams happen. They are not victims of external conditions. Here a person cultivates bravery, tenacity, determination, and dares to know that they have a choice in the decisions they make.

NEUTRALITY 250
Neutrality is a level when people do not have an attachment to a particular outcome. They feel flexible and content with how things are going in their life. They have a sense of being safe and trusting. They see certain possibilities for improvement yet they do not make the necessary changes to realize them.

WILLINGNESS 310
This level involves feelings of being limitless, hopeful, and a state of eagerness. People here are operating successfully in their life pursuits. Others' expectations or judgments do not make an impact on them. It is time to evaluate how energy is spent and if energy can be used in better ways.

ACCEPTANCE 350
This level involves recognition and acknowledgement that people can actively purse the goals they have set for themselves and push beyond any limiting beliefs. They begin to see their potential and take action to be proactive and take control. They are no longer reactive to the balls life throws at them.

REASON 400
People have an unquenchable thirst for knowledge. Their world is based in logic and scientific reasoning and therefore they may not see the forest for the trees. Their lineal thinking may block them in advancing their consciousness. They can see themselves as a force for good in the world.

LOVE 500
At this level, people let their heart instead of their mind be in control. They feel selfless. This is a significant barrier to cross according to Dr. Watkins. It is when a person can leave their ego physical world for a more spiritual realm. They trust their intuition and operate from this place. They embody unconditional love. Dr. Watkins suggests that only 0.4% of the population or $1/250$ will reach this level.

JOY 540
Joy is the realm of compassion, inner joy, bliss, humor, and serenity. At this level, people feel a sense of completeness and oneness with the world. Their sheer presence lifts others in their company. They are in complete harmony with the universe and they are in the flow with their spiritual soul connection to it.

PEACE 600
Peace is a level when people are in total surrender to their higher path and may glow at this level of illumination.

ENLIGHTENMENT 700-1000
The level of spiritual mastery as seen by only the most revered humans who have ever walked on our planet. Some who have attained this level of divinity may include known religious figures like Buddha or Jesus.

HAND MUDRAS

The Sanskrit word, Mudra, means "seal" or "sign"

Mudras are symbolic gestures we make with our body. They are used to reflect, to enhance, or to create a desired state of being. These unique body positions have been taught for thousands of years in the Hindu and Buddhist traditions. But the mudras origins go back to the earliest parts of our human history.

Mudras can be done using the eyes, arms, hands, fingers, and even the whole body. They are mainly a form of body sign language. You do them all the time, whether you are aware or not. You may find yourself doing prayer hands, pointing, flashing the peace sign, or making the open giving hands gesture. So universal are these types of expression, even chimpanzees use similar hand mudra gestures!

Mudras have been known to enrich and enhance one's health and can be targeted to address specific health concerns. They can be used to balance your internal system, boost inner power, activate manifestation, and enhance intuition.

Scholars, spiritual teachers, and practitioners of yoga explain that each mudra hand position creates a unique energy frequency when the fingers and hands connect and touch each other. They claim that the hands reflect and are associated with different parts of the body and brain. Energy circuits are believed to be active in your fingertips that connect to the universal elements.

FINGER ENERGY CIRCUITS

THUMB—SPACE

INDEX FINGER—AIR

MIDDLE FINGER—FIRE

RING FINGER—WATER

PINKY FINGER—EARTH

The Practice

There are over one hundred different mudras. I have selected a variety for you to try with your students. Some mudras are more complex and may even be uncomfortable to practice. Go easy on yourself and release the desire to make it perfect.

- You can do these standing, sitting, or lying down.
- Remember to set an intention before you begin.
- Enjoy good body posture and gentle breathing.
- Keep your fingers, hands, or arms in a relaxed manner while applying light pressure.
- Relax the jaw and soften the eyebrows and forehead.
- Hold each position for 5-10 regular breaths while thinking of the intention of the mudra.

Hand Mudras

ABHAYA VARADA MUDRA

Place your left hand just under the navel in a slightly cupped gesture. Raise the right hand, as in a stop position, next to your head with the palm facing outward. Close your eyes and relax the shoulders. This mudra promotes a sense of security, fearlessness, a trusting heart, limitlessness, and freedom.

Affirmation I am entirely safe and grounded as I journey forward without fear.

ADHI MUDRA
Tuck your thumbs inside of your fist. Promotes a sense of calm, security, relaxation, and trust.

Affirmation I am safe, secure, and trust the awareness of my being.

BHU MUDRA
Make a peace sign by making a fist and extending the forefinger and middle finger outward. Then place the tips of the straight peace sign fingers onto the ground, table, or your thighs. Promotes a sense of grounding, security, and trust.

Affirmation I ground myself into the mother earth.

BUDDHI MUDRA
Touch the tip of the thumb to the tip of the pinky while holding the other three fingers together and straight up. Promotes a sense of calm, security, relaxation, trust, mental clarity, and increased intuition.

Affirmation I am open and receive clear guidance and intuitive communication.

GUPTA MUDRA
Lace fingers downwards and fold the hands down so that the base of the hands touch. The thumbs are outside of the fist with the right thumb crossed over the other. The elbows lift slightly away from the body. Promotes immunity, protection, self-confidence, the release of limiting beliefs, and grounding.

Affirmation I find peace, confidence, tranquility, and balance in my daily actions.

GYAN MUDRA
Touch index fingertip to thumb tip with other fingers relaxed and touching each other. You may rest your hands on the knees if sitting. Place palms upwards to connect you to the universal oneness and knowledge or face the palms and fingers down to ground you into the earth. Promotes good memory, concentration, peace, serenity, and tranquility.

Affirmation I am filled with peace and calm in my body and my mind.

HANSI MUDRA
Make a fist and extend the pinky outward. Promotes a positive mood, wellness, inner smile, bliss, joy, and relaxation.

Affirmation My inner smile awakens my always present bliss and joy within.

JALA MUDRA
Touch the tip of the thumb to the tip of the pinky while holding the other three fingers apart and stretched outward. Promotes energy, feeling uplifted, and expansive.

Affirmation My energy flows with the rhythm of life.

MANDALA MUDRA
Place fingers of the right hand over the fingers of the left and then touch the thumbs gently together forming an oval shape with your hands. Promotes a feeling of togetherness, union, wholeness, balance, and clarity.

Affirmation I am enough, whole, and complete.

MUDRA OF A THOUSAND PETALS
Form a triangle shape with your two hands by placing your thumbs and forefinger tips together. Keep the other fingers extended outwards. Do this mudra about 6 inches above the crown of your head. Promotes a sense of universal consciousness, awareness, and divinity.

Affirmation I honor the light consciousness within me.

PADMA MUDRA
Place hands together as in prayer pose and slowly open wide your fingers, keeping the heels of your hand together, opening your hands keeping pinky to pinky and thumb to thumb together. Promotes a sense of union, integration, connection, wholeness, purity, and open-heartedness.

Affirmation My heart opens like a lotus that connects to the whole of the universe.

PRITHVI MUDRA

Touch the tip of the ring finger to the tip of the thumb with other fingers extended straight up. Promotes centering, trust, security and reduces stress.

Affirmation The earth is abundant and sustains my every breath in life.

PUSHPANJAILI MUDRA

Put the sides of your hands together with the palms facing up as in an offering or receiving position. Promotes generosity, connection, receiving, abundance, love, compassion, openness, and appreciation.

Affirmation I receive every moment in life as a gift and a blessing.

RUDRA MUDRA

Sit comfortably in the lotus position. Bend your arms and elbows and keep them parallel to the floor. Connect the thumb, index, and ring finger while extending outward the middle finger and pinky. Use one or both hands to do this mudra. Promotes self-esteem, clarity, personal will, personal power, and stimulates creativity.

Affirmation I connect and activate my power center.

SHIVALINGAM MUDRA

Hold left hand out with palm facing up. Make a fist with the right hand, extend the thumb upward, and place fist onto the left hand. Promotes a sense of truth, clarity, personal power, ability to reach the highest potential, confidence, centering, and increased physical energy.

Affirmation I trust and embrace the path of my true-life purpose.

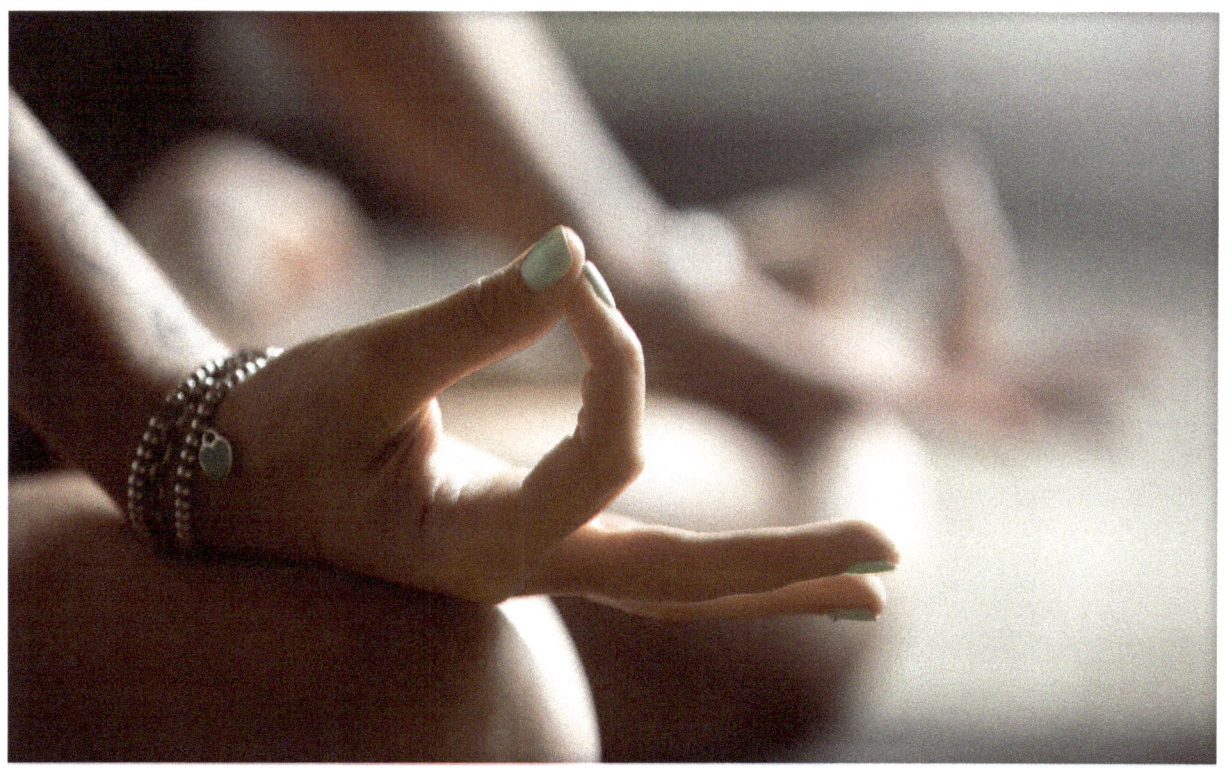

ALTERNATE NOSTRIL BREATHING
Nadi Shodhana

Breathing. We do it all day long but how often do we actually pay attention and bring our awareness to the quality of our breath? We often forget what the ancients knew; how we breathe is directly connected to our emotional, physical, and mental states of being.

One particular type of breathing is a kind of Pranayama or yogic breathing called Alternate Nostril Breathing (Nadi Shodhana). The name implies that through working with our vital life force energy, we can use Nadi, referring to the different pranic channels in the body and Shodhana, meaning to cleanse or purify, as a tool to greater health and wellness.

These techniques are easy and free and can be done anywhere and at any time for your health benefit. I hope you find time to incorporate this breathing practice into your classroom and life.

Benefits of Alternate Nostril Breathing

Considering that 9 out of 10 westerners are chest breathers and so only use the top ⅓ of our lungs, most of us are not fully utilizing our total lung potential. Practicing deep breathing by using all portions of the lungs with pranayama can increase the lung capacity by at least one third. People who suffer from exposure to pollution, smoking, pesticides, and airborne chemicals or have allergies and asthma can increase their oxygen capacity by bringing the breath deeper into the undamaged tissue.

Simple and Effective Antidote to Everyday Stress

Alternate Nostril Breathing boosts brain-power, focus, and attention by correcting the imbalance in the brain. It helps to create a balanced state of being by clearing the mind of chaos, reducing chronic stress, calming the nervous system, alleviating depression, smoothing the emotional state and improving the quality of sleep.

Nadi Shodhana also improves major body functions including increasing metabolism and improving digestion by boosting oxygen capacity in the tissues and organs of all the bodily systems.

How to Perform Alternate Nostril Breathing—Nadi Shodhana

Alternate Nostril Breathing exercises should be done at a comfortable temperature. Before you begin this breathing practice, blow your nose to clear nasal passages. It is also not advisable to do this pranayama if your nasal passageways are congested or if the nose is clogged due to allergies or sickness.

- Sit with your feet crossed or in half lotus or into full lotus if you are feeling flexible, thereby creating an erect spine.
- You can also sit in hero's pose or in a chair with a straight back to keep the spine straight.
- Keep your chin dropped slightly.

To Begin

- Take your right hand and fold down your index and middle finger, keeping your ring and pinky up as best you can.
- Take the thumb on your right hand, plug the right nostril, and inhale up through the left nostril.
- Close the left off with the ring finger, open the right side, and exhale.

- Inhale up the right nostril and close the right with your thumb and exhale through the left nostril.
- Keep your breath smooth and even.
- That is one round.
- Bring your concentration back to the breath if your mind begins to wander.
- Do five or six rounds or repetitions a few times a day.

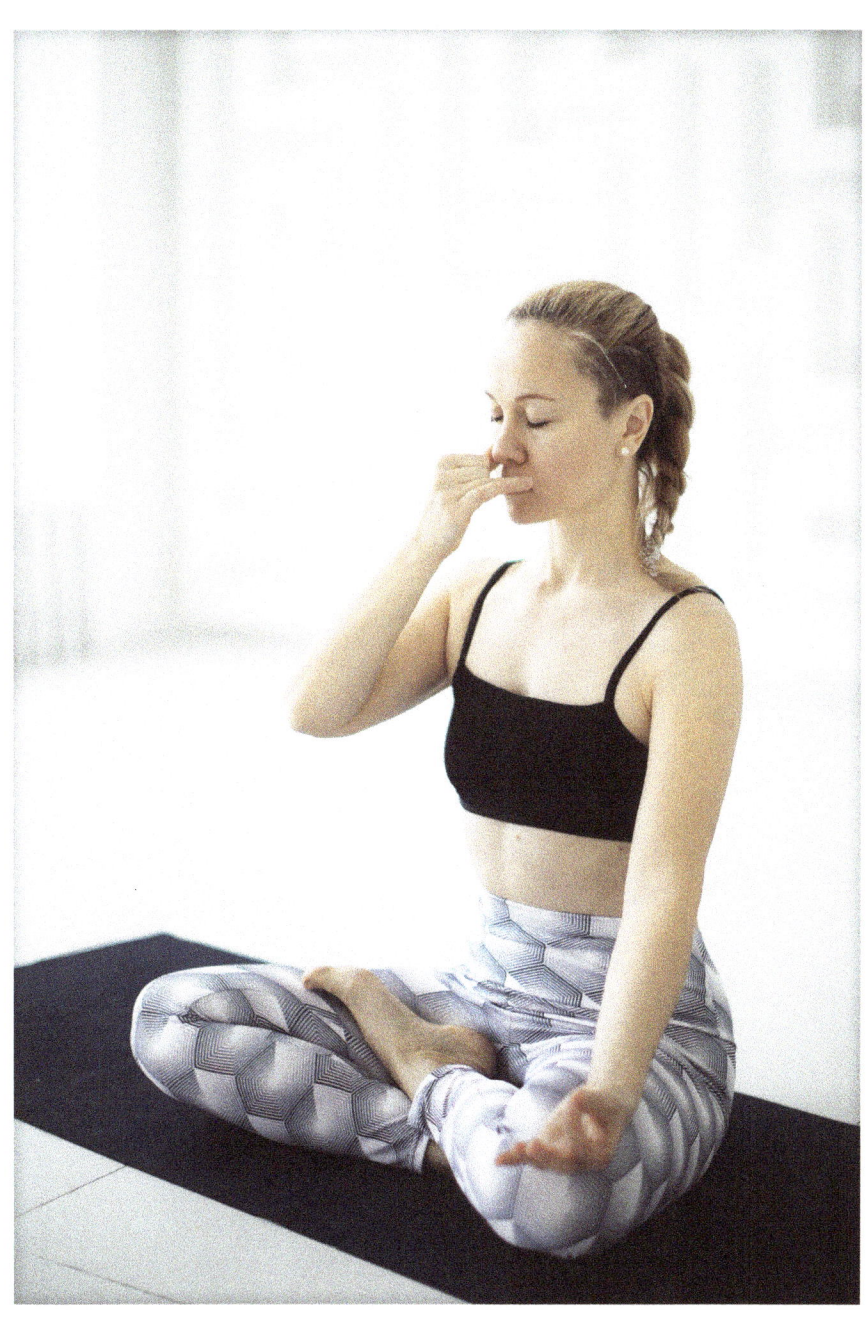

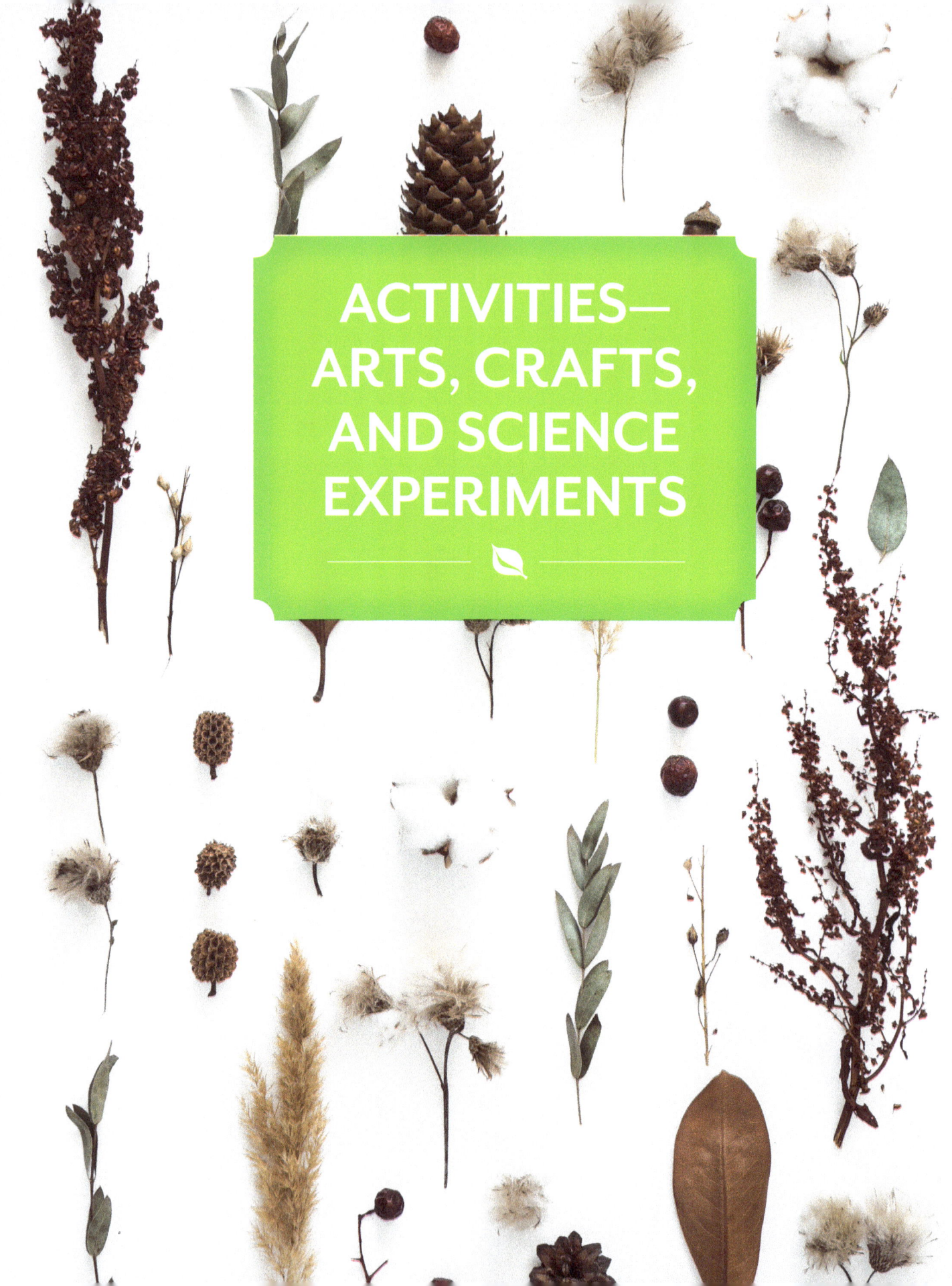

ACTIVITIES—ARTS, CRAFTS, AND SCIENCE EXPERIMENTS

Indian Corn Jewelry

MATERIALS

- Colorful Indian corn cobs, dried. Red, yellow, black, blue, orange are colors grown. Source these husks at farmers markets, grocery stores in the late summer/fall, craft shops, or specialty online stores.
- Fishing line, dental floss, crafting wire, elastic string, or heavy thread
- Heavy duty needles
- Bowl(s) to collect corn kernels
- Warm/hot water for soaking kernels

DESCRIPTION

This activity connects students of all ages to the plant world and to native American culture, while also making something beautiful. Indian corn jewelry makes outstanding gifts for birthdays and holidays and can be a marvelous activity for a Harvest or Earth Day Festival. Students' jewelry can also be used for school auctions or class fundraisers. Have fun and get creative!

BACKGROUND INFORMATION

Indian corn is also known as flint corn because its shell is as "hard as flint." Its botanical name is Zea mays, and is a variety of maize or common corn. Corn has been cultivated by the Native Americans for more than 7,000 years. The early variety of corn originating from Southern Mexico and Central America was known as Teosinte. Since that time, Native Americans have successfully cultivated the corn cob to produce bigger ears, going from just 8 rows of kernels and only a few inches long to today's standard size.

Indian corn grows in beautiful colors like blue, red, white, yellow, and purple/black. It is not as sweet as yellow corn, so it is mostly used ground into flour or popped.

DIRECTIONS

1. Gather a dozen or so dried colorful Indian corn cobs.
2. Remove hardened kernels from the corn cob by picking and pushing them off with your fingers. Place them in bowls. If you desire, keep the different kernel colors separate from each other by putting them into separate bowls.
3. Place the kernels in a bowl of very warm/hot water. Let these kernels sit overnight, or for at least 12 hours, to soften.
4. Strain kernels.
5. Cut a piece of fishing line, dental floss, crafting wire, elastic string, or heavy thread in the desired length to use to string together the kernels into jewelry of your liking.
6. Attach the string to a heavy-duty needle.
7. Create a pattern with the kernels when you string the kernels onto the string.
8. Make a long necklace, a short choker, or a bracelet. You can get as fancy or sophisticated as you so desire. Use clasps to secure the ends or you can simply tie off an elastic string that will fit over the head or wrist.

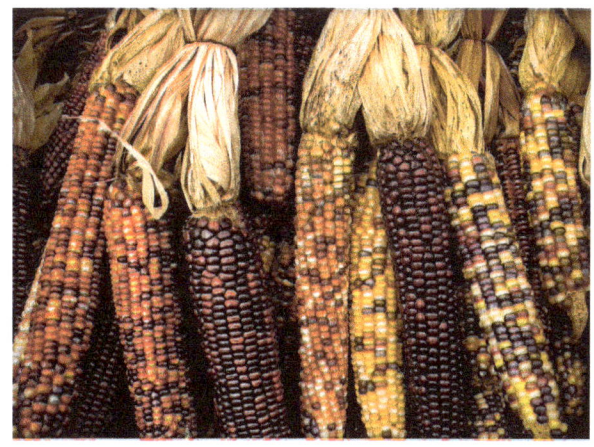

Make Lavender Wands

Lavender flowers are one of the most revered herbs in the botanical world. They have a lovely scent that imbues relaxation and calm in the mind. These cute little wands have been made for hundreds of years to freshen linens and clothes. Enjoy the process and meditative stillness of making these wands and enjoy the lasting gift from this herb.

MATERIALS

- 1 foot long narrow ribbon or raffia strands in the color of your choice
- 15 lavender stems (or some uneven number)

DIRECTIONS

1. Gather 13–15 or other uneven bunch of fresh and nimble lavender stems together.
2. Tie the bunch together tightly with a ribbon below the flowers.
3. Tie the ribbon so one long strand is left.
4. Invert the flowers by bending the stems one by one over the flower head. Use care not to break the stem.
5. Take the long ribbon and begin at the top of the flower bundle, weaving over and under the stems, shaping the cluster as you go along.
6. Pull gently on the ribbon as you go to keep your weave snug.
7. When you get to the bottom of the flower cluster, tie off the ribbon.
8. You can make a loop or a bow.
9. Trim the bottom stems so they are neat.
10. Tuck this nature favor in a clothing drawer, on a night stand, or in a linen closet or hang in any room to add a lovely scent.

DIY Plant Dyes

Explore the rich colors you can make with plant dyes. The different plant parts and techniques you can use to dye clothes, fabrics, and papers naturally are endless. Each piece you create will be one of a kind.

MATERIALS

- Latex or rubber gloves
- Smock
- Large pot for your dye vessel and or separate tub for a fixative bath
- Wooden or stainless-steel spoons
- Stovetop
- Knives, scissors, or pruning tools
- Basket, jars, or paper bags to collect plant materials
- Natural fabrics or clothing; white or light-colored, bamboo, cotton, denim, hemp, muslin, linen, silk, and wool

BEFORE YOU GET STARTED

There are a few steps involved in the dyeing process. Be aware of plant allergies or plants that might be toxic. Use caution and care.

DIRECTIONS

1. Collect fabrics and dyeable materials.
2. Collect plant materials. Gather plants, stems, flowers, bark, seeds, and powders.
3. Make color fixative.
4. Make the dye solution.
5. Dye fabrics.

COLLECT DYEABLE FABRICS AND MATERIALS

Gather a selection of fabric, t-shirts, old clothes, socks, pillow cases, sheets, tablecloths, and paper. For best results, use white or light-colored natural fabrics or clothing. Experiment with dyeing natural materials like bamboo, cotton, denim, hemp, muslin, linen, silk, and wool.

COLLECT PLANT MATERIALS

Collect the stems, leaves, berries, flowers, bark, roots, powders, and lichen that you plan to use.

***Harvest Responsibly

Leave at least half of a stand in the wild when gathering plant materials for dyeing.

Gather enough plant matter (leaves, flowers, etc.) to fill half a 5-gallon water bucket. This is enough water for about a pound to a pound and a half of plant materials. Adjust amounts as needed.

MAKE COLOR FIXATIVE

Fixatives, also known as mordants, are metals or minerals that are added to water that fabrics are soaked in before the dyeing process. This step will allow the dyes to be better absorbed and will help to make the colors brighter and more permanent.

Salt fixative

Add ½ cup of salt to 8 cups cold water.

Vinegar fixative

Add one-part vinegar to 4 parts cold water.

Other fixatives/mordants: lemon juice, baking soda, iron, wood ash, or cream of tartar

DIRECTIONS FOR FIXATIVE

1. Place fabric in the water and fixative solution.
2. Let fabrics soak for 24 hours.
3. Rinse fabrics with clean water and squeeze out excess liquid.

MAKE DYE SOLUTION

1. Wear rubber or latex gloves and a smock or something to protect your clothes during the dyeing process. Plants may stain your hands, cause skin irritation, or allergic reaction. Use caution.
2. Chop or cut plant material into small pieces and place in a large stainless-steel pot.
3. Double the amount of water to plant material.
4. Bring water and plant mixture to a boil and simmer covered for an hour.
5. Strain the plant material and collect dye in a large pot, cool, and store in a glass jar.

DIRECTIONS TO MAKE DYE SOLUTION BATH

1. Place your wet fabric in the hot dye bath and bring mixture to a simmer. Do not boil.
2. Gently swirl the materials around to ensure that the dye evenly absorbs into the fabric.
3. Simmer for at least half an hour and up to 2-3 hours, or until the desired color is obtained. For a stronger shade, allow the material to soak in the dye overnight with the heat turned off.
4. Rinse the material in cool water until water runs clear. The color of the fabric will appear lighter when dry.
5. Launder newly dyed fabrics separately in cold water.

NATURAL PLANT BASED DYE COLORS

Use, bark, berries, flowers, leaves, stems, and roots from plants, trees, and herbs to make natural dye.

Reds
- Beets—roots
- Blackberries—berries
- Cabbage—leaves
- Crab Apple—bark
- Chokecherries—fruit
- Dandelion—roots
- Hibiscus—flowers, dried
- Rosehips—hips
- Safflower—flowers
- St. John's Wort—flowers

Red–Purple
- Artemisia—leaves, stems
- Artichokes—leaves
- Daylilies—flowers, dried
- Hibiscus—flowers
- Huckleberry—berries
- Iris—roots
- Logwood—wood, bark
- Pokeweed—berries

Pink
- Camilla—flowers. For deeper shade, use lemon juice and salt fixative.
- Cherries—fruit
- Elderberry—berries
- Fir—bark
- Strawberry—leaves
- Raspberries—leaves
- Rose—petals. For deep pink, use lemon juice fixative.
- Lavender—flowers. For deep pink, use lemon juice fixative.
- Lichens—leaves
- Oregon Grape—berries
- Toyon—berries

Orange
- Barberry—all parts
- Butternut—seed husks
- Carrot—roots
- Lichen—leaves
- Lilac—twigs
- Onion—skins
- Pomegranate—fruit, rind
- Sassafras—leaves
- Turmeric—roots

Yellow
- Acacia—flowers
- Alfalfa—seeds
- Beet—roots
- Burdock—roots
- Celery—leaves
- Dandelion—flowers
- Daffodil—flower heads, dried
- Dahlia—flowers
- Goldenrod—flowers
- Grapes—leaves
- Heather—foliage
- Hickory—leaves. Use salt as a fixative.
- Marigold—flowers
- Mimosa—flowers
- Mullen—leaves, roots
- Onion—skins
- Oregon Grape—stems, roots
- Oxalis—flower heads
- Paprika—dried spice
- Queen Anne's Lace—flowers
- Red Clover—blossom, leaves, stem. Use alum mordant.
- Safflower—flowers, soaked in water
- Saffron—stigmas
- St. John's Wort—flower, leaves
- Sunflowers—flowers
- Syrian Rue—seeds. Plant dye might glow under black light
- Turmeric—roots, fresh or powdered
- Willow—leaves
- White Mulberry Tree—bark
- Yellow Coneflower—whole flower heads

THE FOOD TREE

Green
- Barberry—roots
- Broom—stems
- Camellia—flowers, pink and red petals
- Coneflower—flowers
- Foxglove—flowers
- Grass—leaves
- Larkspur—flowers
- Lilac—flowers
- Mulga Acacia—seed pods
- Nettles—leaves
- Peach—leaves
- Pigweed—entire plant
- Plantain—roots
- Purple Milkweed—flowers, leaves
- Red onion—skins
- Red Pine—needles
- Spinach—leaves
- Sorrel—roots
- Snapdragon—flowers
- Tea Tree—flowers
- White Ash—bark
- Yarrow—flowers

Blue–Purple
- Black Beans—bean
- Blueberry—berries
- Cabbage, Red—leaves
- Cedar, Red—bark, roots
- Cornflower—flower petals
- Cherry—roots
- Dogwood—fruit
- Elderberries—berries. *The stems and branches are poisonous!
- Grapes—fruit
- Iris—roots, rhizomes
- Longwood—bark, leaves
- Maple Tree, Red—inner bark
- Mulberries—berries
- Oregon Grape—fruit
- Raspberry—fruit
- Saffron—petals
- Hyacinth—flowers

Brown
- Oak—acorns. Need to boil.
- Beet—root
- Broom—bark
- Coffee—grinds
- Dandelion—roots
- Fennel—flowers, leaves
- Fir, Colorado—bark
- Hollyhock—flower petals
- Ivy—twigs
- Amur Maple—dried leaves
- Juniper—berries
- Manzanita—leaves
- Oak—bark
- Yellow Dock—roots
- Sumac—leaves
- Walnut—hulls
- Wild Plum—roots
- White Birch—inner bark

Gray–Black
- Blackberry—fruit
- Carob—pods. Need to boil.
- Oak—galls. Seed cups.

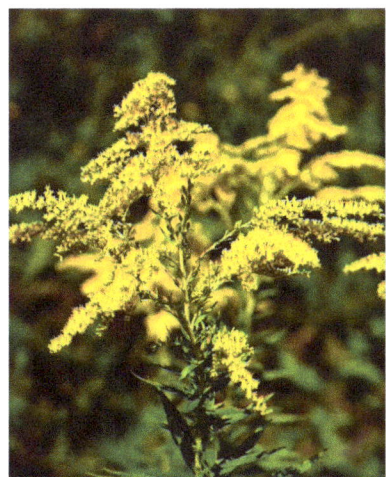
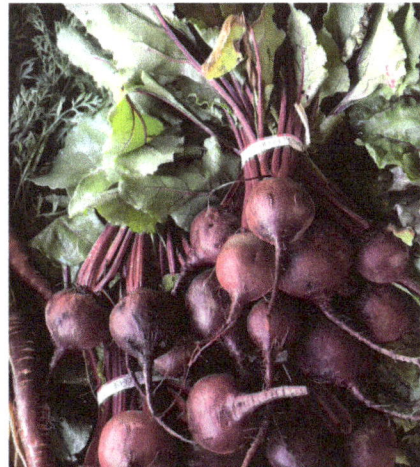
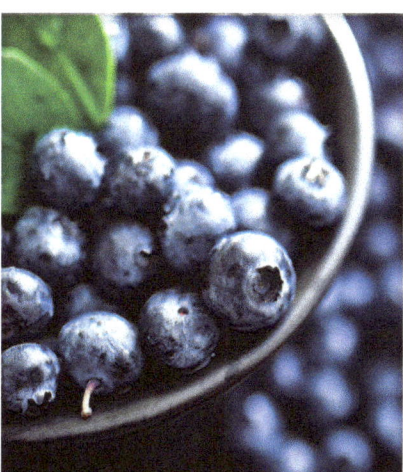

Papier Mâché Fruit and Bowls

Creative, recycled, affordable, and sometimes a bit messy, papier mâché crafts are always fun!

Make fruit, vegetables, insects, animals, bowls, plates, or little trays with newspaper, a simple paste, and brightly colored acrylic paints. When it comes to papier mâché, there are countless things to make.

In this example, I will demonstrate how to make little bowls with the insides painted like the insides of fruits and vegetables. Fun ones to try are orange half, watermelon, lemon slice, kiwi, or any other one you'd like!

If you want to go more free form, you can always build fruits and vegetables. Try making red chili peppers, apples, bell peppers, carrots, grapes, squash, garlic, watermelon wedges, onions, asparagus, bananas, eggplants, and lemons. I recommend you use bright acrylic paint on the dried papier mâché to give your creation a vibrant, shiny finish. Use the finished art as an indoor wreath, table display, or hanging mobiles.

MATERIALS

- Small metal bowls or aluminum pie tins to use as molds
- Newspaper
- Plain white flour, bleached or unbleached. **Whole wheat flour does not work well, so use all-purpose white flour for better stickiness.
- Acrylic paint in a variety of colors
- Large bowl to mix the paste
- Immersion blender (optional)
- Whisk, fork, or large spoon
- Vegetable spray or cooking oil
- Aluminum foil
- Plastic containers to put the paste in for dipping your paper strips into. Use more dipping containers if more than a few people are doing the project.

DIRECTIONS

Newspaper prep

Tear newspaper into one-inch strips.

Paste prep

In a large bowl, mix one-part flour to two-parts hot water. Mix well so that there are no lumps in your batch.

An immersion blender is a good tool to use to make your mix smooth.

Mold prep

If using a mold, like a small bowl, cover the outside with aluminum foil and then wipe or spray a light coating of vegetable oil. Make sure the edges are smooth, as that will be the rim of the bowl.

Now for the fun part!

1. Dip paper strips into the paste and then with your index finger and middle finger, pull the paper through your fingers to remove the excess paste.
2. Apply the strips in different directions so that you cover the entire surface with a nice thick layer of paper strips.
3. Allow your project to dry. Pull off of the mold gently when the paste has completely dried to the touch. Paint as desired.

Do It Yourself Playdough

Playdough is a time-tested material that can be used to make different play foods and other objects.

I include two recipes for your convenience because commercial cream of tartar may contain aluminum.

PLAYDOUGH WITHOUT CREAM OF TARTAR

Makes 1½ cups

Ingredients

- 1 cup flour
- ¼ cup of salt
- 3 tablespoons vegetable oil
- 3 teaspoons vinegar or lemon juice, filtered
- ½ cup of water
- Natural food coloring

PLAYDOUGH WITH CREAM OF TARTAR

Makes 2½ cups

Ingredients

- 2 cups of flour
- 1 cup salt
- 2 cups of water
- 2 tablespoon vegetable oil
- 2 tablespoon cream of tartar (aluminum-free)
- Natural food coloring

DIRECTIONS

1. Add flour and the rest of the ingredients into a medium-sized saucepan and mix.
2. Place on medium heat and stir for 3–5 minutes until you get to the desired texture and feel of playdough.
3. Take the mix off the heat.
4. Roll dough out onto wax paper or on to a greased pan or plate.
5. When the dough is cool to the touch, transfer onto a cutting board.
6. Knead the dough to meet a smooth and even consistency.
7. Divide the dough in the number of colors desired.
8. Add the natural food dye and knead in.
9. Store in an airtight container.

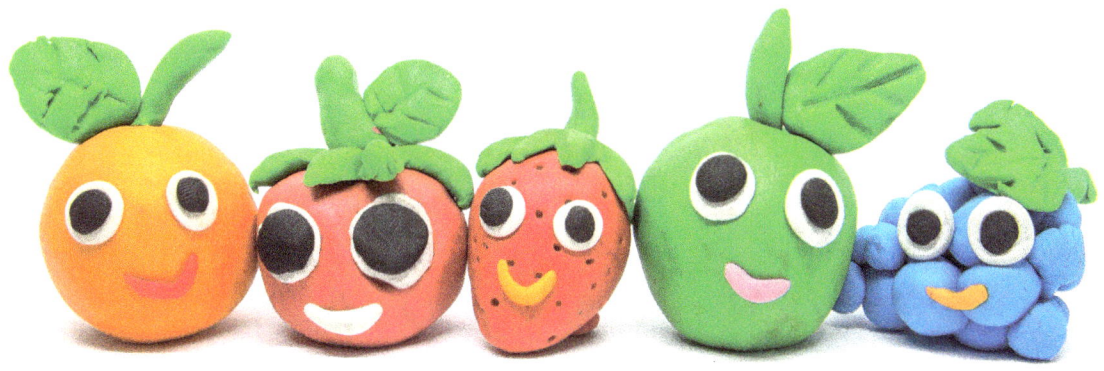

Positive Word Cloud

MATERIALS

- Magic markers, Sharpies, metallic markers
- Paint, tempera or acrylic
- Chalkboard paint
- Cardstock paper, craft paper
- Chalkboard/whiteboard
- Picture frames
- Old magazines
- Scissors
- Glue, glue sticks, Modge Podge

HOW TO CREATE A POSITIVE WORD CLOUD

Create a Positive Word Cloud using positive, life-affirming words, phrases, or sayings. Make Positive Word Clouds individually, as a class, or as an entire school-wide project. Use words that embody and represent who and how you want to be in the world. The goal is to use uplifting and encouraging words. Saying positive words about oneself fosters healthy self-esteem and self-love.

Design the Positive Word Cloud in any shape or size and on virtually any material. Your Positive Word Cloud can be as big or small as you desire. Draw an outline and put the words in a shape like a heart, circle, oval, tree, star, or hand. Or, the Positive Word Cloud can cover the whole surface for a full cloud coverage effect!!

Listed below are a few ideas of art materials to use and fun examples of ways to create a Positive Word Cloud.

- Black cardstock with metallic markers
- Green or black chalkboards with colorful chalkboard markers
- White cardstock with black words cut from magazines
- Paint on windows, picture frame glass, or on a mirror. Use chalkboard paint, washable/permanent markers, or tempera paint with a little dish soap mixed in for easy cleaning
- Cardstock with words from magazines
- Colored cardstock with magic markers or sharpie

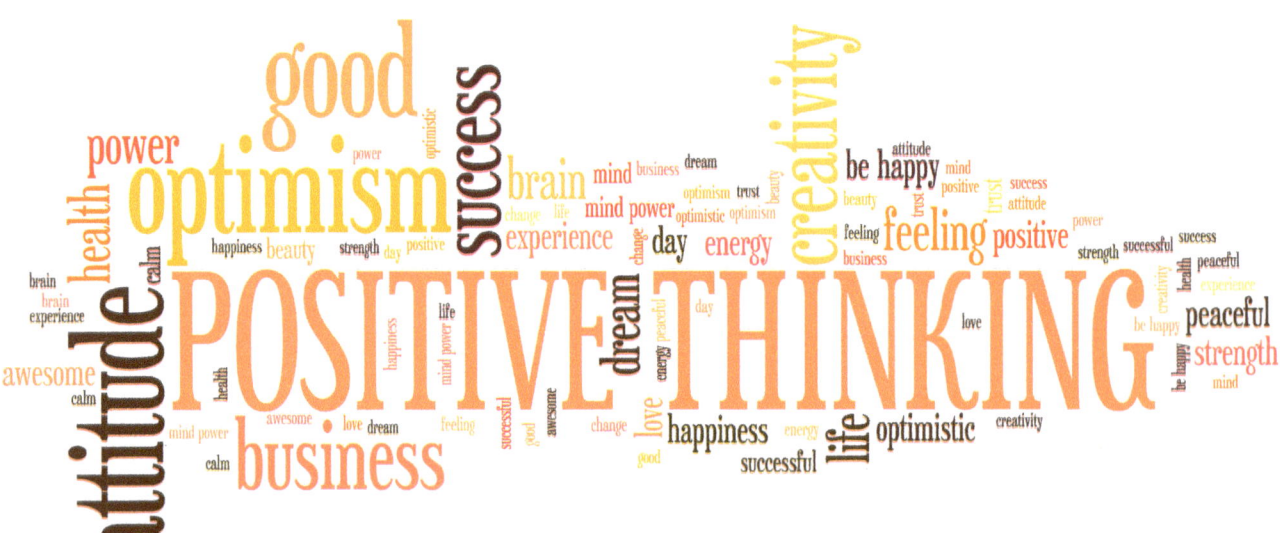

POSITIVE WORDS

Aware	Valued	Successful	Fair-minded
Authentic	Unity	Friendly	Forgiving
Loving	Conscious	Powerful	Enthusiastic
Divine	Driven	Confident	Graceful
Grateful	Good-listener	Humorous	Willing
Tender	Content	Intuitive	Trusting
Oneness	Patient	Graceful	Believing
Beautiful	Nice	Joyful	Stable
Worthy	Determined	Sacred	Loyal
Loving-kindness	Optimistic	Playful	Visionary
Self-love	Good Attitude	Bright	Sincere
Funny	Non-judgment	Light	Altruistic
Cheerful	Strong	Enough	Hopeful
Positive	Helpful	Faithful	Receptive
Sublime	Fortunate	Relaxed	Open-minded
Compassionate	Free-spirited	Well	Abundant
Honorable	Smart	Healthy	Grounded
Generous	Resourceful	Serene	Excited
Enlightened	Competent	Glad	Glowing
Active	Effective	Loving	Natural
Blissful	Independent	Loved	Truthful
Astute	Focused	Inspired	Calm
Affable	Balanced	Empowered	Delightful
Connected	Unity	Clear	Brilliant
Charismatic	Peaceful	Confident	Courageous
Uplifting	Creative	Happy	Imaginative
Genuine	Bright	Motivated	
Passionate	Enjoyable	Brave	
Dreamer	Good	Genuine	
Intention	Gentle	Soulful	

Thank a Farmer, Baker, and Cheese Maker

Thank a farmer, baker, or cheesemaker by writing them a thank you note, drawing them a picture, or making some other gesture that reflects your genuine gratitude. Let them know that you think they are doing exceptional work. There are plenty of farmers and other folks that provide our communities with food who would love to hear from school kids.

The farmers and food producers bring us abundance in variety and quality foods. If you are motivated, you can go on field trips to visit food providers. A visit goes above and beyond as a show of gratitude and is a terrific way of building community awareness.

Start thanking your local farms and food producers from your town or nearby communities. Then spread the love and gratitude to larger food businesses.

WHO TO THANK?

- Local organic farms
- Cheesemakers
- Grocery stores
- Community markets
- Cafes
- Community food banks
- Bakeries
- Coffee roasters
- Dairies
- Chicken ranchers
- Organic cattle ranchers
- Teachers
- Parents
- Friends
- Local businesses
- Restaurants
- …And other wonderful people and places that supply your food.

Draw, Sketch, Paint, and Illustrate Fruits and Vegetables

MATERIALS

- Colored pencils
- Crayons
- Acrylic paints
- Magic markers
- Watercolors
- Pastels
- Canvas
- Paper
- Watercolor paper
- Paintbrushes
- Pencil sharpener
- Paint pallets
- Water for cleaning brushes

STILL LIFE WITH FRUITS AND VEGETABLES

Explore with your class the enormous variety of fruits and vegetables found in our world and the exciting possibilities of capturing their beauty and uniqueness through creating art. View common fruits and vegetables as well as more exotic fruits and vegetables.

Find an image from the internet or magazine, take a photo, arrange a trip to the farmers market or grocery store, or bring in a fresh example.

Choose the medium you will be using, provide instruction on proper use, and then get to creating art!

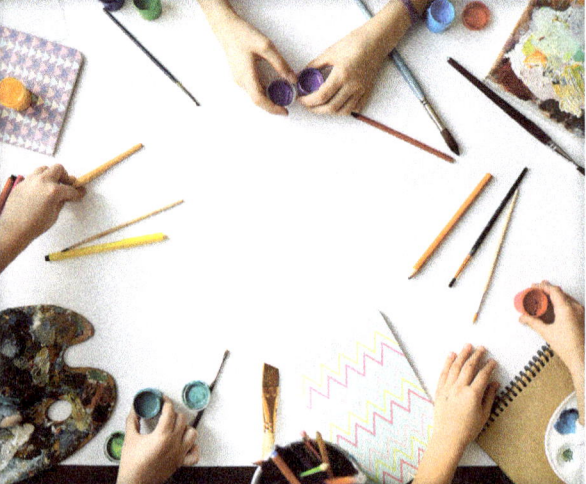

Food Tree Decoupage Collage

Make a collage of The Food Tree with images of what an optimal days-worth of eating looks like. Use photos and graphics that are taken from magazines. Include all meals and snacks based on The Food Tree and The Five Food Groups. Creating a collage is a free and open to interpretation exercise. Students are encouraged to explore what they might want to eat if they could create all of their meals for a day while focusing on positive, healthy choices.

MATERIALS

- Scissors
- Glue sticks, rubber cement, art glue,
- Cooking magazines or other print media to cut out images of healthy foods

DIRECTIONS

1. Cut out images of healthy foods from health and positive lifestyle magazines.
2. Glue images on the tree to represent what a healthy day of eating looks like.

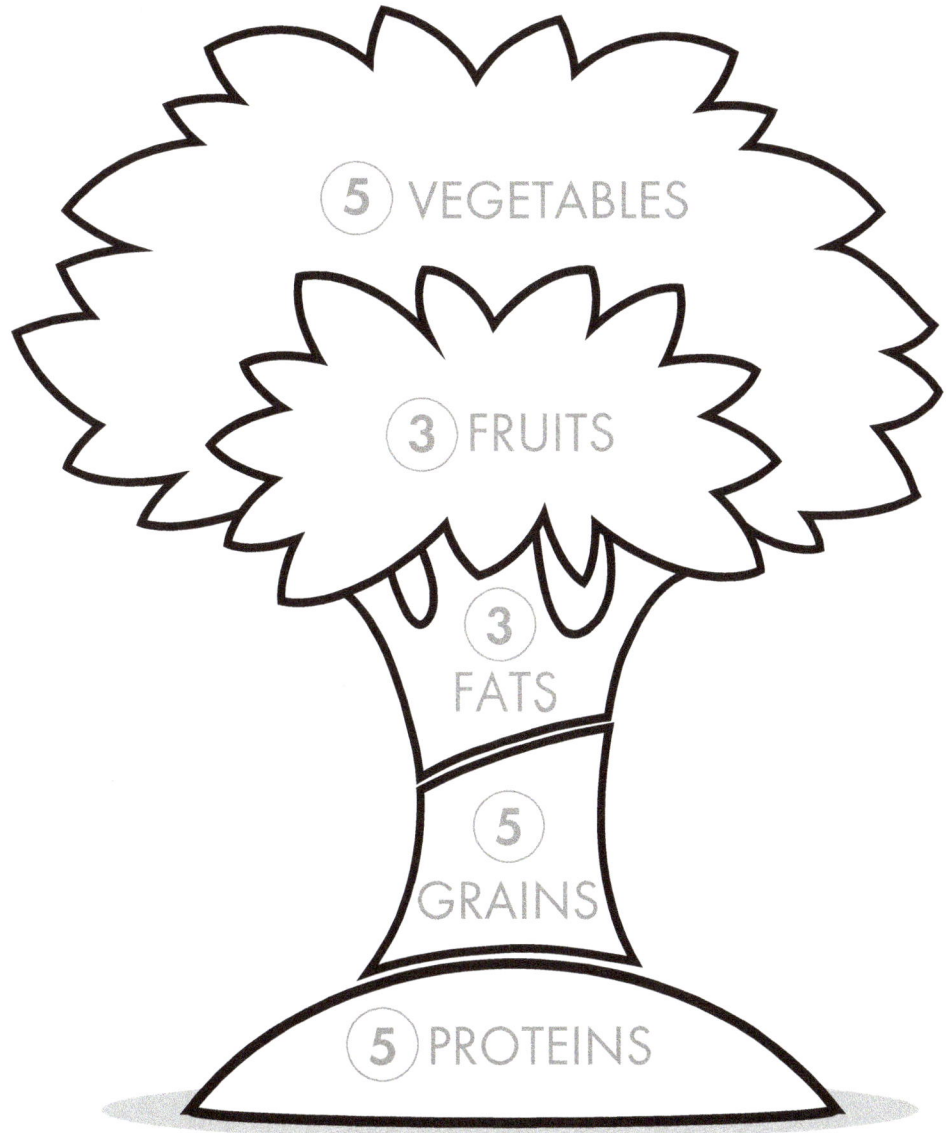

Permission to reproduce. ©The Food Tree

Taste the Rainbow

MATERIALS

- Examples of a variety of fruits and vegetables from all color groups—ROYGBV
- Small cups or plates
- Toothpicks
- Napkins
- Knife
- Cutting board
- Taste the Rainbow Taste Test Sheet

GOALS

Boost knowledge about how different fruits and vegetables taste.

OBJECTIVES

- To sample a variety of fruits and vegetables from each rainbow color group
- To differentiate tastes of fruits and vegetables
- To craft your own rainbow taste test

DISCUSSION

Become a real-life food taster. The best way to grow up healthy and strong is to eat a rainbow of fruits and vegetables every day. Vitamins and minerals are abundant in veggies and fruits. The color in the plants tells you that they have lots of phytonutrients in them.

DIRECTIONS

Encourage your students to choose from a variety of new and favorite colorful fruits and vegetables to include in your tasting. Visit the farmers market or take a trip to your local community grocery store to find fruits and vegetables to try.

Set up a chart on your whiteboard or chalkboard that mimics this reproducible form. Ask students to help fill in the table. You can have them fill in their chart first, or you can fill in the chart together on the board.

Cut fruits and veggies into bite-sized pieces. Provide students with natural toothpicks or dry spaghetti broken into toothpicks size, plates, and napkins.

1. Serve each food by itself, either raw or cooked.
2. Encourage students to look at each piece of food with fresh eyes while leaving behind any past judgments about it.
3. Touch, smell, and taste the food sample.
4. For a twist, have students take a bite with their eyes closed, slowly chewing so that they can concentrate on the taste of the food.
5. Taste and rate the foods.
6. As they talk about various foods, prompt them to use descriptive words such as sweet, crunchy, juicy, tangy, or spicy rather than yucky, okay, or good.
7. After the tasting exercise, lead an informal discussion about the fruits and vegetables the students liked, those they didn't like, and those they would try again.
8. Ask if this exercise helped any of them discover new flavors or foods that they previously thought they didn't like.

VARIATIONS

Grab your friends, classmates, and family and get them involved in the fun food tasting. Some additional ways to experiment with taste testing are by doing a comparing/contrasting session. For instance, compare a granny smith apple to a gala apple, or compare a green bell pepper to a red bell pepper. Or, invite everyone to do taste testing blindfolded.

ASSESSMENT

- After the tasting exercise, lead a discussion about fruits and vegetables the students liked, those they didn't like, and those they've not tried.
- Did this exercise help any of you discover new flavors that you would want to try again?

THE FOOD TREE

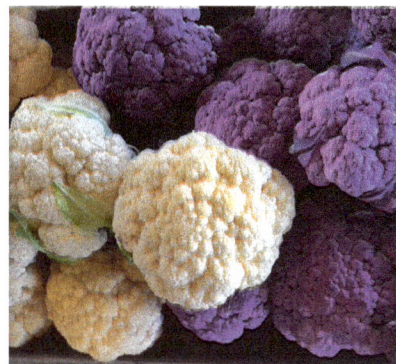 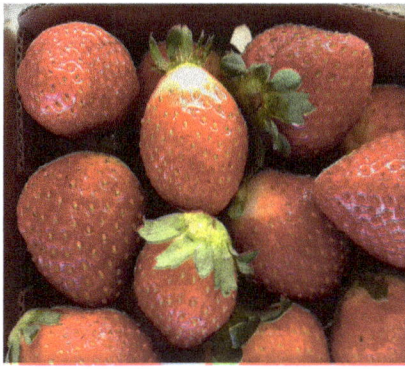 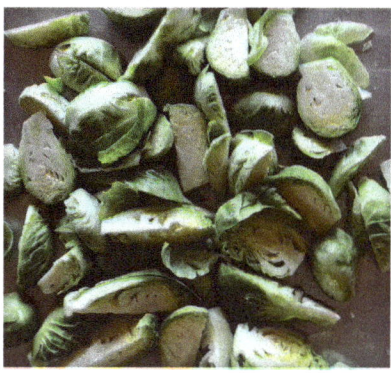

TASTE THE RAINBOW TASTE TEST

COLORFUL FRUITS AND VEGETABLES	RAW OR COOKED?	DESCRIBE THE FLAVOR/TEXTURE	DID YOU LIKE IT?	WILL YOU TRY IT AGAIN?
RED 1. Strawberries 2. Tomatoes				
Orange 1. Orange 2. Carrot/Sweet potato				
Yellow 1. Pineapple 2. Yellow peppers				
Green 1. Kiwi 2. Broccoli/kale				
Blue 1. Blueberries 2. Purple potato				
Purple 1. Fig 2. Purple beets				
White 1. Banana 2. Jicama				

Permission to reproduce. ©The Food Tree

TASTE THE RAINBOW TASTE TEST

COLORFUL FRUITS AND VEGETABLES	RAW OR COOKED?	DESCRIBE THE FLAVOR/TEXTURE	DID YOU LIKE IT?	WILL YOU TRY IT AGAIN?
RED 1. 2.				
ORANGE 1. 2.				
YELLOW 1. 2.				
GREEN 1. 2.				
BLUE 1. 2.				
PURPLE 1. 2.				
WHITE 1. 2.				

Permission to reproduce. ©The Food Tree

THE FIVE FOOD GROUP'S MATCH-UP

	PROTEINS	WHOLE GRAINS	HEALTHY FATS	VEGETABLES	FRUITS
APRICOTS					
SALMON					
OATMEAL					
AVOCADO					
ONION					
BLUEBERRIES					
BROWN RICE					
LENTILS					
YOGURT					
POPCORN					
TOFU					
OLIVE OIL					
KALE					
WHEAT					
CHICKEN					
YAM					

Permission to reproduce. ©The Food Tree

Observing Oxidation

MATERIALS
- Apple, banana, or potato
- A piece of iron, cast iron pan, nail
- Lemon juice
- Worksheet titled "Oxidation."
- Complimentary lesson: Earthing

GOAL
Understand the connection of cellular oxidation in humans to the oxidation of common household items, like fruit or metal.

OBJECTIVE
- To explain the action of oxidation, which is the reaction of materials like fruit or metal when exposed to oxygen

ACTIVATING PRIOR KNOWLEDGE
Discuss a time when students have noticed apple slices or raw potato turn brown. Exposure to oxygen will oxidize fruit, like apples or bananas, and turn them brown.

BACKGROUND INFORMATION
Oxidation is the name of a chemical exchange that occurs when a molecule, like a metal nail or a freshly cut apple, is exposed to oxygen. The element releases an electron molecule, thus becoming vulnerable to rust or in the case of people, a cause of damage to cells. Oxidation forms free radicals that cause a cascade of injury to tissues, cells, and DNA. Oxidation also happens when cooking oils are exposed to air and can then become rancid. Oxidation will change the color of the food or oil and may decrease the food's nutritional values.

PROCEDURE 1
1. Create and hand out the worksheet titled *Oxidation Tally Sheet*.
2. Give students one-fourth of an apple.
3. Ask students to write down the current time.
4. Then, immediately draw the apple section and describe the appearance.
5. Every ten minutes (for a minimum of 1 hour), have students observe their apple and document (draw and write) any changes they see.
6. As a class, have student participate in a discussion based on documented observation.

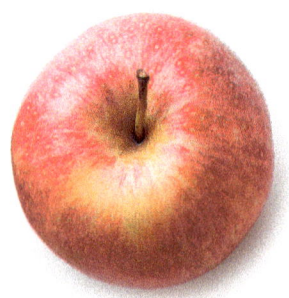
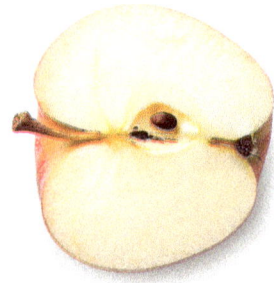
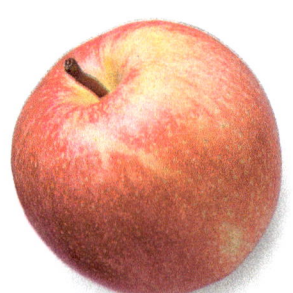
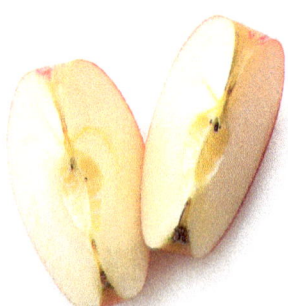

Milk Color Burst Experiment

In this experiment, students explore what happens when dish soap is introduced to milk using food coloring to illustrate the molecular dance!

MATERIALS

- Cow milk: choose at least two types of milk with differing fat contents
  - Half and half
  - Full Fat
  - 2%
  - Skim
  - Fat-Free
- Food coloring or food dye
- Liquid dish soap
- Measuring cups
- Cotton swabs
- Shallow round ceramic dishes, saucers, or shallow sturdy paper plates with a lip
- Scientific Method Sheet located at the end of this section

EXPERIMENTAL PROCEDURE

Discuss the elements found in dairy milk. Talk about what might happen when other elements, like dish soap, are introduced.

Identify Controls

Controls are the materials in the experiment that will stay the same.

Identify Variables

Variables are the materials that will change during each trial.

For example, have students record on the Scientific Method Sheet:

- Amount of milk
- Type of milk
- Type of vessel used
- Type and amount of dish soap used
- Colors used

Write a Hypothesis

Have students create their hypothesis before executing the experiment and write it on the Food Tree Scientific Method Sheet.

Conduct Research

1. Measure the amount of milk you need to cover the bottom surface of your plate completely. Allow the milk to settle so that there are no bubbles.
2. Drop one drop of the food coloring in the milk around the outer edges of the plate. Use four colors in the pattern of 12, 3, 6, and 9 on a clock, or if using five colors, space the dots equidistant apart.
3. Take a cotton swab and dip it into the milk in the center of the vessel.
4. Do not stir the colors around nor disturb the milk in the vessel!!
5. Record observations.
6. Next, add a drop of dish soap onto the end of a clean, dry, cotton swab.
7. Dip the soapy end into the center of the dish. Hold the swab in place for 10-15 seconds.
8. Do not stir or mix the milk and colors around or disturb the vessel.
9. Record observations.
10. Repeat putting the soap on the end of the swab.
11. Record observations.
12. Perform the experiment again using all clean materials with a different type of milk.

Analyze Data

Which type of milk burst the most and under what conditions?

Write a Conclusion

Was your hypothesis correct, partially correct, or totally off base? Explain why or why not. Why did the food coloring move around? What created the changes in the milk when it was exposed to the soap?

WHAT IS REALLY GOING ON!

Milk is made up of different components including:

87%	Water
13%	Proteins
4-5%	Fats (lipids and triglycerides)
5%	Sugar (lactose)

When the soap gets placed in the milk, it alters the chemical bonds of the proteins and fats. The soap molecules, or micelles, distribute the fat molecules around the dish. Soap is both hydrophilic and hydrophobic. It both attracts water and repels it. The soaps water opposing end attaches to the milk fat globule. When the cotton swab inserts into the milk, it causes a break in the surface tension, which prompts the chemical bonds to change and distribute the fat molecules into different and interesting patterns.

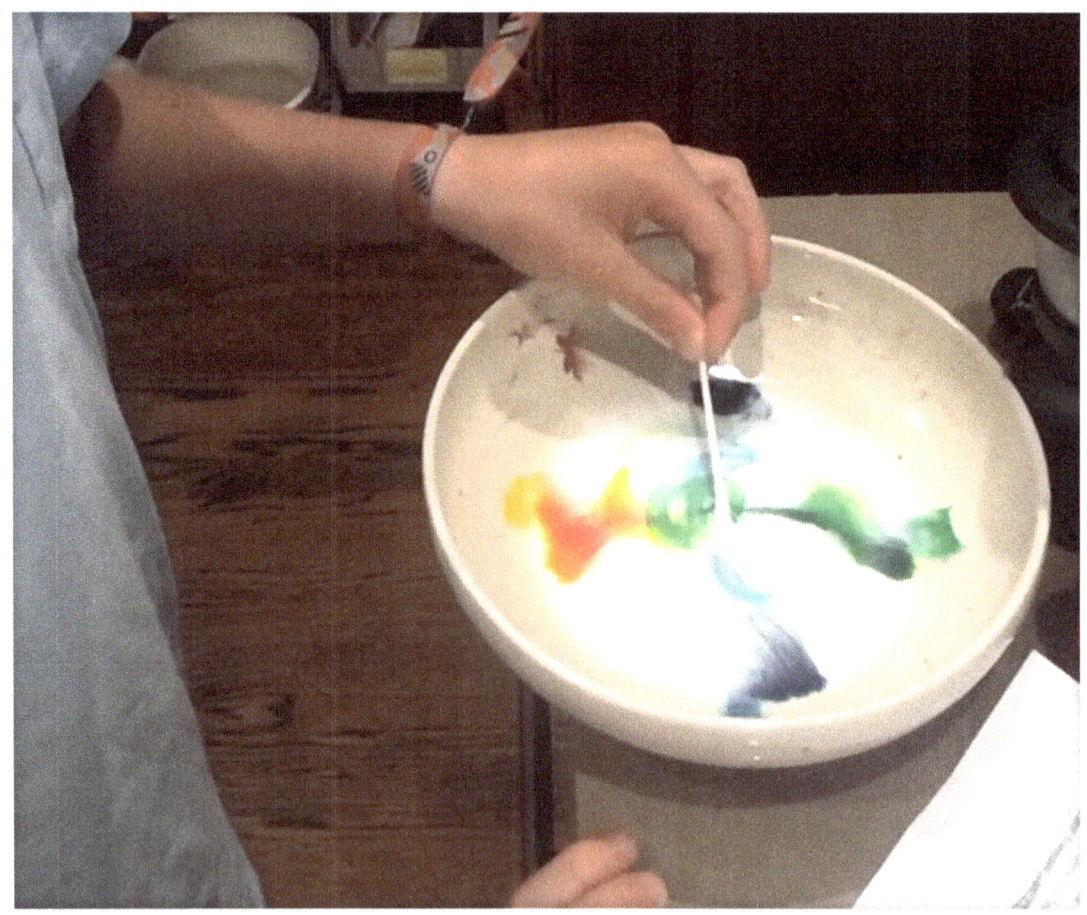

POWER PROTEINS

Circle the names of powerful proteins. Search for the words up, down, forwards, and backwards.

```
B Y B A Z R A J R Y U F O T S J Z X E S
J O W L Q K P M I R H S R R O U B U K D
M S P I R U L I N A A E U M J U V X N E
Z F Y B N S D A M S W U Q K M P Q W K E
K Z F B F Y M T K Z M G U V I S U V Q S
P T Y Y R X E K K O S D N O M L A J M P
I B D J P U F M K W U X Y W K I Z V K M
N B A F K A V Z X B N A U C E T M A V E
T K W J M R P I X K F Q J P A N D V J H
O F B V K L J Z J O L C S G G E E X J Z
B V Z R Q Z F H W P O N F D W L P G J R
E M G S U X D E L Q W L X I A K C W Z A
A H H N I U J P L L E I P G O W P A U O
N W U P N O F M N K R F D S I B W A W N
S V M N O V U E D S S U Y K J I Q P L R
K D G S A Y H T C J E J A J V N S E S F
M I W K D T P E S E E H C I I C Q Z N E
R Q X S B V M M P M D P J S W E H S A C
V S E Z I S C N B R S H E G I C F R E H
A R R Y R D T S W S A Q I T E H H U B C
```

ALMONDS	BEANS	CASHEWS
CHEESE	EGGS	HEMP SEEDS
LENTILS	PINTO BEANS	QUINOA
SHRIMP	SOY	SPIRULINA
SUNFLOWER SEEDS	TEMPEH	TOFU

Permission to reproduce. ©The Food Tree

NUTRITIOUS NUTS AND SCRUMPTIOUS SEEDS

Circle the names of nuts and seeds. Search for the words up, down, forwards, and backwards.

```
M J J M I W B B N U E B T V W S K O N S
R T N L F S J M U F S F I D V G H Y D N
U U Z F B A I M A D A C A M H O O R I W
Z N A C E P M N Z C M N I K P M U P K U
M L K N O Q W N K N E I B Z S Z I N N A
K E A N S S A Q M F O U T D L K B L G B
E Z U Y P W L S N B R A Z I L W P U I T
X A L F G W N V Y I N N L A I M O Y U Q
C H G N M G U E O H E M P L P Q M M L M
V O R Z Q U T F C D B O V M X D E G U V
Q N T M V I A I H C N J H O S M G E R G
E L P J S N E E M L W J B N D N R N R F
A O E Q B Q L D V Z Q N N D G N A G G X
F D A Q A R E W O L F N U S M C N K O P
T U N O C O C F S P U G B K G F A E N K
F Z U F C H E S T N U T B D P J T W V G
W X T X R Q L V X C E T P K U Y E I Y L
Y C Z P O P P Y W S R Y P I N E N U T N
D C A S H E W F R B O I H C A T S I P V
```

ALMONDS	BRAZIL	CASHEW
CHESTNUT	CHIA	COCONUT
FLAX	HAZELNUT	HEMP
MACADAMIA	PEANUT	PECAN
PINENUT	PISTACHIO	POMEGRANATE
POPPY	PUMPKIN	SESAME
SUNFLOWER	WALNUT	

Permission to reproduce. ©The Food Tree

HELLO WHOLE GRAINS

Circle the names of healthy whole grains. Search for the words up, down, forwards, and backwards.

```
Y S O Z B K E F M N L V B O L H F W I J
Y C P X Q Y B K O R A F B P W T W T Q W
C I D C U T E N R I C E G T Q N Y A Z B
D F E W I J S S M X U H U E M A T E H E
M L C D N K B I M S B J E Y L R I H S S
B D O T O J L V V K F J W R M A W W F U
V N O A A P L W I I R V Q A I M E K L O
I Q Z E V C U D X F V D J X N A B C D C
R P D H F B B S R U Y T F G T O K U I S
E S N W D L J R G A P C W U W S P B B U
A U R T W S H Q V Z Z M R L D S T V F O
R B O U Y N V Y O I R C B Q O L M A V C
E F C M I L L E T M L K T C I A G B V V
W J P A R U G L U B Y V S E T K H V L A
H T L K I R T R E E E S P K X I V O P T
J E B F O G B A A V G E B T H M W A X D
D J S O V U V B C L C C Y Z U C O T I Y
Y V F G U W X H D Y E B P W D X W S O P
X M A I F P S P E L T W J Y A F N L E K
S K B G R G R A S D U X N V M C R S R K
```

AMARANTH	BARLEY	BUCKWHEAT
BULGUR	CORN	COUSCOUS
FARO	KAMUT	MILLET
OATS	QUINOA	RICE
RYE	SPELT	WHEAT

Permission to reproduce. ©The Food Tree

FABULOUS FATS

Circle the names of healthy fats. Search for the words up, down, forwards, and backwards.

```
E U K S D E E S A I H C Q W X V U Q U A
D X L L E V V Q K Z W E D C M E M A N L
K L F A X R E T T U B M S Q O I G T H N
Q P G M O O T L H C L W R Z I S I R K U
C E O E H B Z F Y P Q N Z S G G E U R T
X A L F K F G O F L A Z L O T E N G C S
L N O D T Q V G Z E A H F Y Q C J O A S
E U P E M W K R F I W T Z B F P G Y U H
Y T R V K T T A M K M U D E E W A E S A
E S C C F K B P Q Y Z N X A A Z S S N J
H Z D H D Q Q E Y G S O N N C N T L T J
G R L K B T R S P N W C G Z L S G R B U
Z Z K A G L K E X O O O O I A N G D V Q
M M L S H B J E G M D C Q U X E J U X M
A P N Q B O K D E L A O C W Y E Y K Y Z
D E G W V A P O A A C B J A A R N S I I
F O O E G B D I M S O I X A Y G V O H K
Y W I Z P J Z L K U V O L I V E O I L R
Q Q L M I C K T R D A B H K Q C B Z A A
```

AVOCADO	BUTTER	CHIA SEEDS
COCONUT	EGGS	FLAX
GRAPESEED OIL	GREENS	OLIVE OIL
PEANUTS	SALMON	SEAWEED
SOYBEAN	WALNUTS	YOGURT

Permission to reproduce. ©The Food Tree

FRUITS AND VEGETABLES

Circle the names of fruits and vegetables. Search for the words up, down, forwards, and backwards.

```
E Z E Q H Q Z R U L V U V A R Y H C K U
K N O K O X L Y K L U G R H A E H V C O
T C A R R O T L B A G E E H K H I E R Q
W J G G A L K M W P G Z P I R B D D J J
L N M A N U I F Z R N B L U E B E R R Y
V J M M G M W E N I R A T C E N X V I O
F U F X E A I X S C O P Z L Z P O P K X
S X N B N G P X P O P O C E V R A M O J
T N A L P G G E N T N L O L P B G Y N T
R P A P A Y A T N Q T T N P K J W T H D
A E R X U F A I M P Q R S P I N A C H W
W G Q W L H R F T E H Q X A S Y J M I T
B H J T J U B G F A U M A G O N I O N E
E A M I R Q C I H V O C I G B L C W T E
R E N F T S A H J G R I U D V E A D H B
R G S O Z K B X J I C A M A E M K R G Q
Y L P G O K B O Y M G Z F N I O L L G J
N Y B T N W A E X F T R O K Y N T Z Q L
C D O V O L G R E P P E P A N U Y E Y O
W A T E R M E L O N P X F T O M A T O D
```

APRICOT	BEET	CABBAGE
CARROT	EGGPLANT	KIWI
LEMON	NECTARINE	ONION
ORANGE	PAPAYA	PEA
PEPPER	SPINACH	STRAWBERRY
TOMATO	WATERMELON	

Permission to reproduce. ©The Food Tree

PLANT PART MATCHING

Match the fruit or vegetable listed in the column below to the plant part that it comes from. Some fruits and vegetables may have two or even three edible plant parts.

PLANT	FRUIT	FLOWER	LEAF	STEM	ROOT	SEED
Peas						
Arugula						
Asparagus						
Parsley						
Celery						
Cucumber						
Carrot						
Onion						
Artichoke						
Sweet potato						
Kale						
Mango						
Lettuce						
Zucchini						
Broccoli						
Pineapple						
Beet						
Chili peppers						
Strawberry						
Tomato						

Permission to reproduce. ©The Food Tree

DIY pH Papers

Making pH test papers is a fun, affordable, and an easy-to-do science project. The papers test pH levels in liquids, soil, or saliva.

MATERIALS

- Red cabbage
- Cutting board
- Knife
- Pot
- Water
- Purple cabbage
- Blender or Cuisinart (optional)
- Coffee filters or thin porous paper
- Stove or microwave
- Glass bowl
- Cookie sheet
- String
- Clothespins

BACKGROUND INFORMATION

Budding scientists can test different liquid mediums to determine its pH level using paper dyed with red cabbage juice. There is a natural element found in red cabbage, the flavonoid anthocyanin, that happens to be a natural pH indicator. How cool is that?!

The abbreviation pH stands for potential or power of hydrogen. It is a measurement of the hydrogen ions found within a solution and identifies the acidity the acidity or alkalinity within a material. When you drop the test medium onto the pH cabbage paper, it will change color depending on the acidity or alkalinity of the solution. A more acidic solution will turn the anthocyanin in the paper a red color, a neutral solution will appear to turn the paper a blue-purplish color, and a basic pH solution will turn the paper a greenish-yellow color.

THE CHEMISTRY

The changes in color have to do with the juice reacting to changes in its hydrogen ion concentration. Acidic solutions give up hydrogen molecules and alkaline, also known as base, solutions take on hydrogen molecules.

The pH values range in number from 1-14. Acidity is in the lower ranges, with one being the most acidic, and basic being the highest numbers, with seven as the neutral point in the middle of the range.

HOW TO MAKE PH TESTING PAPERS

1. Chop a red cabbage finely or use a blender or food processor.
2. Add the cabbage to a saucepan and heat with just a little bit of water to make a small amount of liquid.
3. Cook over low heat for ten minutes.
4. Let cool for ten minutes.
5. Strain the liquid through a strainer, coffee filter, or cheesecloth.
6. Soak the coffee filter or filter paper in the concentrated cabbage juice liquid for a few hours and hang to dry on a line of string using clothespins or dry on cookie sheets. Note that this may stain clothes, hands, or a white surface.
7. When dry, cut the paper into test strips.
8. Using liquid of your choice, take a dropper or popsicle stick and drop liquid onto the test strips.
9. Tip—do not dip the cabbage strips into your test solution because the juice will get into the material as the paper is not colorfast.

PH TESTING PROCEDURE

Demonstrate how pH balance is impacted by testing saliva with the pH litmus paper. The pH will change depending on if a person is registering as more acidic or alkaline. The minerals found in vegetables will create a more alkaline ash. The pH ash is the result of the food tending towards acidity, balance, or alkaline. Please note that if you tested the pH of lemon juice, it

> ### NEAT FACT!
> Cabbage grown in more acidic soil will have a reddish-purple color, whereas cabbage grown in alkaline soils will have a greenish-yellow color.

would be extremely acidic, yet when eaten, its ash in the human body will be more alkaline.

Have the students test their saliva, then eat a piece of celery or raw kale, and then test again.

Examples of base foods are baking soda and almonds. Examples of acidic foods are vinegar and lemon juice.

OPTIMAL PH SALIVARY RANGES

Optimal saliva pH levels are between 6.75–7.25.

CABBAGE JUICE TEST STRIPS COLOR INDICATORS FOR PH RANGES

PH	2	4	6	8	10	12
COLOR	RED	PURPLE	VIOLET	BLUE	BLUE/GREEN	GREEN/YELLOW

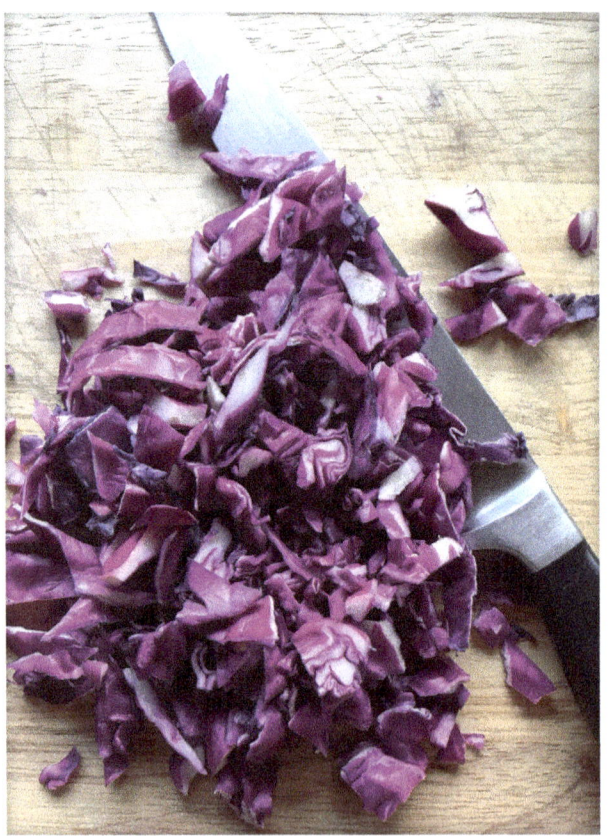

PH RANGES FOR FOODS AND DRINKS

Alkaline-Forming Foods
- Almond
- Amaranth
- Apricot
- Avocado
- Blackstrap molasses
- Brazil nut
- Buckwheat
- Chestnut
- Coconut (fresh)
- Date
- Fig
- Fruits, most
- Grape
- Grapefruit
- Green herbs
- Herbal tea
- Honey
- Leafy greens
- Lemon
- Lima bean
- Maple syrup
- Melon
- Millet
- Mineral or spring water
- Orange
- Quinoa
- Raisin
- Seaweed
- Soaked nuts
- Soy/tempeh
- Sprouted beans
- Sprouted seeds
- Vegetables
- Wheatgrass

Acid-Forming Foods
- Alcohol
- Asparagus
- Bread and Pasta
- Brussels sprouts
- Butter
- Cheeses
- Chickpeas
- Cocoa
- Coffee
- Cornstarch
- Dried beans and peas (most)
- Egg
- Fish
- Flour products
- Fried food
- Fruit (canned/glazed)
- Fruit (dried and sulfured)
- Grain (rye, white rice)
- Ice cream
- Ketchup
- Legumes
- Lentils
- Meat
- Milk
- Mustard
- Noodles
- Nuts (cashew, pecan, peanut)
- Oatmeal
- Olives
- Pepper
- Poultry
- Refined sugar
- Sauerkraut
- Seafood
- Soft drink
- Strawberry, cranberry, pomegranate
- Tea
- Tofu

Neutral Foods
- Almond
- Avocado
- Brazil nut
- Brown rice
- Butter
- Coconut
- Corn
- Cruciferous vegetables
- Flax, hemp, sesame, sunflower, pumpkin seed
- Goat cheese
- Honey
- Nonfat milk
- Raw milk products
- Vegetable oil

Grow Plants from Kitchen Scraps

Growing plants from kitchen scraps is a fun, fascinating, and invaluable activity. This simple gardening act will be sure to impress and create a lasting memory. Save your cuttings, stems, and seeds and grow your kitchen scrap garden.

AVOCADO

Growing an avocado tree from a pit is as easy as making guacamole. Seriously, it IS easy! When you sprout the seed, it will be unclear if it will be a clone of the parent avocado that will produce fruit or if it will be its unique tree, meaning it may not produce fruit. Either way, a lovely tree will grow. Be forewarned that avocado trees do require frequent deep watering.

1. Rinse a fresh avocado pit.
2. Place three toothpicks along the middle of the pit so you can rest the pit in a glass jar or cup of water.
3. Place the pointy side into the water.
4. When there are a few sets of leaves, bring outside in mixed light to acclimate.
5. In one week, plant outside in full sun.
6. Water well.

BASIL

1. Take the stem off a basil plant and gently remove the bottom few leaves.
2. Make sure at least four leaves are remaining on the top of the stem.
3. Place the basil stem in a small glass of water with at least one node (the spot where a leaf grew) submerged underwater.
4. Place in a sunny spot and watch the roots and plant grow.
5. When the stem has a robust cluster of roots, plant in the garden.

CELERY, BOK CHOY, ROMAINE LETTUCE, CABBAGE

1. Cut off two to three inches from the bottom end of the bunch.
2. Place the butt of the vegetable in a shallow dish of water.
3. Leave in a brightly lit area out of direct sunlight.
4. Change water every day.
5. Spray with water every few days to keep fresh.
6. Watch for rootlets to form.
7. Once a nice set of roots form, plant out in the garden or in a pot.
8. Water in and watch new vegetables grow tall and delicious.

GARLIC

1. Break apart a garlic bulb and remove the cloves.
2. Take individual cloves and plant them one inch below the soil surface with the blunt end or root-end facing down into a well-prepared garden bed.
3. Tamp down gently and water in.

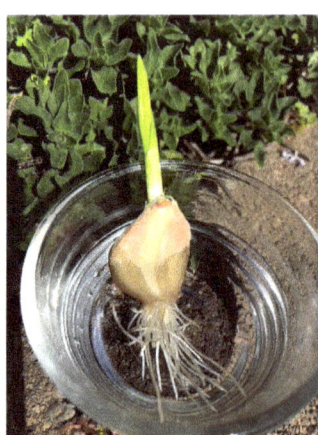

GINGER

1. Prepare a container with organic potting soil.
2. Lay a piece of ginger flat on the soil.
3. Place the root stubs so that any new buds are facing up.
4. Sprinkle with garden soil to anchor in place.
5. Water in and keep in a warm place with indirect sunlight.

GREEN ONIONS

1. Clean off any dead, damaged, or mushy leaves.
2. Cut one inch off the tip, or root-end, of the green onion, leaving the roots.
3. Place the stubs in an inch of water in a small dish, glass, or jar.
4. Make sure the roots are always submerged underwater.

5. Keep onions in bright light but out of direct sunlight.
6. Change water daily.
7. Green onion shoots will start emerging from the tips.
8. When the shoots grow a few inches, they are ready to be planted or eaten!
9. Plant in a pot or plant directly into the garden.
10. Water in gently.
11. They can grow for years.

LEEK

1. Buy leeks at your local grocery store or farmers market.
2. Remove any brown, damaged, or mushy leaves.
3. Cut the bottom inch off of the leek, leaving a good inch, including the roots.
4. Plant the leek in full sun in a well-prepared garden or container that is at least 8-10 inches deep.
5. Water in and watch them grow!

LEMONGRASS

Lemongrass is a tender perennial native to tropical climates, like Thailand. They are easy to propagate.

1. Buy lemongrass from your local grocery store or farmers market.
2. Peel off any dead or damaged leaves.
3. Place the lemongrass stalk in a drinking glass or mason jar with about an inch of water.
4. When a nice cluster of roots form, plant the lemongrass in a well-prepared garden bed or a large pot in full sun.
5. Keep well-watered.
6. Cut back and mulch soil in the fall.
7. In case there is a threat of frost, protect plants by covering with burlap.
8. Or, dig up the cluster, plant in a large container, and bring indoors! Keep plants in a sunny south-facing window.
9. Harvest lemongrass when 12" tall.

FENNEL

1. Clean off any dead, damaged, or mushy leaves.
2. Cut one inch off the root end.
3. Place the fennel bulb in an inch of water in a small dish or jar.
4. Change water daily.
5. Make sure roots are always submerged.
6. Keep in bright light but out of direct sunlight.
7. When roots begin to grow, plant in a deep container or in the garden with well-draining soil. However, planting in a permanent location is best because fennel doesn't fare well when its roots are disturbed
8. Water it gently.
9. This herb likes warm weather.

ONION—RED, WHITE, AND YELLOW

1. Cut off two to three inches from the bottom root end of the onion.
2. Place in the garden, leaving the tip out.
3. Water well.

PINEAPPLE

1. Slice off the top off of the pineapple at the base of the leaves.
2. Pluck off about 5 inches of leaves starting at the cut part and working your way up.
3. Then cut off the end, about 3 inches, removing all of the fruit.
4. Stick 3–4 toothpicks into the side of the plant two inches from the base and place in a jar or plastic container in a little water so that the bottom end is just barely submerged.
5. Leave in a sunny spot.
6. Change the water every two to three days or as needed to keep fresh and bottom submerged.
7. The roots will start to emerge in about ten days.
8. After a total of 30 days, the pineapple is ready to plant in a garden container.
9. Prepare a container with organic potting soil and place the pineapple in a little hole. Backfill with soil and tamp down gently.

10. Water well and then water every few days, allowing the soil to dry out between watering.
11. Leave in a semi-shady spot during the year and bring indoors at any danger of frost.
12. It could take 2-3 years to see any blooms and fruit, so be patient.

POTATOES, SWEET POTATOES, AND YAMS

1. Get your hands on a firm potato. Red potato, yellow potato, blue potato, yam, russet potato, and sweet potato. Any variety will do.
2. Slice off a chunk with a few eyes (the spot where a root would grow from). Let dry for 1–3 days.
3. Plant spuds a few inches below the soil in a large container like a wine barrel, raised bed, or directly in the garden.
4. Watch and wait for new potatoes to grow!

RASPBERRY

1. Remove seeds from a fresh raspberry by smooshing the fruit in a fine-mesh sieve.
2. Carefully rinse off all the flesh to get to the seeds.
3. Dry seeds on a paper towel.
4. Fill a small pot with soil, leaving an inch from the top.
5. Sprinkle seeds on the soil and cover with ¼ inch of soil.
6. Leave the container in a warm, sunny spot.
7. Water and keep lightly moist.
8. When plants grow a few true leaves, transplant outside in a sunny location.

STRAWBERRY

1. Pick the seeds out of a fresh strawberry by removing them with a toothpick. You can also push the fruit through a fine mesh sieve.
2. Carefully rinse off all the flesh to get to the seeds.
3. Dry the seeds on a paper towel.
4. Fill a small pot with soil, leaving an inch reservoir from the top.
5. Sprinkle the strawberry seeds on top of the soil and cover with ¼ inch of soil.
6. Water and keep lightly moist.
7. Leave the container in a warm sunny spot.
8. Watch the plants grow!
9. When the seedling grows a few true leaves, transplant outside in sunny location.

TOMATO

1. Fill a garden container ¾ with damp potting soil.
2. Slice tomato into thirds, horizontally.
3. Place the slice of tomato in the container and cover with an inch of potting soil.
4. Water in well.
5. Leave the container in a warm, sunny spot.
6. Keep lightly watered.
7. Watch for little sprouts to come up in a few days.
8. When each plant has a few true leaves, divide very carefully and plant each seedling separately in containers or plant directly into a well-prepared garden bed in full sun.

DIY: Sprouts and Microgreens

A simple, fun, and cost-effective way to grow nutrient-dense foods is to grow sprouts and microgreens. Growing sprouts is one of the simplest and satisfying food and garden projects you can do with children. It may lead them to actually like little green things! I mean, come on! Who wouldn't want to nibble on home-grown spouts?

Sprouts are a perfect snack to eat with lunches, for snacks, and anytime you want a quick energy boost. Microgreens, like sunflower seeds, are super crunchy and have a sweet, nutty taste. They grow best in a soil medium in a shallow tray, unlike sprouts that grow best in a glass jar.

And, would I be remiss if I didn't say that microgreens and sprouts are so good for you? Yes! They are power-packed with antioxidant phytochemicals that add longevity to your life. They thwart the ravages of time.

My vision at The Food Tree includes seeing little trays of sprouts and micro greens sitting on desks across the U.S. for students to have as a quick and immediate snack. Can you see it now?

There are dozens of seeds you can sprout in just a few days that are delicious on salads and sandwiches. Buy a pack of seeds from a reputable organic supplier like Botanical Interests. Grab a packet of alfalfa and sunflower seeds right now and get sprouting today!

MATERIALS

- Seeds
- Wide-mouth quart jar
- A pie tin or shallow dish
- Newspaper
- Cheesecloth
- Muslin, nylon netting, or metal or plastic mesh lid
- Water
- Rubber band or string

DIRECTIONS

For Sprouts

1. Put one tablespoon of seeds in a pint mason jar.
2. Cover seeds with water.
3. Place cheesecloth or metal sprouting screen over the mouth of the jar and secure it with a rubber band or metal lid ring.
4. Place the jar on a windowsill or countertop out of direct sunlight and soak overnight or for 4–12 hours.
5. Continue to rinse and drain seeds twice a day for one week or less (depending on seed variety and conditions).
6. Rinse seeds thoroughly and drain well to avoid mold and to prevent rot.
7. If the sprouts start to smell bad, toss them out and try again.

In 3-5 days, your sprouts will be ready to eat and enjoy!! Store in fridge, well-drained, in an airtight container or moistened cotton bag for 3-7 days.

FOR MICROGREENS: SUNFLOWER SEEDS, AND MORE!

Sunflower seeds grow best in a potting medium, unlike sprouts that are best to grow without soil in a jar with only water. Once the sprout puts out its first set of leaves and leaf's out, they are ready to snip and eat. You can eat the sprouts fresh on a sandwich, on a salad, or over a stir-fry.

MATERIALS

- Sunflower seeds, garbanzo beans, adzuki beans
- Baking trays, pie tins, shallow dish
- Potting soil
- Water
- Scissors

TRY GROWING

- Adzuki Beans
- Alfalfa
- Broccoli
- Chickpea
- Mung Beans
- Peas
- Sunflower Seeds
- White Radish
- Wheat Berries

DIRECTIONS

Striped Sunflower Seeds

1. Soak seeds overnight or for 6-8 hours in a bowl of cool water to enhance the germination rate.
2. Rinse very carefully when you see little sprouts of green popping out.
3. Prepare the growing container.
4. Cover the bottom of a dish with an inch of organic non-fertilized potting soil.
5. Sprinkle one even layer of sunflower seeds on the soil and then cover with another inch of soil.
6. Spritz with water and keep the soil moist. Cover with another dish or tray for 1- 2 more days until the sprouts start to poke out of the soil; at that time, remove the cover and allow them to be in full sunlight. Keep the soil hydrated.
7. Cut sprouts right above the soil.
8. EAT and ENJOY!!
9. Compost the soil and rootlets when all the sprouts are eaten.

*The microgreens are ready to harvest when they grow to around 3 inches tall and develop one set of leaves. Estimate approximately 12 days to harvest.

Bazillions of Beans

There are over 40,000 different kinds of bean varieties in the world. To that, we have to say, WOW. Beans, lentils, and peas are all part of the legume family. Legumes are an easy vegetable to grow, they are very easy to cook, and there are endless numbers of dishes to make.

I have included this activity on beans because I believe they are an important part of many peoples' diets. It is a staple food for many in the United States and around the world, especially for those that are vegan and vegetarian. There is a big movement to eat more plant-based. Therefore, it is beneficial if we can all learn a bit more about these nutritional dynamites.

One cup of uncooked sprouted lentils contains just about 18 grams of protein, 40 grams of carbohydrates, 230 calories, and 1 gram of fat.

Some of the most common beans eaten in the United States are the black bean, garbanzo bean (chickpea), lentils (black, brown, green, orange, yellow), pinto bean, red kidney bean, soybean, and white bean. However, there are so many, many more to check out!

ACTIVITY
Bean Identification!

Engage your senses in the beautiful world of beans, lentils, and peas. Gather as many types and varieties from the grocery store as you desire and share them with your class. Make sure to check out the bulk food sections to find unique beans. Pass them around in little jars.

Do a fun test to see how many names of beans, lentils, and peas they can remember. Bean identification is encouraged! You can share recipes that feature beans and even do a taste test of a few beans to see how your students like them. Talk about how often they eat beans and the kinds of beans they would like to try more.

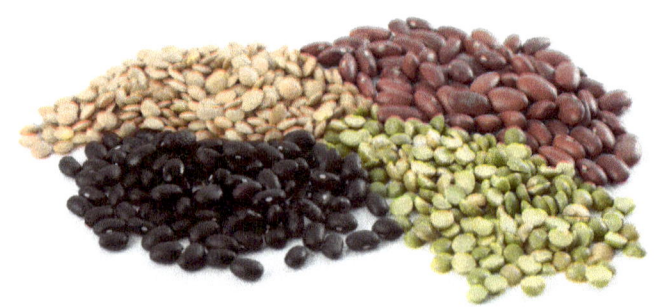

BEAN, LENTIL AND PEA LIST

- Adzuki Bean (Red Oriental Bean)
- Anasazi Bean
- Appaloosa Bean
- Black Bean
- Black-eyed Pea
- Bolita Bean
- Brown Speckled Cow Bean
- Cannellini Pole Bean (White Bean)
- Calypso Bean
- Cherokee Trail of Tears Bean
- Christmas Lima Bean
- Chili Bean (Pink Bean)
- Chickpea (Garbanzo Bean)
- Cranberry Bean
- Fava Bean
- Gandules (Pigeon Peas)
- Garbanzo Bean (Chickpea)
- Great Northern Bush Bean
- Good Mother Stallard Bean
- Hidatsa Shield Figure Bean
- Jackson Wonder Bean
- Kidney Bean
- Lablab Bean
- Lentils (black, brown, green, orange, yellow)
- Lima Bean (Wax Bean)
- Lingot Bean
- Lupini Bean
- Madagascar Bean (Lima Bean)
- Maicoba Bean
- Marrow Bean
- Mountain Pima Pinto Pole Bean
- Mortgage Runner Bean
- Mung Bean
- Navy Bean
- Painted Pony Bush Bean
- Pink Bean (Chili Bean)
- Red Ball Bean
- Pinto Bean
- Rattlesnake Bean
- Red Bean
- Red Eye Bean
- Red Kidney Bean
- Red Oriental Bean (Azuki Bean)
- Rice Bean
- Scarlet Runner Bean
- Soybean
- Spanish Tolosana Bean (Tolosana Bean)
- Split Pea
- Steuben Yellow Bean
- Swedish Brown Bean
- Tarbais Pole Bean
- Tepary Bean
- Tolosana Bean (Spanish Tolosana Bean)
- Tongues of Fire Bean
- Trout Bean
- Turtle Bean (Black Bean)
- Wax Bean (Lima Bean)
- White Kidney Bean (Cannellini Bean)
- Yellow Indian Woman Bean

Take A School Field Trip

Take your class on a trip to interesting places that are related to food. Go to unique spots that supply foods, package foods, distribute foods, sell foods, talk about foods, and make foods. Whether you live near the "salad bowl" of Central California or near a vegetable packing facility of an inner city, our world is teeming with exciting food-related places to visit.

Here are a few ideas to get you started. I realize every school, town, city, or state will have many diverse things to offer your students. Get out there and explore your community's awesomeness.

- Farms and Gardens
- Seed collection bank
- Restaurants offering farm to table, organic, vegetarian, or ethnic foods
- Dairy farm
- Bee keeper
- Egg farm
- Bakery
- Canning facility
- A homesteader
- Boat harbor
- Fish hatchery
- Slaughterhouse (umm… may turn people into vegetarians!)
- Community kitchen
- Food pantry
- Cheesemaker
- Cider house
- Tortilla factory
- Water sanitation facility
- Tree farm
- Plant nursery
- Farmers market
- Homeless shelter
- Soup kitchen
- Orchard
- Food packing plant
- Government offices—Mayor, City Council, and other food policy offices

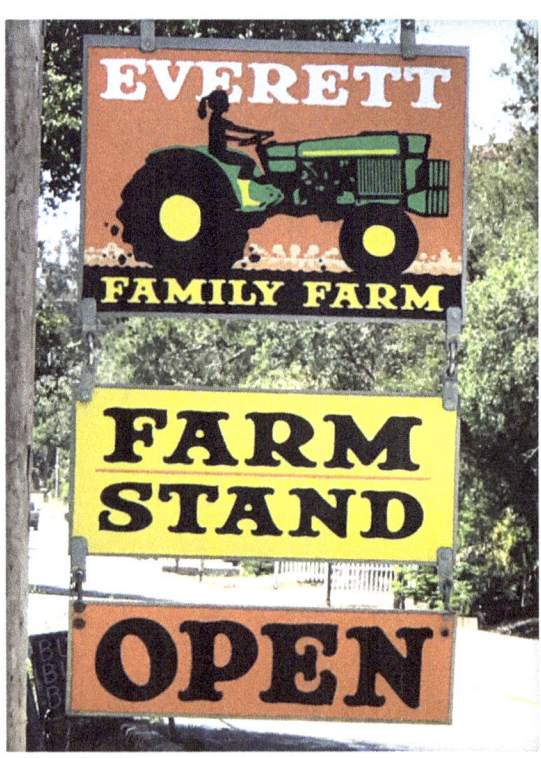

THE FOOD TREE SCIENTIFIC METHOD SHEET

Ask a question.	
Do background research.	
Construct hypothesis.	
Experiment to test your hypothesis.	
What materials do you need?	
What are your controls?	
Analyze your data and draw a conclusion.	
Share your results.	

Permission to reproduce. ©The Food Tree

RECIPE FOR HEALTH

How to grow the healthiest _____!

Ingredients:

1.

2.

3.

4.

5.

6.

7.

8.

9.

10.

Permission to reproduce. ©The Food Tree

THE FOOD TREE DAILY FOOD JOURNAL

5 PROTEINS   5 WHOLE GRAINS   3 HEALTHY FATS   5 VEGETABLES   3 FRUIT

Breakfast	
Snack	
Lunch	
Snack	
Dinner	

Permission to reproduce. ©The Food Tree

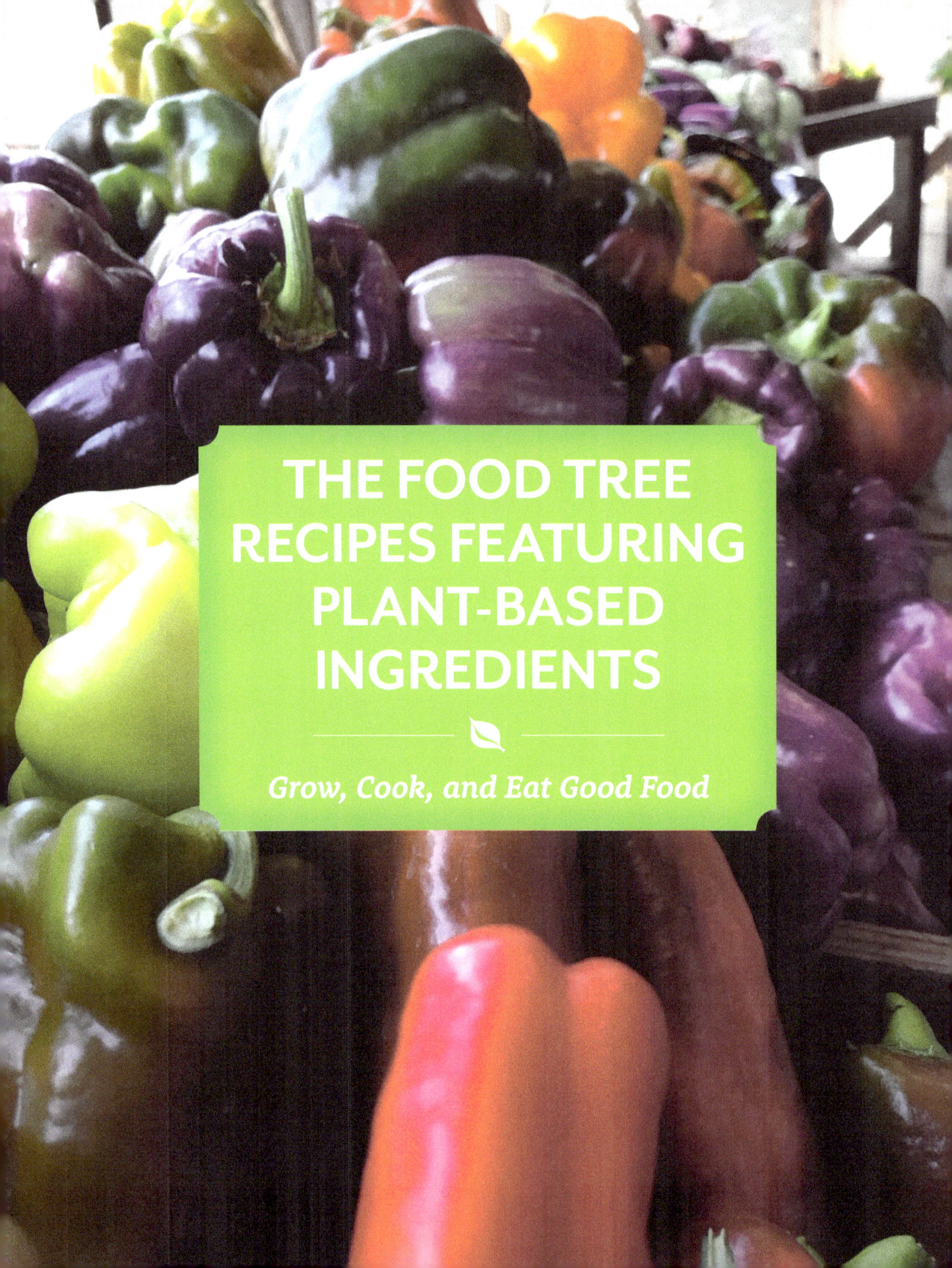

THE FOOD TREE RECIPES FEATURING PLANT-BASED INGREDIENTS

Grow, Cook, and Eat Good Food

Educate, empower, and inspire children to cook and enjoy eating healthy, tasty foods! Children and students of all ages can have fun bringing nutritious meals to the table. The more exposure that they have helping in the kitchen, the more confidence and proficiency they will gain. And in no time, they will be able to make breakfast, lunch, snacks, dinner, and the best desserts ever. You will be delighted at the enthusiasm you get from your young chefs and be amazed at what children can do while creating a precious bond with your students.

The Food Tree highlights the importance of enjoying being physically active in growing and preparing food. Connect children to where food comes from by bringing in the natural process. If it is possible, take your class and visit a farm. Turn kids on to the experience of picking strawberries or making jam. Grow a lemon tree and make homemade lemon-aid. Take food scraps and toss them into your compost pile. Then, spread compost around the lemon tree and in your garden. These are concrete, tangible ways children learn about the cycles of life and from where food comes.

I encourage teaching kids how to slow down and enjoy the actual act of eating. The Food Tree supports organizations like The Slow Food Movement and The Psychology of Eating that teach about adopting a healthy relationship to food and eating. The goal is for the child to feel successful in the kitchen, to learn and master new skills, and to create a healthy and respectful connection to food and cooking. Explore the wide variety of recipes and get the kids into the garden and kitchen. Experiment with different ingredients, smells, tastes, food combinations, and textures. Create a safe and encouraging environment with adult supervision. Don't worry about the mess because cleaning up together is part of the process. Wearing chef hats and aprons are encouraged!

Being active in the kitchen is one of the best and most rewarding ways to do this. Have fun exploring the tastes of traditional foods while mixing it up with modern twists. The Food Tree supports buying locally grown, in-season, organic, fair trade, and homegrown foods as much as possible. Get out cookbooks with your class, students, and parents, or find recipes that people want to try.

Get kids involved and interested in cooking!

- Start an afterschool or weekend cooking club.
- Make healthy snacks ahead of time so you are prepared when hunger strikes.
- Ask students to go shopping with their parents.
- Visit the farmers market.
- Grow a garden at home or at school.
- Create and publish a class or schoolwide cookbook.
- Have students prepare lunch for the rest of the whole class after checking for any allergies.
- Make cooking part of the curriculum.
- Teach your students to listen to what their bodies want and need. Counting calories is one way but if you listen to signals your body sends, you are quite capable of making choices that are beneficial without counting.
- Eat in-season. Make a plan with yourself not to buy grapes or watermelon in the middle of winter from Chile.
- Start a cooking business preparing foods for busy new moms or the elderly.
- Keep the language around food and eating neutral and positive.
- Discuss who cooks in their family. Where and when do people eat? How often do people eat out?
- Have awareness as this is a sensitive topic for many of our youth. Use discretion on how you discuss food awareness and accessibility.
- Try the recipes listed here.
- Ask your class to share their favorites or their family's special traditional foods and recipes.

Tamari Toasted Pepitas

Pepitas, or "little seed of squash", are the Spanish name for pumpkin seeds. We love, love, love these simple, tasty, and oh so very healthy big flavored treat that is packed with big nutrition! These green seeds are loaded in vitamins and minerals, including selenium and zinc. They are very high in protein, so they are perfect for taking with you for a quick energy boost. You can enjoy them raw but many people like them toasted, too.

Ingredients

1 cup of pumpkin seeds or sunflower seeds

2 tablespoons tamari sauce, Bragg Liquid Amino Acids, or soy sauce

Directions

In a medium-hot cast iron skillet or stainless-steel pan, add one cup of pumpkin seeds.

Stir the seeds frequently to avoid them sticking and burning.

The pumpkin seeds will pop and crackle in the pan.

Toss around for one more minute and then turn off the flame and move the seeds to another dish.

Add a few dashes of Bragg Liquid Aminos, tamari, or soy sauce to the seeds and toss to coat evenly.

Eat by the handful, sprinkle in a salad, soup, sandwich, burrito, or stir fry. Store in an airtight container.

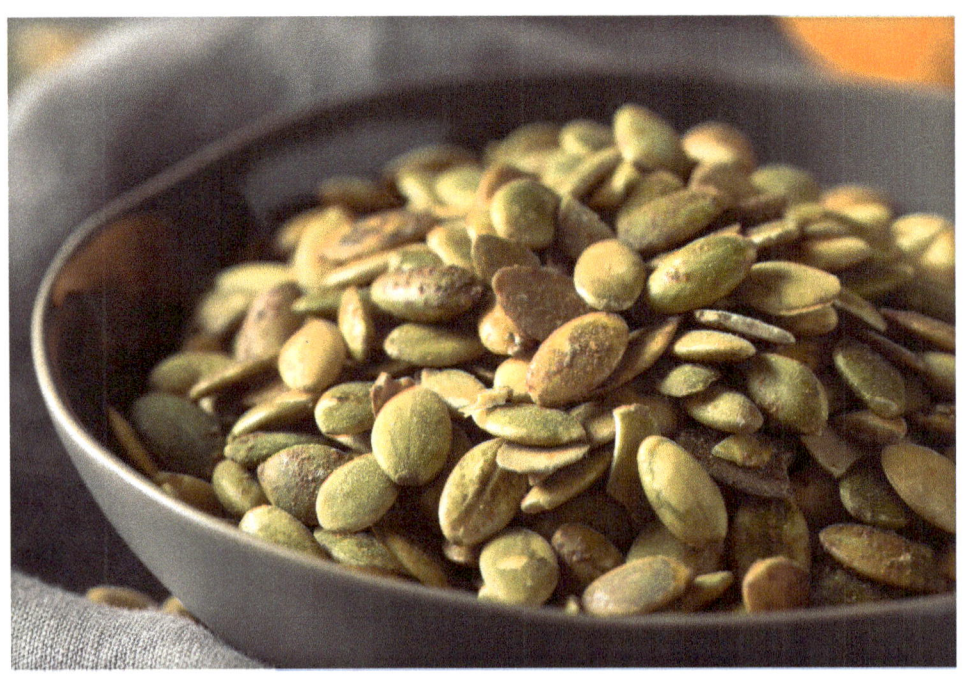

Toasted Nori Sheets

Warning! These are addictive! Kids love them. Teachers can't get enough. Nori is a type of seaweed that is dried and made into very thin sheets, often used in sushi rolls. Here, I show you how to make nori sheets into highly nutritious, irresistibly tasty snacks!

Ingredients

3 nori seaweed sheets
1 tablespoon sesame oil
Sea salt

Directions

Preheat oven to 400°F.

Coat one side with sesame oil using your fingers or a brush.

Sprinkle lightly with sea salt.

Bake for 1–2 minutes.

Watch nori carefully as they cook fast and you want them to retain their green color.

Share with your friends and loved ones!!

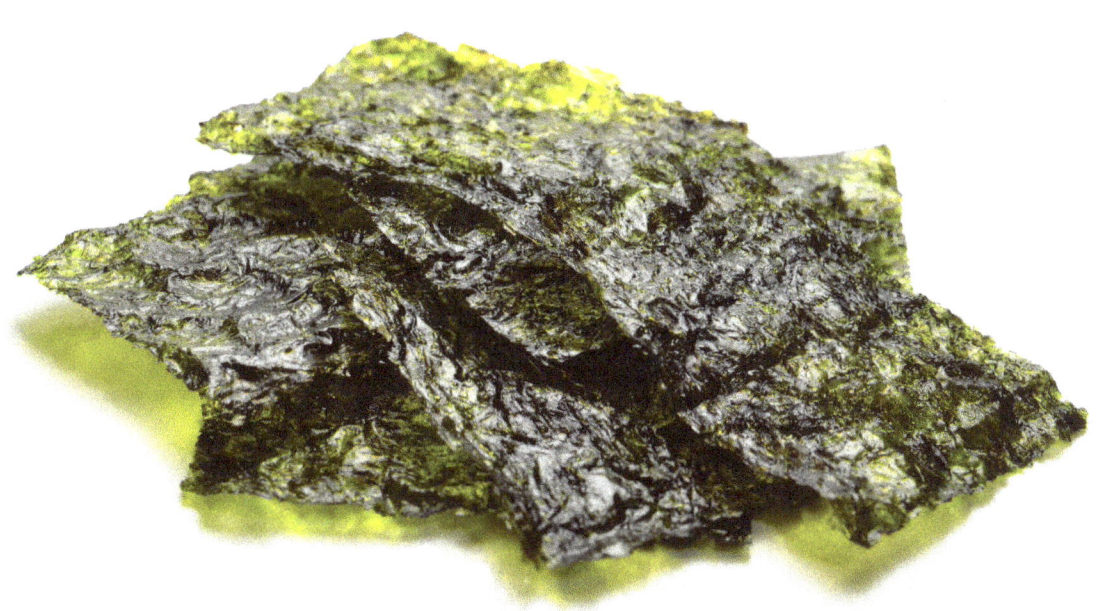

Roasted Chickpeas

Simple, easy to make, and tasty.

Ingredients

15 ounces cooked chickpeas (garbanzo beans)

1½ tablespoons olive oil

Salt

Spice blend of your choice

Directions

Preheat oven to 400°F.

Drain garbanzo beans in a strainer and rinse with water.

Spread the beans over a paper towel or dishtowel. Use another cloth to press gently to absorb the water on the beans.

Remove the thin skin from the beans by rolling them around on a towel.

Pour beans on to the baking sheet.

Drizzle the olive oil over the beans and toss to coat.

Bake for 30–40 minutes.

Remove halfway through baking and stir. Continue baking until the beans are golden brown and crunchy.

Season with Himalayan salt, sea salt, or any spice blend.

Cool, then store in an airtight container.

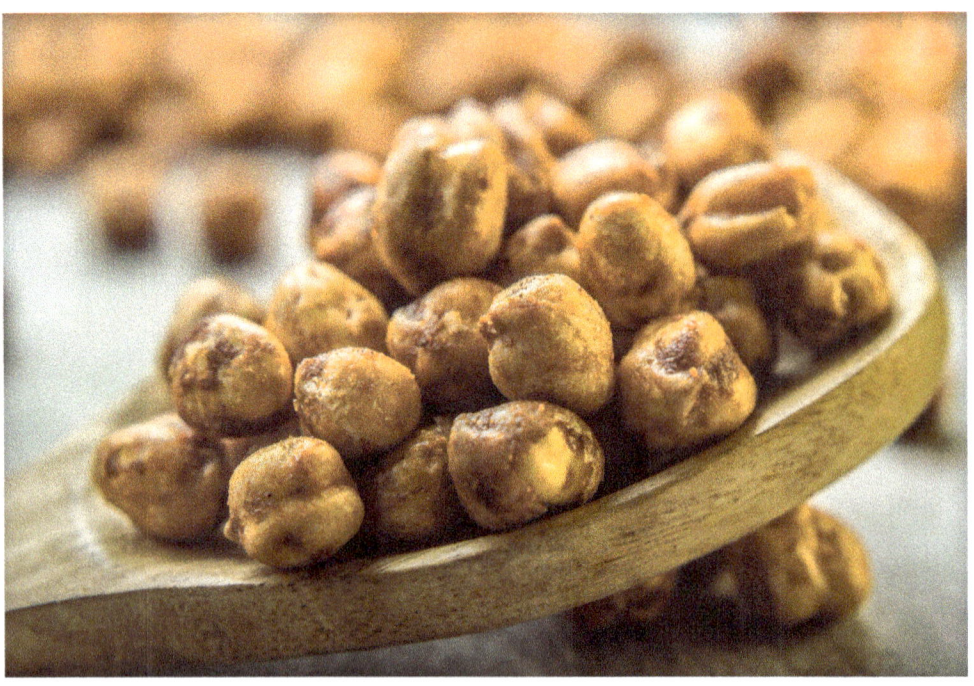

Kale Chips

Of course, I had to include a kale chip recipe. What kind of holistic nutrition curriculum would this be without one? Kale chips are easy to make and even easier to gobble up! You can bake them in a regular oven set on a very low temperature, or you can dehydrate them in a dehydrator. Either way you go, they are delicious and nutritious.

Here I offer up a basic kale chip recipe that is perfect for the kale chip beginner. However, there are many different seasonings you can always add to your kale chip repertoire. I encourage exploration.

Ingredients

3 bunches of kale, curly or Lacinato (Tuscan, dinosaur kale)

3 tablespoons olive oil

Sea salt or pink Himalayan salt

Additional Toppings

4 tablespoons nutritional yeast

Cayenne pepper to taste

2 tablespoons maple syrup or honey

2 tablespoons Bragg Liquid Aminos

1 tablespoon almond butter

1 teaspoon garlic powder

Directions

Tear the kale leaves off of the center midrib and rip into smaller pieces.

Wash kale in a salad spinner and spin dry.

Place kale in a bowl and add olive oil and salt.

Mix around well to coat all of the leaves.

Distribute kale on a baking sheet or dehydrator tray one layer thick.

Oven

Preheat oven to 250° F. Dehydrate for 20–40 minutes, flip the leaves and turn the baking sheets twice during dehydrating.

Dehydrator

Start at 145° F then lower the temperature to 115° F for 6–7 hours.

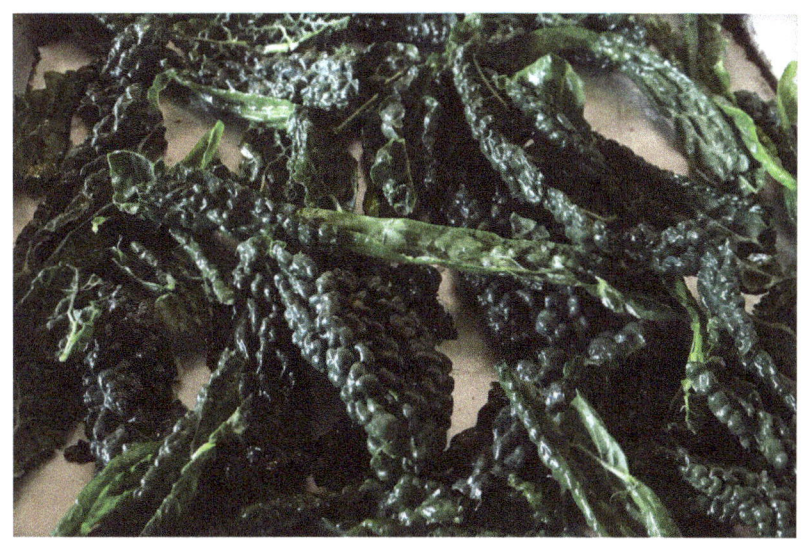

Brussels Sprouts Chips

Enjoy these tasty morsels as a nutritious and satisfying snack.

Ingredients

1 lb. Brussels sprouts, use big sprouts with big leaves

2 tablespoons olive oil

Garlic powder

Sea salt

Black pepper

Nutritional yeast

Directions

Preheat oven to 400° F.

Wash Brussels sprouts and pat dry with a clean cotton dishtowel.

Peel off any damaged or brown outer leaves.

Cut the nubs off of the bottom of the sprout with a paring knife.

Pull off all of the leaves or slice very thinly.

Toss the leaves with the oil, garlic powder, salt, and pepper.

Arrange them in a single layer on a baking sheet.

Bake for ten minutes.

Remove and shake them around, continue cooking for another five to ten minutes, or until the leaves start to crisp up and turn golden on the edges.

Observe them carefully to make sure that you do not overcook or burn.

Season more if needed with salt, pepper, or nutritional yeast.

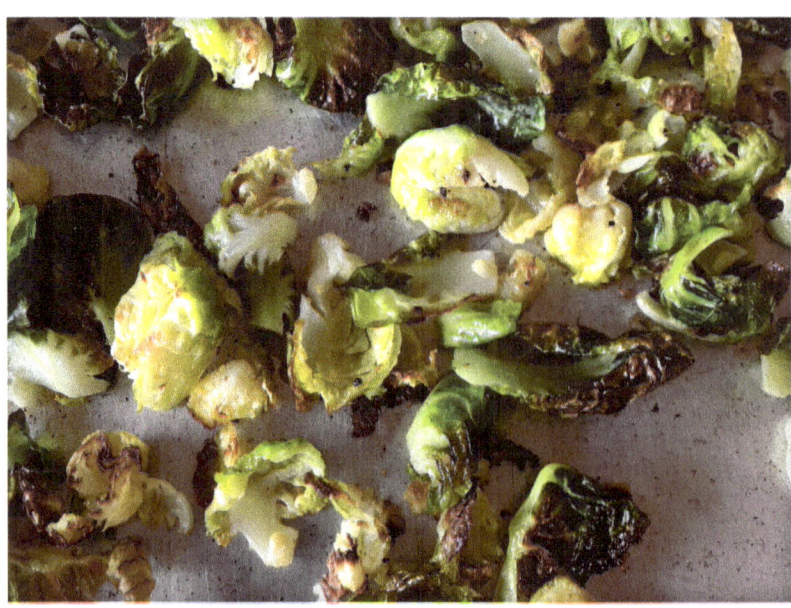

Power Nut Balls

Power Nut Balls are little balls of goodness that are simple to make. The ingredients provide excellent sources of fiber, healthy fats, proteins, and minerals.

Ingredients

1 cup rolled oats

1 cup almond butter or peanut butter

1 cup almonds or peanuts, chopped

2 teaspoons maple syrup

4 teaspoons hemp seeds

1 cup coconut flakes

Optional

1 cup dried chopped fruit of your choice—mulberry, raisins, apricot, cranberry, and date

2 teaspoons cocoa powder

Spirulina or blue-green algae powder

Directions

In a large mixing bowl, add all of the ingredients including cocoa powder, if desired, except the coconut flakes.

Mix well.

Roll the mix in the palm of your hand into two-inch balls.

Then roll the balls in the coconut flakes to cover. You might need to press the coconut into the ball.

Place the balls on a baking sheet, cover with foil, and place in the fridge for an hour to chill.

Put the chilled balls into a sealed container. They will store in the fridge for one week or freeze for up to two months.

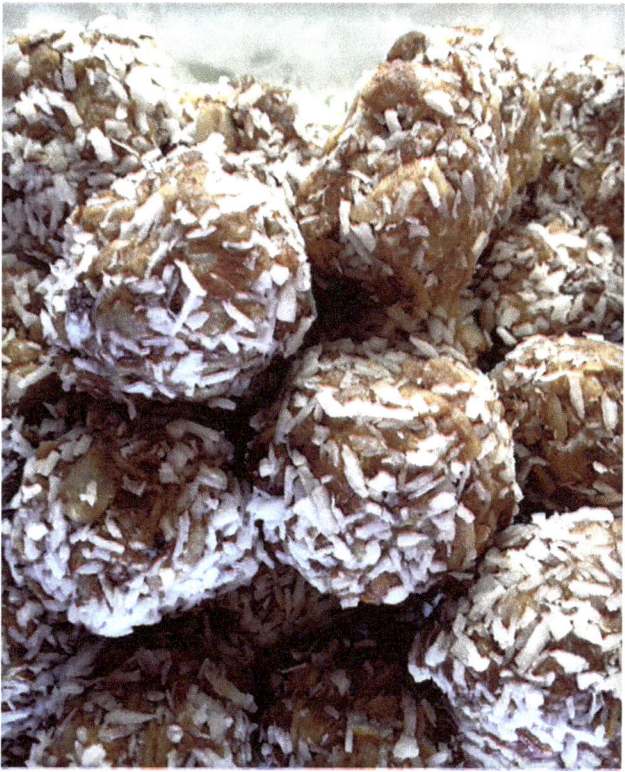

Dill Pickles

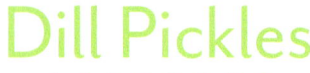

Materials
32-ounce glass jar with tight fitting lid

Ingredients
1 pound pickling cucumbers

1½ tablespoon sea salt or Himalayan salt (do not use iodized salt)

1 bunch fresh dill, picked over, washed, dried, chopped

2 cloves garlic, peeled and minced

2 fresh grape leaves or bay leaves

1 teaspoon black peppercorn

32 ounces of water

Directions
Wash and scrub cucumbers well to remove any dirt.

Soak them for two hours in a large bowl of ice water to plump them up before pickling.

Sterilize a glass quart jar and lid.

Prepare brine:

Dilute 1½ tablespoons salt with 1 cup of boiled water. Then add the rest of the water.

Put cucumbers in a large jar or crock.

Pour brine, herbs, and seasonings over cucumbers to cover them completely.

If using a crock, make sure pickles are submerged entirely under the brine. To do so, you can use a plate with a weight (cans, rock, or brick) on top to push down cucumbers. If using a jar, put the lid on tightly and make sure cucumbers are completely covered with the brine. If you need more brine, use a bit under 1 tablespoon of salt to 1 cup of water and add to the jar as needed.

Check your pickles every day. Look for signs of spoiling. Skim any mold off the surface or the plate, if there is any. Wash the plate and put it back on the crock.

The pickles will be ready anywhere in one to four weeks, depending on the temperature. Taste them to see if they are to your liking.

When they are ready, put them into clean jars and refrigerate. Enjoy!!

Nut and Seed Butters

Nut butter is fun to make and definitely worth all of the sticky mess. You can jar them up and give them as gifts or keep them in the freezer or fridge to eat as a ready to go nutritious snack.

Materials

Rubber spatula

Food processor or high-speed blender

Ingredients

16 ounces (1 lb.) of nuts or 8 ounces of seeds—almond, cashew, hemp seeds, peanut (skinned, raw), sesame seeds, sunflower seeds

Optional Additions

1 tablespoon honey

½ teaspoon cinnamon

1–2 tablespoons cocoa powder or melted semi-sweet or dark chocolate chips

¼ cup dates

1 teaspoon vanilla extract

1 teaspoon soy sauce or Bragg Liquid Aminos

Few dashes of sea salt

Directions

Add 1–2 cups of nuts or half of the seeds into the food processor, pulse, stopping often to scrape down the sides.

Once the nuts and seeds look like they are almost all blended, add any additional ingredients and pulse for a few more moments.

Scoop nut butter into a clean jar and refrigerate for up to 2 months.

Try these nut butter combinations

Peanut butter, cinnamon, honey, with raisins on toast, or apple slices

Cashews, coconut flakes, and coconut powder over toast or crackers

Sesame seeds or tahini with lemon juice, garlic, and salt for a savory spread on raw vegetables

Sunflower seeds, tamari, and maple syrup

Hazelnuts and chocolate

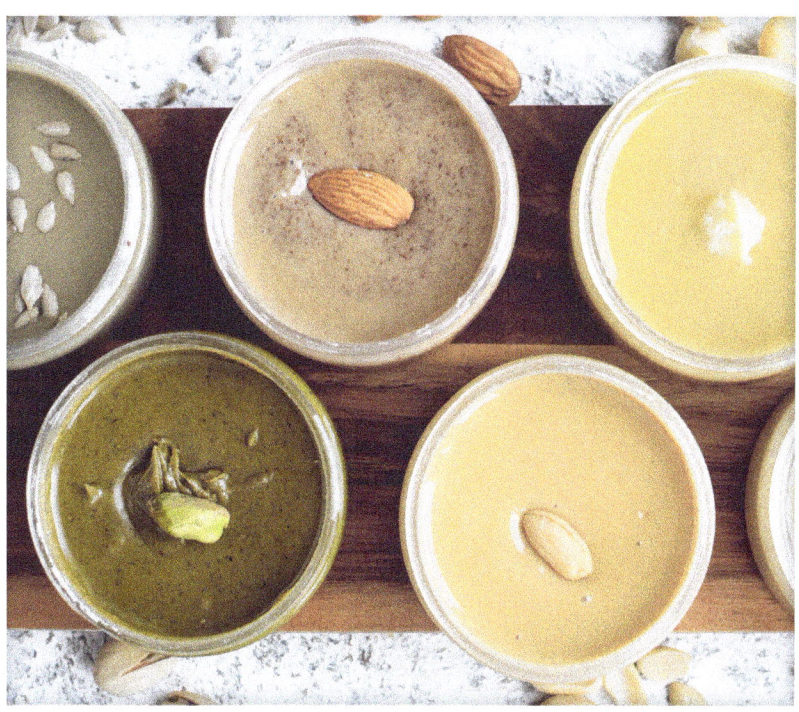

Steel Cut and Rolled Oat Oatmeal

Oatmeal is known to be a staple breakfast food but it can also be a perfect energy boosting snack.

Ingredients

1 cup rolled oats

2 cups whole milk, soy milk, rice milk, almond milk, or water

Pinch of sea salt

Delicious toppings

1 teaspoon cinnamon

Fresh fruit, like berries, banana slices, chopped apples

¼ cup raisins or dates

¼ cup nuts and seeds

2 teaspoons coconut flakes

Maple syrup

Honey

Butter

Milk

Directions

Bring water to a boil in a medium-sized saucepan. Add oats and a pinch of salt, and then turn down to a simmer.

Add banana, raisins, or dates.

Stir and cover.

Cook rolled oats for 5 minutes and steel cut oats for 10–20 minutes.

Remove from heat, cover, let stand for 2–3 minutes.

Spoon into bowls and add the remaining ingredients.

Serve with butter, yogurt, milk, cream, nuts, fresh fruit, and dried fruit. You can sweeten with honey or maple syrup, as desired.

Quinoa Hot Cereal

Ingredients

1 cup milk, nut milk, soymilk, rice milk, or cow milk

1 cup of water

1 cup quinoa

2 cups fresh berries

½ teaspoon ground cinnamon

½ cup chopped pecans, walnuts, almonds

1 teaspoon honey or maple syrup

Directions

Combine milk, water, and quinoa in a medium saucepan and bring to a boil.

Reduce heat to medium-low, cover, and simmer 15 minutes or until most of the liquid is absorbed.

Turn off heat and let stand, covered, for 5 minutes.

Add cinnamon and mix well.

Spoon cereal into four bowls and top with mixed berries, nuts, and honey.

Broccoli Soup

Ingredients

3 tablespoons butter, or avocado oil room temperature

1½ pounds fresh broccoli

1 large onion, chopped

1 carrot, chopped

Salt and freshly ground black pepper

4 tablespoons whole wheat flour

4 cups vegetable broth

½ cup cream: dairy, soy, or almond milk

Optional

Homemade croutons

Cheddar cheese

Pepitas

Crunchy bread

Directions

Melt 4 tablespoons butter in a heavy medium-sized pot over medium-high heat.

Add broccoli, onion, carrot, salt, and pepper and sauté until onion is translucent, about 6 minutes.

Add the flour and cook for 1 minute until the flour is lightly browned.

Add stock and bring to a boil.

Lower the heat to a simmer and cook uncovered until broccoli is tender, about 15 minutes.

Turn off heat and pour in cream.

Puree the soup in a blender or use an emersion blender.

Add salt and pepper, to taste, and then add the soup back to the pot and heat.

Serve hot and top with croutons, crunchy bread, shredded cheddar cheese, or pepitas.

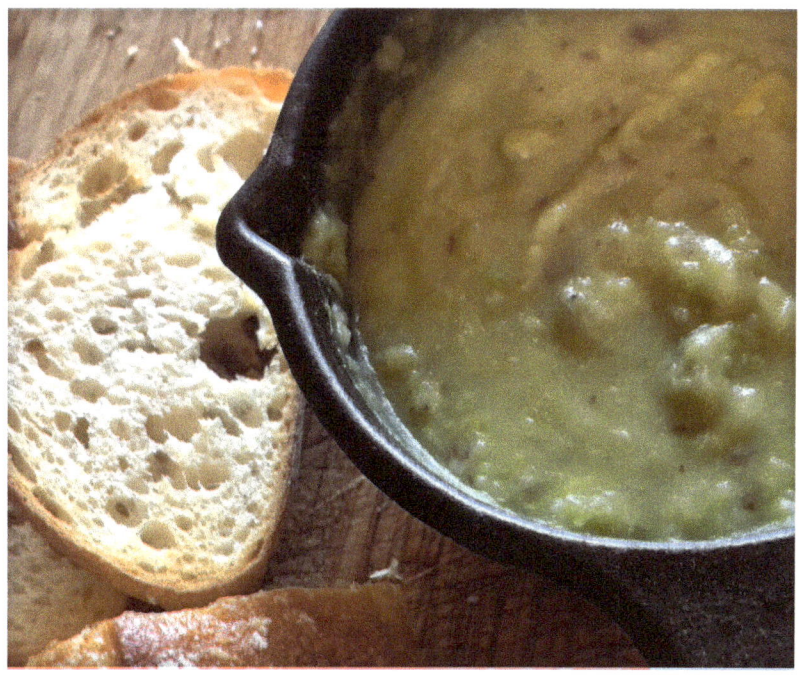

Lentil and Greens Soup

Ingredients

1 cup dried brown lentils, rinsed

2 tablespoons olive oil

2 cups yellow onion, diced

1 tablespoon garlic, minced

1 cup carrots, diced

4 cups vegetable broth or stock

1 bunch kale, stems removed, and sliced

Directions

Add oil, onions, and garlic to a pot and cook over medium heat until onions are translucent.

Add the kale and then the carrots and cook down for a few minutes.

Add stock and stir.

Add lentils and cover for 30–40 minutes on simmer.

Add more vegetable stock or water if needed.

Add sea salt and pepper to taste.

Cheddar Cheese Whole Wheat Muffins

Cheddar cheese surrounded by savory green onion bits melted together and nestled in a warm muffin …..mmmm. How good does that sound? It is best to make more muffins than you think in case people forget how to share!!

Ingredients

2 cups whole wheat pastry flour

3 teaspoons baking powder

½ teaspoon salt

1 teaspoon turbinado sugar

3 eggs, lightly beaten

1 cup buttermilk

¼ cup light vegetable oil (grapeseed, safflower, sunflower)

1 cup green onions, chopped

1 cup sharp cheddar cheese, finely diced

Directions

Preheat oven to 400° F.

Fill muffin tin with paper liners or lightly grease.

Sift the flour, baking powder, salt, and sugar together and set aside.

In a large bowl, combine eggs, milk, and oil.

Stir flour mixture quickly into the wet ingredients and blend in green onions and cheese.

Spoon into muffin tins, filling halfway.

Bake muffins until golden brown, about 15 minutes.

Serve warm.

Watermelon and Arugula Salad

The combination of ingredients in this salad taste so incredibly good. I am not sure why the flavors are so wonderful together, but trust me, it is delicious.

Ingredients

6 cups arugula

6 cups watermelon, seeded and off the rind, cut into 1-inch cubes

½ red onion, thinly sliced

Dressing

⅓ cup olive oil

¼ cup balsamic vinegar

2 teaspoons honey

1 teaspoon sea salt

Fresh ground black pepper to taste

Optional

1 cup feta cheese crumbles

½ cup pan toasted pumpkin seeds

Directions

Dressing

In a small bowl, whisk together the oil, vinegar, honey, salt, and pepper.

Salad

In a large bowl, add the arugula, watermelon, and onion and toss together.

Drizzle the dressing over the salad and toss it gently until coated.

Add feta crumbles and pepitas, if desired, and serve.

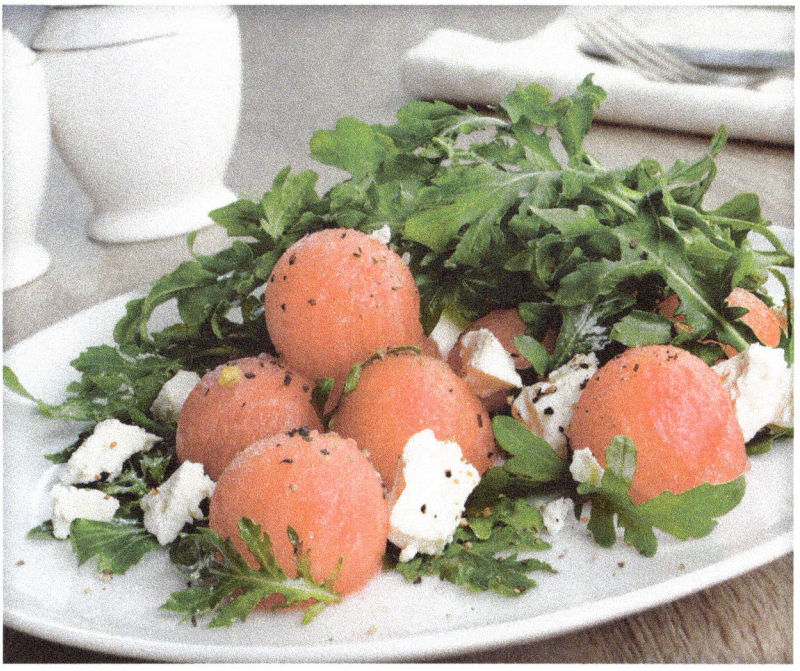

Corn Tortillas

Materials

Mixing bowl

Wax paper or plastic freezer bag

Tortilla press or glass pie dish (you can also use hands to form tortillas)

Dishtowel

Basket

Ingredients

4 cups masa harina, available in Latin grocery stores or use fresh corn masa.

2½ cups hot water

½ teaspoon salt, optional. Salt is not used in traditional recipes.

Directions

In a large bowl, add the masa harina and hot water.

Mix dough with your hand or a spoon and knead into a large ball.

Make sure to incorporate water evenly.

Cover unused dough with a damp dishtowel to prevent the dough from drying out.

If the dough is too dry, add more water. If it is too wet, add more masa harina.

Form dough into 18 balls (the size of a golf ball).

Press dough using the tortilla press to form a 6-inch tortilla.

Use plastic or wax paper to prevent sticking.

If edges crack, use a little water to smooth them out.

To cook

Heat a cast iron skillet or pan and cook the tortilla on one side for 30 seconds, flip, then cook for another 45 seconds to one minute. Then flip one more time for another quick 15 seconds.

Stack on a clean dish towel in a basket made of natural fibers and cover to keep warm.

The uncooked fresh dough can be stored in an airtight container for up to one day.

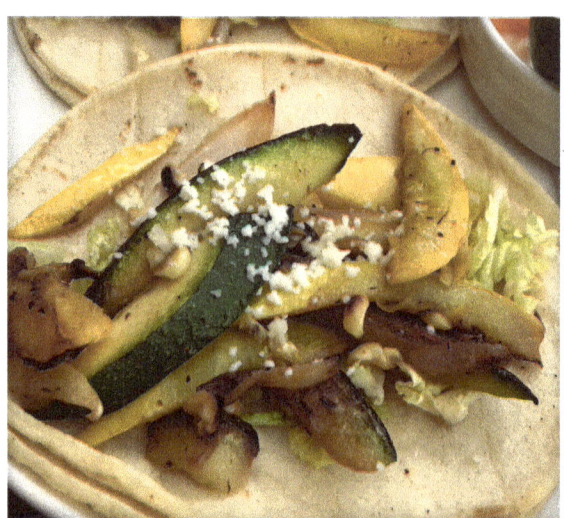

Broccoli with Garlic and Walnuts

This soup is a simple yet so very delicious way to enjoy beautiful broccoli. This recipe is adapted from a favorite vegetarian cookbook, *The Passionate Vegetarian* by Crescent Dragonwagon. And yes, this broccoli dish is as wonderful as her name! Don't you love it?!

Ingredients

1 head of broccoli, cut into florets and steamed

¼ cup olive oil or butter

3–5 cloves garlic, peeled and chopped

⅓ cup walnuts, chopped into little bits

Sea salt and fresh ground black pepper to taste

Directions

Steam broccoli and set aside.

Heat the oil or butter in a small skillet over medium-high heat.

Add the garlic and cook, continually stirring, until garlic is light golden brown.

Add the walnuts and cook until fragrant and infusing nicely with the garlic oil, about 2 minutes.

Pour the hot garlic walnut sauce, and pinch of sea salt, over the steamed broccoli, adding more oil if needed.

Nutty Raw Soft Tacos

Make wrappers with a lettuce leaf or use your favorite soft corn tortilla. These are easy to make and kids love the taste and crunchy texture.

Ingredients

1 cup raw cashews

1 cup sunflower seeds

8–16 ounces fresh salsa

3 tomatoes, ripe or canned, diced

1 red onion, diced

1 cup sunflower or bean sprouts

8 lettuce leaves or corn tortillas

1 avocado, sliced

Directions

Place cashews and sunflower seeds in a food processor and grind to a fine meal.

Slowly add salsa until the consistency is like a moist spread.

Place tortilla or lettuce leaf in your hand, taco-style, and fill with pate mix.

Top with tomatoes, avocado, sprouts, red onion, and more salsa, if desired.

Most Excellent Refried Beans

Refried beans aren't refried at all! Refried beans are mashed pinto or black beans with savory items like garlic and onions added, plus a little liquid, to make them smooth.

Ingredients

2 cups of cooked pinto beans

3 tablespoons olive oil or butter

½ medium onion, chopped

4 cloves garlic, minced

1 teaspoon ground coriander

½ teaspoon ground cumin

⅔ to 1 cup vegetable broth or stock

Sea salt and freshly ground pepper to taste

Directions

In a medium-sized mixing bowl, mash ⅔ of the cooked beans with a large fork and set aside.

Heat oil in a heavy skillet or frying pan over medium heat.

Add the onion and sauté until lightly browned, about 3–4 minutes.

Add the garlic and continue to cook, stirring often, until fragrant.

Add cumin and coriander, stir, and cook another minute.

Add the mashed beans and half the broth, cook, frequently stirring, until slightly thickened, about 5 minutes.

Add the rest of the beans and enough broth to create a batter-like consistency.

Simmer until the beans are thick but not too pasty, about 2 minutes.

Season with salt and pepper to taste.

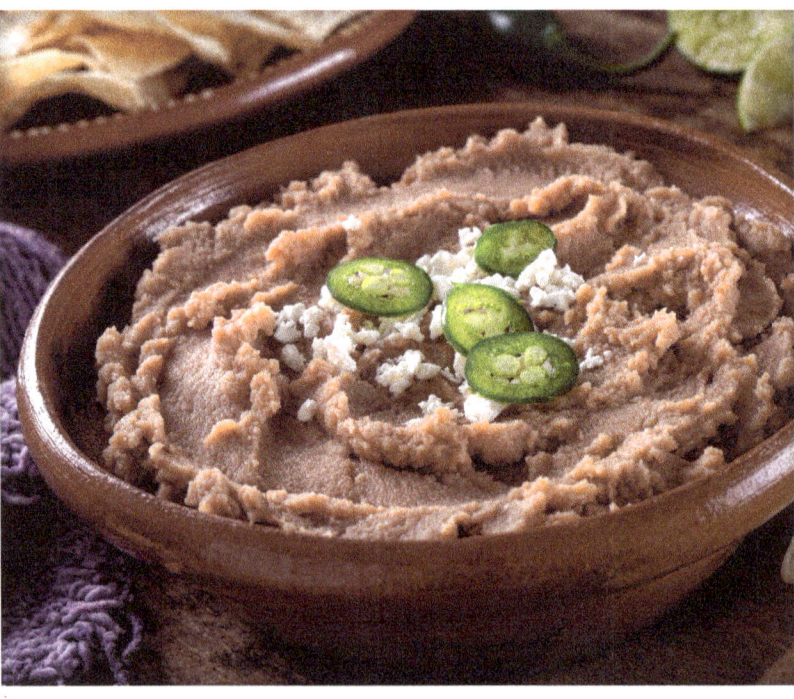

Rainbow Rolls

Choose any colorful fruit, vegetable, or protein of your choice to make a savory or sweet roll.

Ingredients

Wrappers—choose any wrapper to roll up your fixin's.

Large lettuce leaf, romaine lettuce or butter leaf lettuce, washed and dried

Rice paper

Whole wheat tortilla

Nori sheet (seaweed sheets)

Chapati

Fillings

Red

Red cabbage

Red onions

Salsa

Strawberry

Orange

Apricot, dried, thinly sliced

Carrot, raw or steamed

Mandarin oranges, peeled and sectioned

Sweet potato/yam, baked

Yellow

Nectarines

Yellow bell peppers

Green

Avocado

Broccoli, steamed

Green onions

Kiwi

Kale, raw rubbed with oil or steamed

Pickles, bread and butter or dill

Blue and Purple

Black beans

Blueberries

White/Brown

Almond butter

Banana

Brown rice

Coconut flakes

Dates

Jicama

Miso paste

Nuts, chopped: almonds, cashews, walnuts

Peanut butter

Directions

Place lettuce leaf, nori sheet, or rice wrapper on a flat surface.

Spread your fruits, vegetables, and other ingredients in a thin layer on the lettuce leaf.

Add as many ingredients as you can roll-up without everything falling out.

Roll snuggly.

Cut into one-inch slices.

Enjoy the rainbow you created!

Make a dipping sauce to go with the different flavors you created.

Roll Examples

Asian Fusion Roll

Nori wrapper + brown rice + avocado + red bell pepper + sweet potato

South of the Border Roll

Lettuce leaf + black beans + avocado + yellow bell pepper + jicama + salsa

Fruit and Nut Roll

Rice wrapper + almond or peanut butter + strawberries + sliced apricots + banana + coconut flakes

Vegetable Sushi Rolls

Ingredients

Nori sheets

1 cup short grain brown rice or brown sticky rice

Soy sauce or Bragg Liquid Aminos

1 cup water (1:1 ratio of water to sushi rice)

2 tablespoons plus 1 teaspoon rice vinegar

1 tablespoon turbinado sugar

2 teaspoons mirin or sherry

Dash of sea salt

The Fixings! *Prepare the desired amount of vegetables and other ingredients.*

Carrot strips

Cucumber strips

Scallions sliced the long way

Sweet potatoes baked or steamed

Broccoli, steamed

Cashews, peanuts, macadamia nut pieces

Avocado

Cream cheese

Tofu

Gobo—burdock root

Daikon radish sprouts

Umeboshi plum paste

Sesame seeds

On the Side

Wasabi

Pickled ginger

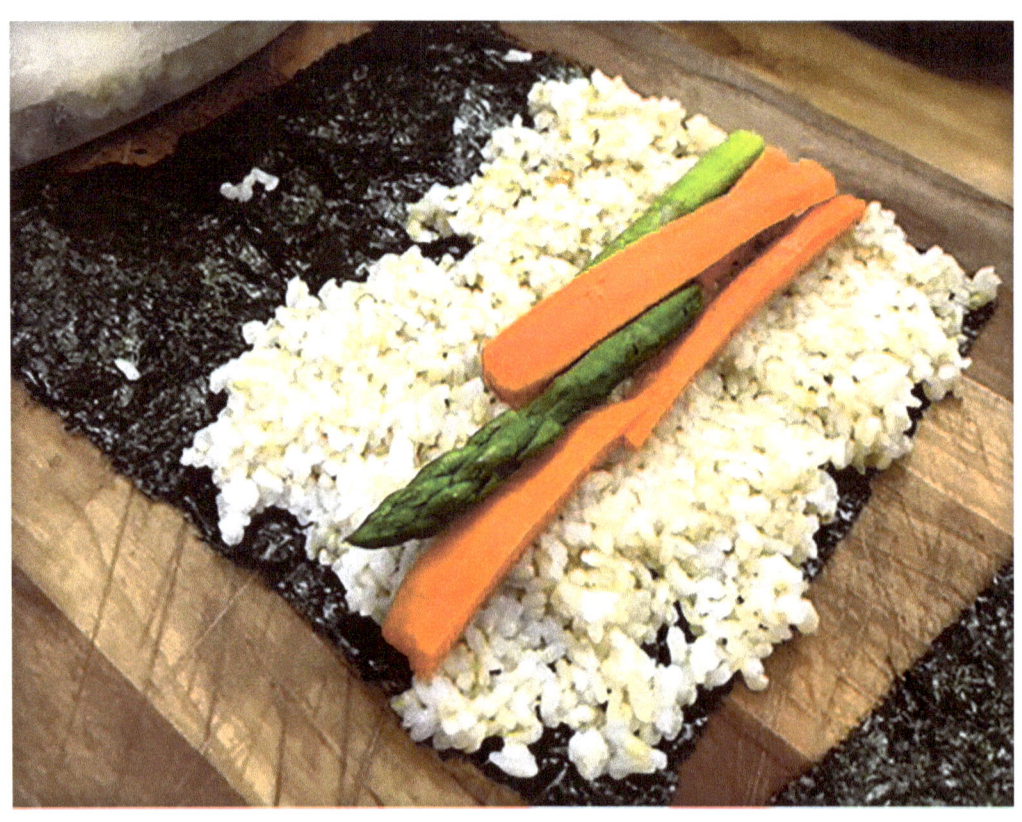

Directions

To make sushi rice:

Use brown rice and either rinse under cold water until water is clear to release starch or soak in 1⅓ cups water for 6 hours or overnight. Drain well, rinsing a few times.

Cook rice in 1¼ cups cold water, stir and bring to a boil then turn down to a low simmer, cover the pot, and cook for 40 minutes or until all water is gone. Do not stir. Or, cook in a rice cooker, Instant Pot, or pressure cooker.

When done, turn rice onto a wide, flat bowl, and turn gently with a wooden spoon or paddle to cool off.

In a medium-sized saucepan, combine sugar, vinegar, and a little salt. Heat over medium heat.

Add 2 teaspoons mirin or sherry and take off heat.

Sprinkle rice with sauce.

Carefully break up clumps, being careful not to mash the rice.

Stir and fan rice with an actual fan, potholder, or folded magazine for 3–5 minutes to cool down.

Let rice stand until it has reached room temperature. Cover. Do not refrigerate rice. Use within 2 hours.

To make sushi rolls:

Lay nori on a flat surface and then paddle and press rice onto ⅔ of the sheet about ½ inch thick.

Lay assortment of vegetables and nuts across the rice.

Roll up sushi and seal with a dab of water across the end and press roll closed.

Slice roll into 1-inch rounds.

Dip sushi pieces into soy sauce, add pickled ginger slices and wasabi, and enjoy.

Tofu Scramble

Ingredients

1 block of firm tofu, cubed and drained

1 tablespoon coconut oil or other high heat oil

2 teaspoons curry powder

1 cup chopped broccoli

2 carrots, washed, peeled, diced

2 cups sliced kale with the midribs removed

2 tablespoons green onions, chopped

4 cloves garlic, minced

2 teaspoons Bragg Liquid Aminos or soy sauce

½ cup cashews, halved or whole

Salt and black pepper to taste

Directions

In a pan, add coconut oil and tofu and cook over medium heat until lightly brown on all sides. Let the tofu brown before flipping over.

Add a few dashes of Bragg Liquid Aminos and a dusting of curry powder to the tofu and mix well.

While the tofu is cooking, sauté onions and garlic in a cast iron pan until onions become translucent.

Add the broccoli, kale, and carrots and cook until they turn bright in color. Turn off heat.

Add the vegetable mix and the green onions to the tofu, stir and heat together.

Serve over brown basmati rice with cashews on top.

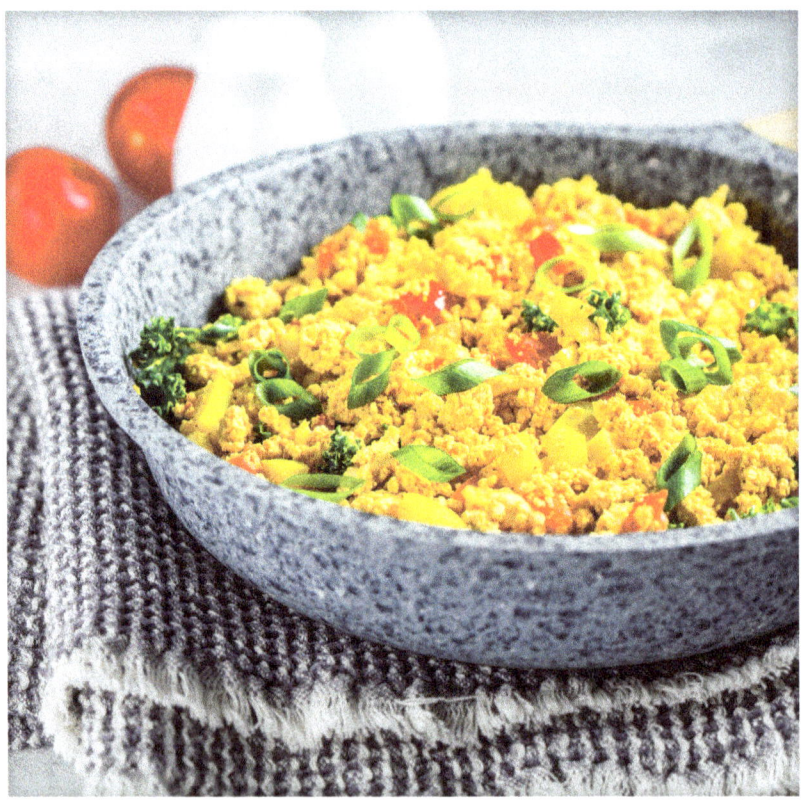

Curried Sweet Potato Latkes

Celebrate Hanukkah, or any day, with Curried Sweet Potato Latkes! If you haven't ever tried a sweet potato latke, this recipe is the one to try. These flavorful latkes are great even when it's not Hanukkah. The sweetness from the potatoes combined with the rich curry flavor blend together into something memorable. They are wonderful with toppings, too. They are traditionally served with apple sauce or sour cream. But, anything from a yogurt-based dip to a thick chutney will make these treats even more delish.

Ingredients

1 pound sweet potatoes, peeled

½ cup whole wheat flour

2 teaspoons turbinado sugar

1 teaspoon baking powder

¼–½ teaspoon cayenne powder

2 teaspoons curry powder

1 teaspoon cumin powder

1 teaspoon sea salt

Ground black pepper to taste

2 large eggs, beaten

½ cup milk (soy milk)

Peanut oil for frying

Paper towels and newspaper for draining latkes

Directions

Wash and scrub potatoes.

Prepare plates or cookie sheets lined with newspaper and paper towels.

Grate the sweet potatoes coarsely.

In a separate bowl, mix the flour, sugar, baking powder, curry powder, cumin, salt, and pepper.

Add eggs and milk to the dry ingredients to make a stiff batter.

Add the potatoes. The batter should be moist; if too stiff, add more milk.

Heat ¼ inch of peanut oil in a frying pan until very hot, do not allow to reach smoking point. Drop 1 tablespoon of batter into the oil and fry over medium heat. Fry on both sides until golden. Drain on paper towels and serve hot with topping of your choice.

Recipe adapted, courtesy of Epicurious.com.

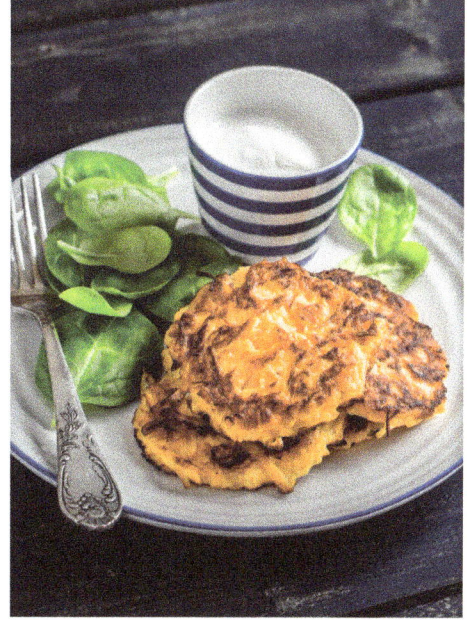

Frozen Ice Pop Favorites

Crafting the tastiest and most tempting ice pop is such a fun and eclectic art! The flavor combos you can make are quite endless. It's pretty hard not to create something satisfying, especially if you start with whole and delicious fruits and juices.

Orange Creamsicle—The 70's Classic

This delicious ice pop will be a familiar and nostalgic taste that everyone born in the last century will still love. And the kids today will too!

Combine in a blender or mixing bowl:

1½ cups orange juice

½ cup plain yogurt, whole milk

1–2 tablespoons honey

2 teaspoon vanilla extract

Pour slurry into ice pop molds and freeze for at least 4 hours.

Mango Madness

Mangoes are the world's most popular fruit. Need I say more?

Combine in a blender:

1 cup mango, fresh or frozen

1 cup of orange juice

1 cup strawberry, fresh or frozen

½ cup pineapple juice

Pour slurry into ice pop molds and freeze for at least 4 hours.

Berry Blast

This frozen pop captures a warm summer day in the cold freezer.

Combine in a blender:

1 cup strawberry, fresh or frozen

1 cup blueberry, fresh or frozen

½ cup raspberries, fresh or frozen

1 cup mixed berry juice

½ cup of soy milk

Pour slurry into ice pop molds and freeze for at least 4 hours.

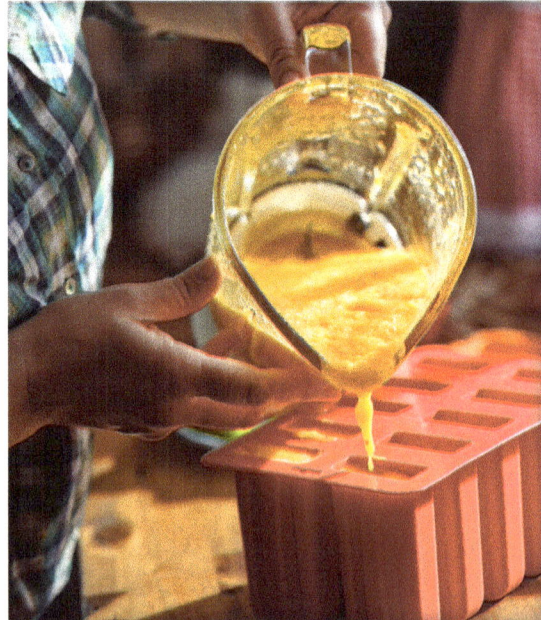

Ice-pop History

"In 1905 in San Francisco, 11-year-old Frank Epperson was mixing powdered flavoring for soda and water out on the porch. He left it there, with a stirring stick still in it. That night, temperatures reached a record low, and the next morning, the boy discovered the drink had frozen to the stick, inspiring the idea of a fruit-flavored 'Popsicle.'" Wikipedia

Herbal Infused Water

Enjoy this lovely deliciousness of herbal infused water with any thirsty summertime crowd. Infused water is one of the easiest ways to incorporate herbs into your daily life. There are countless possibilities of combinations to create. The blend of fragrant herbs along with the refreshing hints of fruit is oh-oh so good and does quench your thirst. People will think this is a magical elixir on a warm day, and that's what makes infused water so special.

Materials
Pint or quart sized mason jars

Ingredients
Water

Flavorful herbs, flowers, and fresh fruit

Directions
In a quart-sized mason jar, fill ¼ full with fresh herbs, flowers, and fruit, washed, with leaves pulled off stems.

Try spearmint, peppermint, rose geranium flowers and leaves, lemon balm, and orange slices.

Discard stems and damaged or bruised leaves.

Fill the rest of the jar with water and refrigerate for 2 hours or up to 2 days.

Strain and enjoy!

Variations
Combine common garden variety herbs like lemon balm, chamomile, mints, lavender, rosemary, and sages in a bowl.

Explore using flowers like rose geranium, rose petals, rose hips, lavender, and borage that will add color, flavor, and whimsy to your water.

Adding fruit like citrus, berries, and cucumber will add nutrients, and kids love the taste.

You can never go wrong with using mint. It is easy to grow, resilient in many climates, and is nutritious. Mint is good for digestion and adds cooling qualities, which are especially beneficial on hot days.

Stevia Lemonade

Enjoy this delicious naturally sweetened lemonade, using the amazing herb, stevia. Stevia is an incredibly sweet plant that doesn't interfere with blood sugar regulation nor does it have any calories.

Ingredients

½ cup fresh lemon juice

⅛ teaspoon white stevia powder

4 cups cold water or chilled carbonated water

Create your own drink with these snazzy additions.

Lemon zest

Fresh strawberries or raspberries

Sprig of mint

Splash to ⅓ cup unsweetened cranberry juice

Seltzer or carbonated water

Directions

Mix the juice and stevia until the stevia dissolves completely.

Mix in seltzer water for a fizzy drink, or add chilled water and serve.

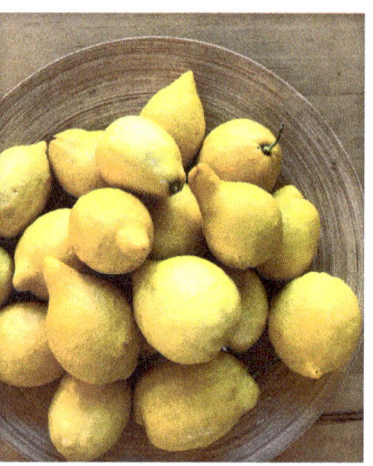

Coconut Turmeric Smoothie

A Coconut Turmeric Smoothie is a refreshing nutrient-rich drink that is perfect for dessert and works wonders as an anti-inflammatory elixir. Or freeze and enjoy it as a popsicle!

Ingredients

1 cup of coconut milk

½ cup of frozen pineapple and or mango

1 fresh or frozen banana

1 teaspoon turmeric root powder

½ teaspoon cinnamon powder

½ teaspoon fresh grated ginger or ⅛ tsp dried ginger

⅛ teaspoon black pepper

Directions

In a blender, add all the ingredients, blend until smooth. Or, freeze and turn them into popsicles!

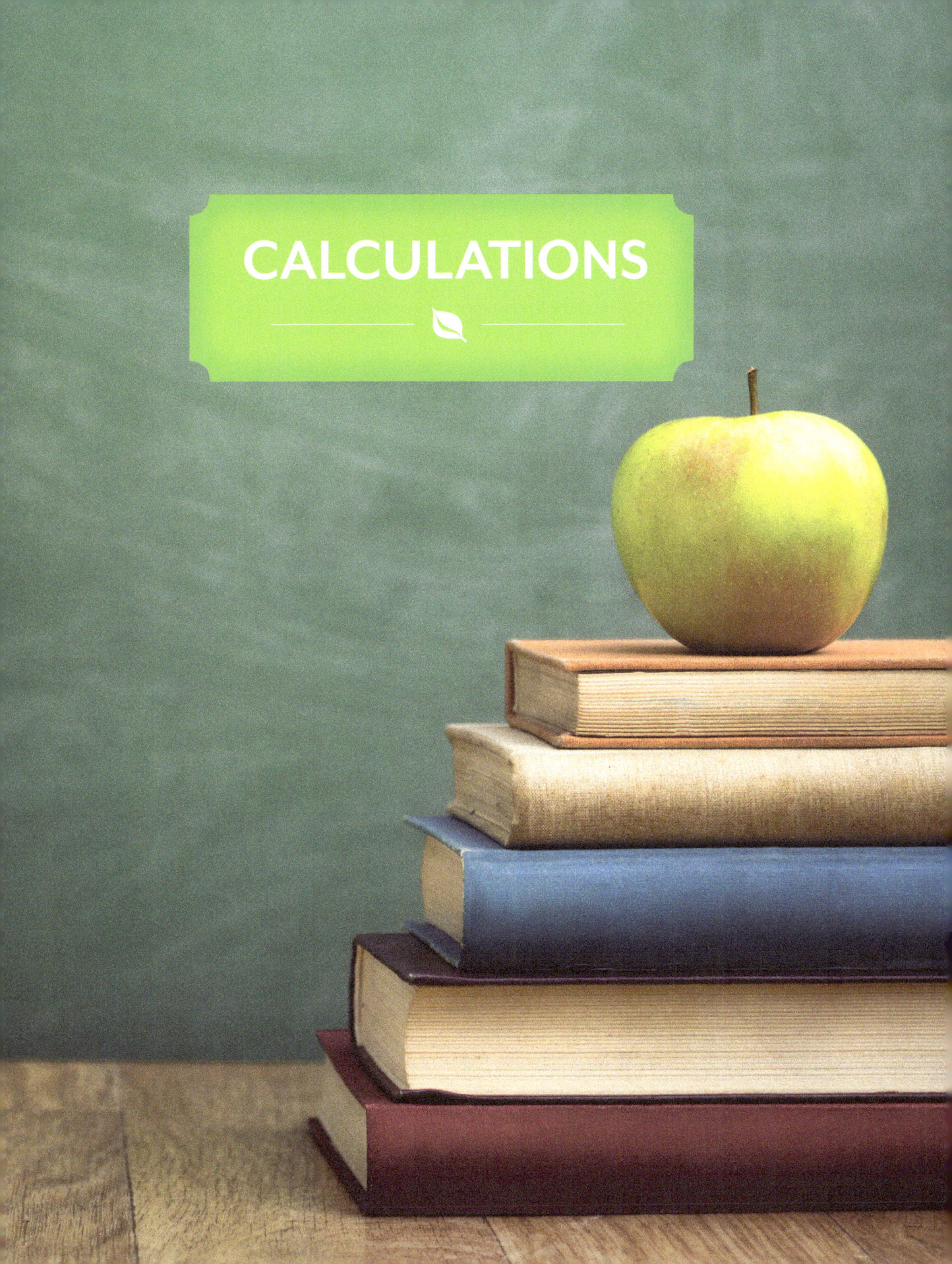

MACRONUTRIENT CALORIE, PERCENTAGE, AND GRAM CALCULATIONS

People receive their nutrients from the three macronutrient food groups: proteins, fats, and carbohydrates. Within these groups, a person will find all the nutrients as needed to live, including vitamins, minerals, phytonutrients, fiber, amino acids, and fatty acids.

People wonder how many servings they need of macronutrients. People wonder if fats are good or bad. They wonder if "carbs" are bad or whether they are getting enough protein foods. The bottom line is, all three macronutrients are necessary for human health. The only thing you need to figure out is the right percentages to eat. Many holistic nutritionists suggest an average balanced diet should include 50% carbohydrates, 25% proteins, 25% fats. (1)

1. What are your caloric needs per day?
2. How many calories are in a serving of food?
3. What percentage of proteins, carbohydrates, and fats do you require for a day?
4. How many grams of food do you need per macronutrient?

Use the following calculations to figure out the answers to those questions. Good luck and have fun.

Convert Grams to Calories

How Many Calories are in Proteins, Carbohydrates, and Fats?

The calculation enables you to determine how many calories there are in a macronutrient food.

Take the grams of macronutrient in the food, meal, or diet and multiply by the calories per gram of macronutrient.

Carbohydrate = 4 calories per gram

Proteins = 4 calories per gram

Fat = 9 calories per gram

Ex: One slice of bread = 13 grams of carbohydrate x 4 = 52 calories from carbohydrate.

Ex: 1 apple = 25 grams of carbohydrate x 4 = 100 calories from carbohydrate.

Ex: 1 egg = 5 grams of fat x 9 = 45 calories from fat.

Convert Calories to Grams Calculation

To convert calories to grams, divide macronutrient calories by its unit of energy.

4 for Carbohydrates

4 for Proteins

9 for Fats

Calorie Counting Equation with Food Grams

Fat (g) x 9 + carb (g) x 4 + protein (g) x 4 =

Examples:

75 fat calories divided by 9 = 18 grams of fat

268 carbohydrate calories divided by 4 = 67 grams of carbohydrate

Daily Protein, Carbohydrate, and Fat Recommendations

Protein Calorie Percentages Recommendation Calculation

For protein grams and calorie calculations for optimal daily nutrition, this formula will estimate the daily grams of protein needed based on a person's weight and activity level.

1. Weight in pounds divided by 2.2 = _____
2. Multiply that number by the person's activity level (.6 -1.5).

    .6 = Sedentary

    1. = 30 minutes average daily activity

    1.5 = School or professional athlete

The number you get is the recommended number of grams of protein to eat in a day.

Carbohydrate Calorie Percentage Recommendation Calculation

The USDA Dietary Guidelines for Americans recommends 45-65% of a person's diet should come from carbohydrates.

Fats Calorie Percentage Requirement Recommendation Calculation

A healthy balanced diet will include around 25% -30% fats a day. Fats can be broken down into sub-groups called Polyunsaturated, Monounsaturated, and Saturated fats. Holistic nutrition professionals recommend 40% Polyunsaturated, 40% Monounsaturated, and 20% Saturated Fat daily as an average.

MACRONUTRIENT CALCULATIONS

If your goal is to have 50% of your diet to be carbohydrates and you want to eat 1,500 calories a day total, multiply 1,500 by 0.50 = 750 calories from carbohydrates.

To calculate the percentage of a macronutrient in a food, a meal, or the diet:

Take the grams of the macronutrient and divide by calories = Macronutrient Percentage

$$21 \text{ grams}/140 = 0.15 = 15\%$$

Percentage of Calories from Macronutrients Formula

To find the percentage of macronutrients, take the total calories in the food or diet and divide by the macronutrient calories.

If you consume 1,500 calories per day, what is the % of calories from that macronutrient?

$$\frac{450 \text{ calories from carbohydrate?}}{1{,}500 \text{ total calories}} = 0.30 = 33\% \text{ of total daily calories from carbohydrate}$$

$$\frac{500 \text{ calories from fat?}}{1{,}500 \text{ total calories}} = 0.33 = 33\% \text{ of total daily calories from fat}$$

$$\frac{375 \text{ calories from protein?}}{1{,}500 \text{ total calories}} = 0.25 = 25\% \text{ of total daily calories from protein}$$

MACRONUTRIENTS—WHAT PERCENTAGE IS BEST FOR YOU?

CARBOHYDRATES • PROTEINS • FATS

Macronutrients in the Diet

A balanced diet refers to a diet that is 50% carbohydrate, 25% protein, and 25% fat. These percentages are intended as a rough gauge and a moderate baseline. Please consider that these numbers will fluctuate during a person's life based on differing needs.

Directions: Draw a line down the middle and then draw a line dividing the half-circle into two quarters. Label the half-circle carbohydrates and label one-quarter fats and one-quarter proteins.

Permission to reproduce. ©The Food Tree

THE FOOD TREE

MACRONUTRIENT CALORIE CALCULATIONS EXAMPLE

	CARBOHYDRATES	PROTEINS	FATS
GRAMS	400 x 4 Calories	120 x 4 Calories	65 x 9 Calories
CALORIES	1600	480	585
DIVIDE BY			
= PERCENTAGE	60%	18%	22%

Total calories = 2665

MACRONUTRIENT CALORIE CALCULATIONS PRACTICE

	CARBOHYDRATES	PROTEINS	FATS
GRAMS	x 4 Calories	x 4 Calories	x 9 Calories
CALORIES			
DIVIDE BY			
= PERCENTAGE			

Total calories =

Permission to reproduce. ©The Food Tree

BMI
Basal Metabolic Index

BMI (Basal Metabolic Index) is a tool used to screen people for weight issues. It is based on a simple calculation using a person's weight and height. The formula for adults, teens, and children are the same. However, the children's and teen's numbers are expressed as a percentage and plotted on a graph. The numbers were derived relative to other children of the same age and same gender. The CDC (Centers for Disease Control) provides BMI charts online for boys and girls ages 2-20.

Plotting the number on the chart will determine the weight category of the child or teen. Since children have rapid growth spurts, their bodies change quickly and may have more muscle mass at different times. A higher BMI may not necessarily indicate a high measurement of body fat or be indicative of overweight or obesity. Use the BMI accordingly.

Underweight	Less than the 5th percentile
Healthy weight	5th percentile to less than the 85th percentile
Overweight	85th to less than the 95th percentile
Obese	Equal to or greater than the 95th percentile

(Centers for Disease Control, 2015)

ADULT RANGES

Normal 18.5—24.9

Overweight 25—29.9

Obese 30—40

Super morbid obese ^50

BMI CALCULATION FOR CHILDREN, TEENS, AND ADULTS

Weight in pounds, divided by height in inches divided by height in inches, multiplied by 703, equals the BMI.

Or look at it this way…

$$(W \div H (in) \div H (in)) \times 703 = BMI$$

BMR

Basal Metabolic Rate

The Basal Metabolic Rate (BMR) determines the number of calories that are needed per day to support the body's work, including the heartbeat, respiration, body temperature, and while at rest. A person can calculate their BMR using their weight and a factor known as Activity Level. The activity level is determined by how physically active you are.

Activity Level

For mild daily activity, use an activity level of 1.1

For moderate daily activity, use an activity level of 1.3

For strenuous daily activity use an activity level of 1.5–1.7

The formula to calculate the BMR is:

Determine weight in kilograms (weight in pounds ÷ 2.2) x 24 = BMR at rest

Then, multiply BMR at rest by the Activity Level = total calories needed

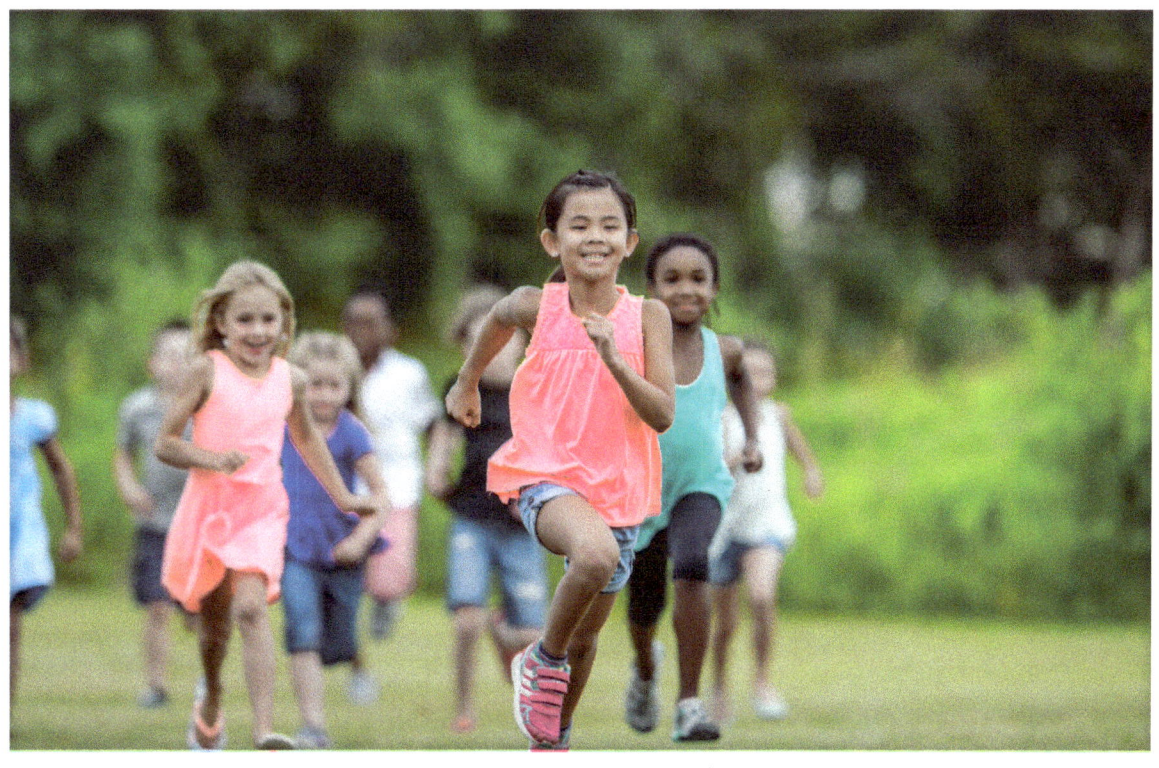

IDEAL DAILY WATER INTAKE
Water, The Elixir of Life

Staying hydrated is an essential part of keeping and staying healthy. Water is critical to life and survival. We are made up mostly of water, 60%! A person would only live between two to four days without water.

The wonders of water include:

- Filters out waste and toxins via urine
- Forms saliva
- Aids in digestion
- Controls body temperature
- Lubricates the joints
- Essential for every cell in your body to function
- Carries and delivers oxygen
- Used by the brain to make neurotransmitters and hormones
- Adds moisture to the mucous membranes
- Keeps skin plump and youthful looking

Drinking water is good for your body!

To figure out how much water a person needs to drink a day, take the persons weight and divide in half. The number you get will equal the amount of water in ounces that is optimal to drink every day. Always take into consideration that your water and hydration needs can change rapidly. Pay attention to keeping well hydrated especially on hot days, during increased physical exertion, while under stress, upon waking, and in other unique situations. As well, we get water in fruits and vegetables, herbal teas, and juices.

Be an eco-warrior and remember to bring your own reusable stainless steel, glass, or ceramic water bottle where ever you go!

Daily Water Requirement Calculation

Weight (lbs.) ÷ 2 = optimal daily intake of water in ounces.

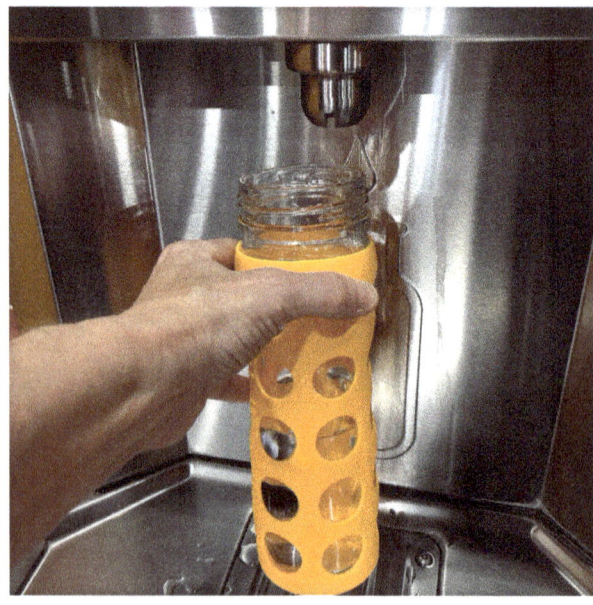

APPENDIX

THE FOOD TREE NUTRIENT SCROLL
The Long List of the Nutrients People Need

Print out the list below and tape together to make one long scroll. Attach a dowel or pencil at the top and roll up the paper. Release the scroll, so it drops down for a dramatic effect! This visual is a fun way to show the list of micronutrients necessary to eat daily or over a 3 to 4-day period for optimal health. (1)

Vitamins

Vitamin A	Vitamin B2 (riboflavin)	Inositol
Carotenoids	Vitamin B3 (niacin)	Vitamin C (ascorbic acid)
Alpha carotene	Vitamin B5 (pantothenic acid)	Vitamin D
Beta carotene	Vitamin B6 (pyridoxine)	Vitamin E (tocopherol)
Cryptoxanthin	Vitamin B7 (biotin)	Vitamin K
Lutein	Vitamin B8 (ergadenylic acid)	Dietary fiber
Lycopene	Vitamin B9 (folic acid)	Soluble fiber
Zeaxanthin	Vitamin B12 (cyanocobalamin)	Insoluble fiber
Vitamin B1 (thiamine)	Choline	Starch

Sugars

Monosaccharides	Glucose	Maltose
Fructose	Disaccharides	Sucrose
Galactose	Lactose	

Amino Acids

Alanine	Histidine	Serine
Arginine	Isoleucine	Theanine
Asparagine	Leucine	Threonine
Aspartic acid	Lysine	Tryptophan
Cysteine	Methionine	Tyrosine
Glutamic acid	Ornithine	Valine
Glutamine	Phenylalanine	
Glycine	Proline	

Fats

Polyunsaturated
    Linoleic acid
    Linolenic acid
    Stearidonic acid
    Eicosatrienoic acid
    Arachadonic acid
    EPA—eicosapentaenoic acid
    DHA—docosahexaenoic acid
Monounsaturated fats
    Myristol
    Pentadecanoic acid
Palmitic acid
Heptadecenoic acid
Oleic acid
Eicosyl
Erucic acid
Nervonic acid
Saturated fats
    Butyric acid
    Caproic acid
    Caprylic acid
    Capric acid
Lauric acid
Myristic acid
Pentadecanoic acid
Palmitic acid
Heptadic acid
Stearic acid
Arachidonic acid
Behenic acid
Tetracos acid
Cholesterol

Minerals

Boron
Calcium
Chloride
Chromium
Copper
Fluoride
Iodine
Iron
Magnesium
Manganese
Molybdenum
Phosphorus
Potassium
Selenium
Sodium
Sulfur
Zinc

Organic Acids

Acetic acid
Citric acid
Lactic acid
Malic acid

2 to 20 years: Girls
Body mass index-for-age percentiles

NAME ____________________

RECORD # ____________

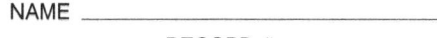

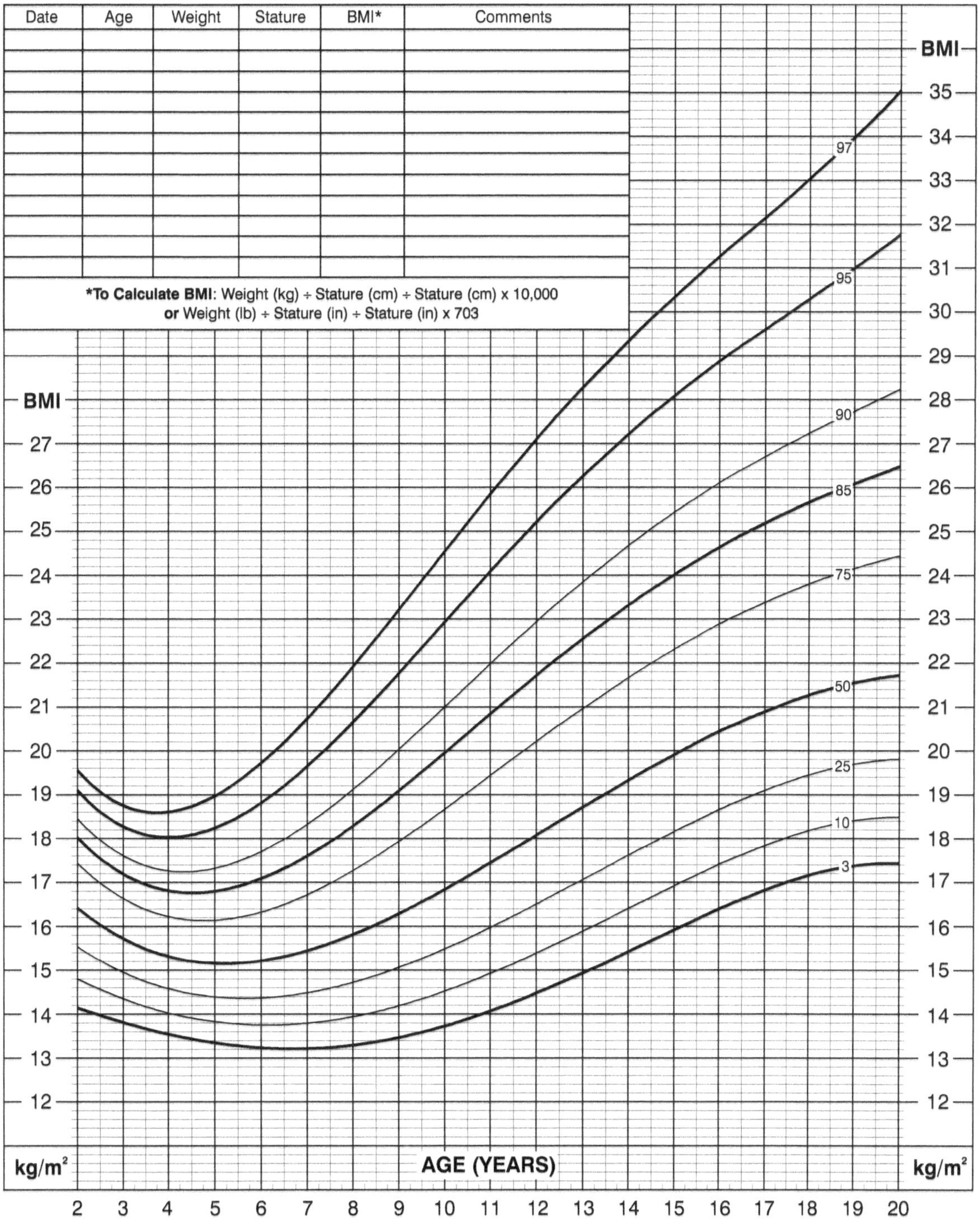

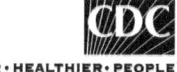

Published May 30, 2000 (modified 10/16/00).
SOURCE: Developed by the National Center for Health Statistics in collaboration with
the National Center for Chronic Disease Prevention and Health Promotion (2000).
http://www.cdc.gov/growthcharts

CDC
SAFER • HEALTHIER • PEOPLE™

2 to 20 years: Boys
Body mass index-for-age percentiles

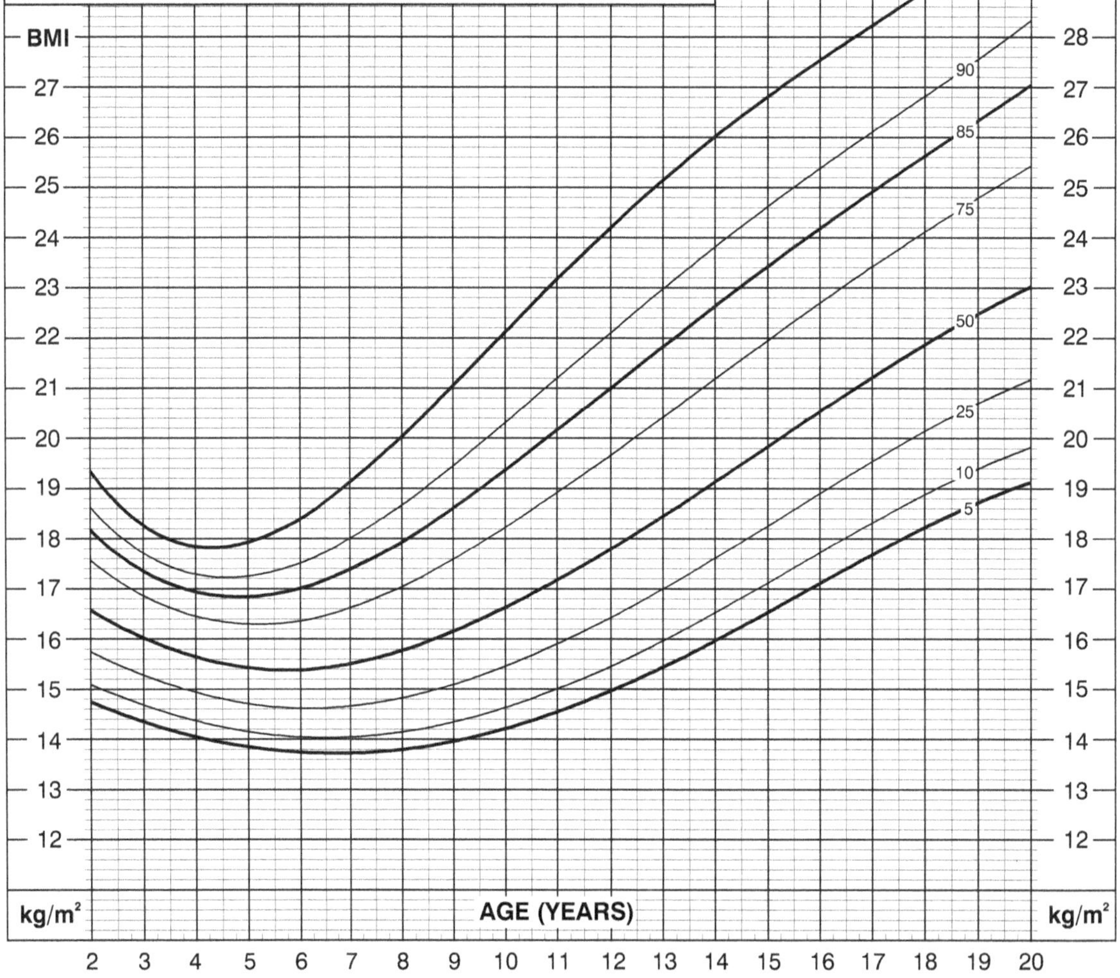

NAME _____

RECORD # _____

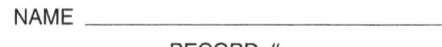

BODY MASS INDEX CHART FOR ADULTS

	Normal						Overweight					Obese									Extreme Obesity														
BMI	19	20	21	22	23	24	25	26	27	28	29	30	31	32	33	34	35	36	37	38	39	40	41	42	43	44	45	46	47	48	49	50	51	52	53	54
Height (inches)														Body Weight (pounds)																						
58	91	96	100	105	110	115	119	124	129	134	138	143	148	153	158	162	167	172	177	181	186	191	196	201	205	210	215	220	224	229	234	239	244	248	253	258
59	94	99	104	109	114	119	124	128	133	138	143	148	153	158	163	168	173	178	183	188	193	198	203	208	212	217	222	227	232	237	242	247	252	257	262	267
60	97	102	107	112	118	123	128	133	138	143	148	153	158	163	168	174	179	184	189	194	199	204	209	215	220	225	230	235	240	245	250	255	261	266	271	276
61	100	106	111	116	122	127	132	137	143	148	153	158	164	169	174	180	185	190	195	201	206	211	217	222	227	232	238	243	248	254	259	264	269	275	280	285
62	104	109	115	120	126	131	136	142	147	153	158	164	169	175	180	186	191	196	202	207	213	218	224	229	235	240	246	251	256	262	267	273	278	284	289	295
63	107	113	118	124	130	135	141	146	152	158	163	169	175	180	186	191	197	203	208	214	220	225	231	237	242	248	254	259	265	270	278	282	287	293	299	304
64	110	116	122	128	134	140	145	151	157	163	169	174	180	186	192	197	204	209	215	221	227	232	238	244	250	256	262	267	273	279	285	291	296	302	308	314
65	114	120	126	132	138	144	150	156	162	168	174	180	186	192	198	204	210	216	222	228	234	240	246	252	258	264	270	276	282	288	294	300	306	312	318	324
66	118	124	130	136	142	148	155	161	167	173	179	186	192	198	204	210	216	223	229	235	241	247	253	260	266	272	278	284	291	297	303	309	315	322	328	334
67	121	127	134	140	146	153	159	166	172	178	185	191	198	204	211	217	223	230	236	242	249	255	261	268	274	280	287	293	299	306	312	319	325	331	338	344
68	125	131	138	144	151	158	164	171	177	184	190	197	203	210	216	223	230	236	243	249	256	262	269	276	282	289	295	302	308	315	322	328	335	341	348	354
69	128	135	142	149	155	162	169	176	182	189	196	203	209	216	223	230	236	243	250	257	263	270	277	284	291	297	304	311	318	324	331	338	345	351	358	365
70	132	139	146	153	160	167	174	181	188	195	202	209	216	222	229	236	243	250	257	264	271	278	285	292	299	306	313	320	327	334	341	348	355	362	369	376
71	136	143	150	157	165	172	179	186	193	200	208	215	222	229	236	243	250	257	265	272	279	286	293	301	308	315	322	329	338	343	351	358	365	372	379	386
72	140	147	154	162	169	177	184	191	199	206	213	221	228	235	242	250	258	265	272	279	287	294	302	309	316	324	331	338	346	353	361	368	375	383	390	397
73	144	151	159	166	174	182	189	197	204	212	219	227	235	242	250	257	265	272	280	288	295	302	310	318	325	333	340	348	355	363	371	378	386	393	401	408
74	148	155	163	171	179	186	194	202	210	218	225	233	241	249	256	264	272	280	287	295	303	311	319	326	334	342	350	358	365	373	381	389	396	404	412	420
75	152	160	168	176	184	192	200	208	216	224	232	240	248	256	264	272	279	287	295	303	311	319	327	335	343	351	359	367	375	383	391	399	407	415	423	431
76	156	164	172	180	189	197	205	213	221	230	238	246	254	263	271	279	287	295	304	312	320	328	336	344	353	361	369	377	385	394	402	410	418	426	435	443

Source: Adapted from *Clinical Guidelines on the Identification, Evaluation, and Treatment of Overweight and Obesity in Adults: The Evidence Report.*

REFERENCES

THE FOOD TREE HOLISTIC NUTRITION CURRICULUM PHILOSOPHY, GUIDELINES, AND STANDARDS

1. "About OCA." *About OCA*, www.organicconsumers.org/about-oca.
2. "Organic Standards." *Organic Standards | Agricultural Marketing Service*, www.ams.usda.gov/grades-standards/organic-standards.
3. McEvoy, Miles. "Organic 101: Allowed and Prohibited Substances." National Organic Program Director in Food and Nutrition." *Research and Science USDA*, 25 January, 2012, www.usda.gov/media/blog/2012/01/25/organic-101-allowed-and-prohibited-substances.
4. Fair Trade International (www.fairtrade.net) Fair Trade Certified, www.fairtradecertified.org.

PROTEINS FOOD GROUP

Introduction to the Protein Food Group

1. "Recommended Dietary Allowances: 10th Edition, Protein and Amino Acids." National Research Council (US) Subcommittee on the Tenth Edition of the Recommended Dietary Allowances. Washington (DC): National Academies Press (US); 1989.
2. Kummerow, Fred. "Protein: Building Blocks of the Body." Health Topics, The Weston A. Price Foundation, 4 October, 2011, westonaprice.org/health-topics/abcs-of-nutrition/protein-building-blocks-of-the-body/.

Lesson: Serving Sizes and Daily Recommendations for Proteins

1. "Recommended Dietary Allowances: 10th Edition, Protein and Amino Acids." National Research Council (US) Subcommittee on the Tenth Edition of the Recommended Dietary Allowances. Washington (DC): National Academies Press (US); 1989. ncbi.nlm.nih.gov/books/NBK234922/.
2. Benachour N, Séralini GE. Glyphosate formulations induce apoptosis and necrosis in human umbilical, embryonic, and placental cells. Chem Res Toxicol. 2009 Jan;22(1):97-105. doi: 10.1021/tx800218n.
3. Taetzsch T, Block ML. "Pesticides, Microglial NOX2, and Parkinson's Disease". J Biochem Mol Toxicol. 2013 Feb;27(2):137-49. doi: 10.1002/jbt.21464. Epub 2013 Jan 24.

Lesson: Benefits and Function of Protein Foods

1. Kubala, Jillian. "Essential Amino Acids, Benefits and Food Sources." 12 June 2018 Healthline, healthline.com/nutrition/essential-amino-acids.
2. Van De Walle. "9 Important Functions of Protein in your Body." 20 June 2018, Nutrition, Healthline, healthline.com/nutrition/functions-of-protein.
3. Schmidler, Cindy. "Endocrine System Glands and Hormones." 13 April 2018, Anatomy and Function, Healthpages, healthpages.org/anatomy-function/endocrine-system-gland/.
4. "A Simple Guide to Neurotransmitters." 30 July 2015, Compound Interest, compoundchem.com/2015/07/30/neurotransmitters.
5. Insel, Thomas. "Post by Former NIMH Director Thomas Insel: Are Children Overmedicated?" 6 June 2014, National Institute of Mental Health, nimh.nih.gov/about/directors/thomas-insel/blog/2014/are-children-overmedicated.shtml.
6. Pompili, Maurizio et al. "Antidepressants and Suicide Risk: A Comprehensive Overview." *Pharmaceuticals (Basel, Switzerland)* vol. 3,9 2861-2883. 30 Aug. 2010, doi:10.3390/ph3092861.
7. Coupland, Carol, et al. "Antidepressant use and risk of suicide and attempted suicide or self-harm in people aged 20 to 64: cohort study using a primary care database." 18 February 2015, BMJ 2015; 350: h517.
8. "Measuring Neurotransmitter Levels." Neurotransmitters, Integrative Psychiatry, integrativepsychiatry.net/neurotransmitter.html.
9. "What are proteins and what do they do?" 2 April 2019, Genetics Home Reference, U.S. National Library of Medicine, ghr.nlm.nih.gov/primer/howgeneswork/protein.

Classification of Amino Acids

1. Kubala, Jillian. "Essential Amino Acids: Definition, Benefits and Food Sources." 12 June 2018, Nutrition, Healthline, healthline.com/nutrition/essential-amino-acids.

Lesson: Exploring Plant Based, Vegetarian, Vegan Diets and Lifestyles

1. Figus, Cinzia. "375 million vegetarians worldwide. All the reasons for a green lifestyle." 27 October 2014, Expo Net, Expo, expo2015.org/magazine/en/lifestyle/375-million-vegetarians- worldwide.html.
2. Palmer, Ashley. "2011 Vegetarian and Vegan Stats." 30 October 2013, PETA peta.org/living/food/2011-vegetarian-vegan-stats/.
3. Robbins, John. "Healthy at 100." 2019, Food Revolution Network, foodrevolution.org/videos/john-robbins-healthy-at-100/.
4. "Countries With The Highest Rates of Vegetarianism." 2019, Society, World Atlas, worldatlas.com/articles/countries-with-the-highest-rates-of-vegetarianism.html.
5. Flynn, Mary, M. "Economical Healthy Diets (2012): Including Lean Animal Protein Costs More Than Using Extra Virgin Olive Oil." 23 Sep 2015, Journal of Hunger & Environmental Nutrition, pages 476-482 https://doi.org/10.1080/19320248.2015.1045675.
6. "Cowspiracy", The Sustainability Secret, Film, 2014, cowspiracy.com/.

Lesson: Protein Deficiencies

1. "Recommended Dietary Allowances: 10th Edition, Protein and Amino Acids." National Research Council (US) Subcommittee on the Tenth Edition of the Recommended Dietary Allowances. Washington (DC): National Academies Press (US); 1989.
2. Institute of Medicine (US) Committee on Military Nutrition Research; Marriott BM, editor. Food Components to Enhance Performance: An Evaluation of Potential Performance- Enhancing Food Components for Operational Rations. Washington (DC): National Academies Press (US); 1994. 14, Performance-Enhancing Effects of Protein and Amino Acids.
3. Yoshida, Shohei. Role of dietary amino acid balance in diet restriction mediated lifespan extension, renoprotection, and muscle weakness in aged mice." Aging Cell, Anatomical Society, 2018 Jun 25 17(4): e12796, PMCID: PMC6052467, doi: 10.1111/acel.12796.
4. Kubala, Jillian. "Essential Amino Acids: Definition, Benefits and Food Sources." Nutrition, Health Line, 12 June 2018, https://www.healthline.com/nutrition/essential-amino-acids.
5. Arnarson, Atli. "8 Signs and Symptoms of Protein Deficiency." 31 October 2017, Nutrition, Healthline, https://www.healthline.com/nutrition/protein-deficiency-symptoms.

Lesson: Protein Foods to Avoid

1. Sharma, Sanjay. "Food Preservatives and their harmful effects." April 2015, International Journal of Scientific and Research Publications, Volume 5, Issue 4, A, ijsrp.org/research- paper-0415/ijsrp-p4014.pdf.
2. "Q & A on the carcinogenicity of the consumption of red processed meat." World Health Organization, October 2015, www.who.int/features/qa/cancer-red-meat/en/.
3. "WHO report says eating processed meat is carcinogenic: Understanding the findings.", The Nutrition Source, Harvard T.H. Chan School of Public Health, 3 November 2015, www.hsph.harvard.edu/nutritionsource/2015/11/03/report-says-eating-processed-meat-is- carcinogenic-understanding-the-findings.
4. Uribarri, Jaime et al. "Advanced glycation end products in foods and a practical guide to their reduction in the diet." *Journal of the American Dietetic Association* vol. 110,6 (2010): 911-16.e12. doi:10.1016/j.jada. 2010.03.018.
5. Carvalho, AM. "High intake of heterocyclic amines from meat is associated with oxidative stress." 28 April 2015, Br J Nutr., 113(8):1301-7. doi: 10.1017/S0007114515000628. Epub. ncbi.nlm.nih.gov/pubmed/25812604.
6. Robey, Ian Forrest. "Examining the relationship between diet-induced acidosis and cancer." *Nutrition & Metabolism* vol. 9,1 72. 1 Aug. 2012, doi:10.1186/1743-7075-9-72.
7. Rosenburg, Martha. "Turkey Bacon Products Recall Puts Focus on Dangerous Chemicals Used In Meat Production." 27 August 2015, Food and health, Food Revolution, https://foodrevolution.org/blog/meat-production-dangerous-chemicals/.

WHOLE GRAINS FOOD GROUP

Introduction to the Whole Grains Food Group

1. "What are carbohydrates (carbs)?" Diabetes, WebMD, 26 June 2016, webmd.com/diabetes/qa/what-are-carbohydrates-carbs.

2. Levy. Jillian. "3 Macronutrients You Need & Top Food Sources." Dr. Axe, 26 March 2017, draxe.com/macronutrients/.

Lesson: Getting to Know Whole Grains

1. Gunnars, Kris. "Grains: Are They Good For You, or Bad?" 4 June 2017, healthline.com/nutrition/grains-good-or-bad#section1.
2. "Why is it important to eat grains, especially whole grains?" Choose My Plate, USDA, 12 June 2016, https://www.choosemyplate.gov/eathealthy/grains/grains-nutrients-health.
3. "Nutrients and Health Benefits." *Choose MyPlate*, 12 June 2015, www.choosemyplate.gov/grains-nutrients-health.
4. "How Highly Processed Foods Liberated 1950s Housewives." *National Women's History Museum*, www.womenshistory.org/articles/how-highly-processed-foods-liberated-1950s-housewives.
5. "Dietary Reference Intakes for Energy, Carbohydrate, Fiber, Fat, Fatty Acids, Cholesterol, Protein, and Amino Acids." Health and Medicine, The National Academies of Sciences Engineering Medicine, http://www.nationalacademies.org/hmd/Reports/2002/Dietary-Reference-Intakes-for-Energy-Carbohydrate-Fiber-Fat-Fatty-Acids-Cholesterol-Protein-and-Amino-Acids.aspx.
6. Campbell-McBride, Natasha. Gut and Psychology Syndrome: Natural Treatment for Autism, Dyspraxia, A.D.D., Dyslexia, A.D.H.D., Depression, Schizophrenia. Rev. and expanded ed. United Kingdom: Medinform, 2010.
7. Seneff, Stephanie. "Roundup: The 'Nontoxic' Chemical That May Be Destroying Our Health." *The Weston A. Price Foundation*, 30 Oct. 2013, www.westonaprice.org/health-topics/environmental-toxins/roundup-the-nontoxic-chemical-that-may-be-destroying-our-health/.

Lesson: Serving Sizes and Daily Recommendations for Whole Grains

1. 1. "Whole grains vs. regular grains: What's the difference?" The Mayo Clinic Diet, The Mayo Clinic, 2019, diet.mayoclinic.org/diet/eat/whole-grains-vs-regular-grains?xid=nl_MayoClinicDiet_20160421.

Lesson: Benefits and Functions of Whole Grains

1. Food Search, Nutrient Database for Standard Reference Legacy Release, USDA Food Composition Databases, 2019, https://ndb.nal.usda.gov/ndb/nutrients/index.
2. Rimm EB, Ascherio A, Giovannucci E, Spiegelman D, Stampfer MJ, Willett WC. Vegetable, fruit, and cereal fiber intake and risk of coronary heart disease among men. JAMA. 1996; 275:447-51.
3. Fuchs CS, Giovannucci EL, Colditz GA, et al. Dietary fiber and the risk of colorectal cancer and adenoma in women. N Engl J Med. 1999; 340:169-76.
4. McKeown NM, Meigs JB, Liu S, Wilson PW, Jacques PF. Whole-grain intake is favorably associated with metabolic risk factors for type 2 diabetes and cardiovascular disease in the Framingham Offspring Study. Am J Clin Nutr. 2002; 76:390-8.

Lesson: Take a Poll on Grain Diversity

1. "Why Refined Carbs Are Bad for You." Healthline. www.healthline.com/nutrition/why-refined-carbs-are-bad.
2. Seneff, Stephanie. "Roundup: The 'Nontoxic' Chemical That May Be Destroying Our Health." *The Weston A. Price Foundation*, 30 Oct. 2013, www.westonaprice.org/health-topics/environmental-toxins/roundup-the-nontoxic-chemical-that-may-be-destroying-our-health/.
3. "Is Corn Oil Healthy? Benefits, Uses and Side Effects." *Mercola.com*, articles.mercola.com/herbal-oils/corn-oil.aspx.

Lesson: History and Trade Route of Grains in the U.S.

1. "All About Sorghum." *United Sorghum Checkoff*, www.sorghumcheckoff.com/all-about-sorghum.

FATS FOOD GROUP

Lesson: Getting to Know Fats

1. Enig, Mary G. *Know Your Fats: The Complete Primer for Understanding the Nutrition of Fats, Oils and Cholesterol*. Bethesda Press, 2010.
2. Liu, Ann G et al. "A healthy approach to dietary fats: understanding the science and taking action to reduce consumer confusion." *Nutrition journal* vol. 16,1 53. 30 Aug. 2017, doi:10.1186/s12937-017-0271-4.

Classification of Fats and Oils

1. "Is Corn Oil Healthy? Benefits, Uses and Side Effects." *Mercola.com*, articles.mercola.com/herbal-oils/corn-oil.aspx.

Lesson: Serving Sizes and Daily Recommendations for Fats

1. Udo Erasmus, *Fats that Heal Fats that Kill*. 1994. Alive Books, Canada.
2. Know Your Fats. Mary G Enig, Ph.D. 2000. Bethesda Press.

Lesson: Benefits and Functions of Fats

1. "The Biology of Fats in the Body." *ScienceDaily*, ScienceDaily, 23 Apr. 2013, www.sciencedaily.com/releases/2013/04/130423102127.htm.Ricciotti, Emanuela.
2. "Prostaglandins and inflammation." *Arteriosclerosis, thrombosis, and vascular biology* vol. 31,5 (2011): 986-1000. doi:10.1161/ATVBAHA.110.207449.
3. Derbyshire, E. "Do Omega-3/6 Fatty Acids Have a Therapeutic Role in Children and Young People with ADHD?" *Journal of Lipids* vol. 2017 (2017): 6285218. doi:10.1155/2017/6285218.
4. "Laboratory rodents that consumed an EFA mixture before being administered either cortisol or saline to induce "cold stress" their cortisol and cholesterol levels did not rise as much in response. Additionally, their ability to maneuver a maze was not impaired by stress inducers." Yehuda et al., 2000; 73-87 Intern J Neuroscience.
5. Küllenberg, Daniela et al. "Health effects of dietary phospholipids." *Lipids in health and disease* vol. 11 3. 5 Jan. 2012, doi:10.1186/1476-511X-11-3.
6. Kresser, Chris. "The Diet-Heart Myth: Cholesterol and Saturated Fat Are Not the Enemy." *Chris Kresser*, Chriskresser.com, 16 Mar. 2019, chriskresser.com/the-diet-heart-myth-cholesterol-and-saturated-fat-are-not-the-enemy/.
7. "Essential Fatty Acid Deficiency—Nutritional Disorders." *Merck Manuals Professional Edition*, Merck Manuals, www.merckmanuals.com/en-ca/professional/nutritional-disorders/undernutrition/essential-fatty-acid-deficiency.

Lesson: Benefits of Essential Fatty Acids Omega 3 and Omega 6

1. "The Importance of the Ratio of Omega-6/Omega-3 Essential Fatty Acids." *Biomedicine & Pharmacotherapy*, Elsevier Masson, 11 Sept. 2002, www.sciencedirect.com/science/article/abs/pii/S0753332202002536?via=ihub.
2. "Office of Dietary Supplements—Omega-3 Fatty Acids." *NIH Office of Dietary Supplements*, U.S. Department of Health and Human Services, ods.od.nih.gov/factsheets/Omega3FattyAcids-HealthProfessional/.

Lesson: Problems Associated with Eating Fats and Oils

1. Morris, S.G. "Fat Rancidity, Recent Studies on Mechanism of Fat Oxidation in Its Relation to Rancidity." *J. Agric. Food Chem.*, 1954, 2 (3), pp 126–132 DOI: 10.1021/jf60023a004, Publication Date: February 1954.
2. "Executive Summary." *EWG*, www.ewg.org/research/ewgs-good-seafood-guide/executive-summary.
3. Center for Food Safety and Applied Nutrition. "Food Additives & Ingredients—Final Determination Regarding Partially Hydrogenated Oils (Removing Trans Fat)." *U S Food and Drug Administration Home Page*, Center for Food Safety and Applied Nutrition, www.fda.gov/food/ingredientspackaginglabeling/foodadditivesingredients/ucm449162.htm.
4. Chen, Chun-Lin et al. "A mechanism by which dietary trans fats cause atherosclerosis." *The Journal of nutritional biochemistry* vol. 22,7 (2010): 649-55. doi:10.1016/j.jnutbio.2010.05.004.
5. Dhaka, Vandana et al. "Trans fats-sources, health risks and alternative approach—A review." *Journal of food science and technology* vol. 48,5 (2011): 534-41. doi:10.1007/s13197-010-0225-8.

VEGETABLES FOOD GROUP

Introduction to the Vegetable Food Group

1. Harvard Health Publishing. "The Best Foods for Vitamins and Minerals." *Harvard Health*, www.health.harvard.edu/staying-healthy/the-best-foods-for-vitamins-and-minerals.

Getting to Know Vegetables

1. 1. "How Many Calories Are in One Gram of Fat, Carbohydrate, or Protein?" *United States Department of Agriculture*, www.nal.usda.gov/fnic/how-many-calories-are-one-gram-fat-carbohydrate-or-protein.
2. "Fruits and Vegetables." *The Harvard School of*

Public Health State of Ohio, Ohio, ship.oh.networkofcare.org/ph/library/article.aspx?id=1205.

3. Lobo, V et al. "Free radicals, antioxidants and functional foods: Impact on human health." *Pharmacognosy reviews* vol. 4,8 (2010): 118-26. doi:10.4103/0973-7847.70902.

4. "Progress on Children Eating More Fruit, Not Vegetables." VitalSigns |CDC." *Centers for Disease Control and Prevention*, Centers for Disease Control and Prevention, www.cdc.gov/vitalsigns/fruit-vegetables/index.html.

Lesson: Serving Sizes and Daily Recommendations for Vegetables

1. "Fruits and Vegetables." *The Harvard School of Public Health State of Ohio, Ohio*, ship.oh.networkofcare.org/ph/library/article.aspx?id=1205.

2. *Shopping*, www.naturalhealthyconcepts.com/resources/infographics/phytonutrients.

Lesson Benefits and Functions of Vegetables

1. Beck, M A. "Antioxidants and Viral Infections: Host Immune Response and Viral Pathogenicity." *Journal of the American College of Nutrition*, U.S. National Library of Medicine, Oct. 2001, www.ncbi.nlm.nih.gov/pubmed/11603647.

2. Aghajanpour, Mohammad et al. "Functional foods and their role in cancer prevention and health promotion: a comprehensive review." *American journal of cancer research* vol. 7,4 740-769. 1 Apr. 2017.

3. Wang, Li-Shu, and Gary D Stoner. "Anthocyanins and their role in cancer prevention." *Cancer letters* vol. 269,2 (2008): 281-90. doi:10.1016/j.canlet.2008.05.020.

4. Pavan, Rajendra et al. "Properties and therapeutic application of bromelain: a review." *Biotechnology research international* vol. 2012 (2012): 976203. doi:10.1155/2012/976203.

5. Higdon, Jane V et al. "Cruciferous vegetables and human cancer risk: epidemiologic evidence and mechanistic basis." *Pharmacological research* vol. 55,3 (2007): 224-36. doi:10.1016/j.phrs.2007.01.009.

6. "How to Add More Fiber to Your Diet." *Mayo Clinic*, Mayo Foundation for Medical Education and Research, 16 Nov. 2018, www.mayoclinic.org/healthy-lifestyle/nutrition-and-healthy-eating/in-depth/fiber/art-20043983.

7. Morowitz, Michael J et al. "Contributions of intestinal bacteria to nutrition and metabolism in the critically ill." *The Surgical clinics of North America* vol. 91,4 (2011): 771-85, viii. doi:10.1016/j.suc.2011.05.001.

8. "The Pancreas and Its Functions." *The Pancreas and Its Functions | Columbia University Department of Surgery*, columbiasurgery.org/pancreas/pancreas-and-its-functions.

Lesson: Problems Related to Low Dietary Intake of Vegetables

1. "Dietary Guidelines for Americans 2015–2020 8th Edition." *2015-2020 Dietary Guidelines*, health.gov/dietaryguidelines/2015/guidelines/.

2. *Mineral Deficiency, Definition and Patient Education*. www.healthline.com/health/mineral-deficiency.

3. Why Is Fiber Important in Digestive Health?" *EverydayHealth.com*, 19 Feb. 2016, www.everydayhealth.com/digestive-health/experts-why-is-fiber-important.aspx.

4. *Dealing with Gum Disease—Ship.oh.networkofcare.org*. ship.oh.networkofcare.org/ph/library/article.aspx?id=1211.

5. Brown, Susan E. "Key Minerals for Bone Health—Magnesium." *Better Bones*, Center for Better Bones, 21 Jan. 2019, www.betterbones.com/bone-nutrition/magnesium/.

6. 5. Song K and Milner J A. **The influence of heating on the anticancer properties of garlic**. Journal of Nutrition 2001;131(3S).1054S-1057S.

7. 6. Vallejo F, Tomas-Barberan F A, and Garcia-Viguera C. Phenolic compound contents in edible parts of broccoli inflorescences after domestic cooking. Journal of the Science of Food and Agriculture (15 Oct 2003).

FRUITS FOOD GROUP

Getting to Know Fruit Group

1. "Fruits and Vegetables." The Harvard School of Public Health State of Ohio, Ohio, ship.oh.networkofcare.org/ph/library/article.aspx?id=1205.

2. "Why Is Fiber Important in Digestive Health?" EverydayHealth.com, 19 Feb. 2016, www.everydayhealth.com/digestive-health/experts-why-is-fiber-important.aspx.

Benefits and Functions of Fruits

1. "Fruit Archives." *Healthy Concepts with a Nutrition Bias*, blog.naturalhealthyconcepts.com/tag/fruit/.

2. "Top 12 Trace Mineral Rich Foods." *DrJockers.com*, 12 Feb. 2019, drjockers.com/top-12- trace-mineral-rich-foods/.

3. Mangge, Harald, et al. "Antioxidants, Inflammation and Cardiovascular Disease." *World Journal of Cardiology*, Baishideng Publishing Group Inc, 26 June 2014.

4. "How to Add More Fiber to Your Diet." Mayo Clinic, Mayo Foundation for Medical Education and Research, 16 Nov. 2018, www.mayoclinic.org/healthy-lifestyle/nutrition-and- healthy-eating/in-depth/fiber/art-20043983.

SUPPORT LESSONS

Lesson: Rainbow Food Phytonutrients and Antioxidants

1. Krebs-Smith, Susan M et al. "Americans do not meet federal dietary recommendations." *The Journal of nutrition* vol. 140,10 (2010): 1832-8. doi:10.3945/jn.110.124826.

2. Duthie, Susan J et al. "Effect of increasing fruit and vegetable intake by dietary intervention on nutritional biomarkers and attitudes to dietary change: a randomised trial." *European journal of nutrition* vol. 57,5 (2018): 1855-1872. doi:10.1007/s00394-017-1469-0.

3. Wang, Li-Shu, and Gary D Stoner. "Anthocyanins and their role in cancer prevention." *Cancer letters* vol. 269,2 (2008): 281-90. doi:10.1016/j.canlet.2008.05.020.

Lesson: Focus on Fiber

1. "What Foods Contain Cellulose?" LIVESTRONG.COM, Leaf Group, www.livestrong.com/article/464063-what-foods-contain-cellulose/.

2. "Soluble vs. Insoluble Fiber: MedlinePlus Medical Encyclopedia." MedlinePlus, U.S. National Library of Medicine, medlineplus.gov/ency/article/002136.htm.

3. "How Much Fiber Is Found in Common Foods?" Mayo Clinic, Mayo Foundation for Medical Education and Research, 17 Nov. 2018, www.mayoclinic.org/healthy- lifestyle/nutrition-and-healthy-eating/in-depth/high-fiber-foods/art-20050948.

4. High-Fiber Foods—Helpguide.org. www.helpguide.org/articles/healthy-eating/high-fiber- foods.htm?pdf=13288.

5. "How to Add More Fiber to Your Diet." Mayo Clinic, Mayo Foundation for Medical Education and Research, 16 Nov. 2018, www.mayoclinic.org/healthy-lifestyle/nutrition-and- healthy-eating/in-depth/fiber/art-20043983.

6. "How Much Fiber do You Need?", Ask Dr. Sears, 2019, https://www.askdrsears.com/topics/feeding-eating/digestive-health/how-much-fiber-do-you-need.

7. "Why You Need to Eat More Fiber", Weil, 2019, https://www.drweil.com/blog/bulletins/why-you-need-to-eat-more-fiber/.

Lesson: The Delicate Dynamic Digestive Tract

1. Masters, Rachel C et al. "Whole and refined grain intakes are related to inflammatory protein concentrations in human plasma." The Journal of nutrition, vol. 140,3 (2010): 587-94. doi:10.3945/jn.109.116640.

2. Samsel, Anthony, and Stephanie Seneff. "Glyphosate, pathways to modern diseases II: Celiac sprue and gluten intolerance." *Interdisciplinary toxicology* vol. 6,4 (2013): 159-84. doi:10.2478/intox-2013-0026.

3. Myers, Amy. "This Is Your Gut On Gluten." *Amy Myers MD*, 14 Mar. 2019, www.amymyersmd.com/2016/05/your-gut-on-gluten/.

4. Azzouz, Laura. "Physiology, Large Intestine." ncbi.nlm.nih.gov/books/NBK507857/.

5. "Digestive Tract Health." Health Library, Cleveland Clinic, 22 Nov 2016 my.clevelandclinic.org/health/articles/14122-digestive-tract-health.

Lesson: Developing Critical Thinking Skills; Food, Diet, Eating, and the Media

1. "Time Flies: U.S. Adults Now Spend Nearly Half A Day Interacting with Media." Nielsen Newswire Newsletter, Global Nielsen, 31 July 2018. https://www.nielsen.com/us/en/insights/news/2018/time-flies-us-adults-now-spend-nearly- half-a-day-interacting-with-media.html.

2. "Children eating more fruit, but fruit and vegetable intake still too low." CDC, CDC Newsroom, 2014, https://www.cdc.gov/media/releases/2014/p0805-fruits-vegetables.html.

3. "Fast Food Nation (Around the World), Center for Innovation, 2007, https://blog.centerforinnovation.mayo.edu/2016/04/07/fast-food-nation-around-the-world/.

NUTRITION VAMPIRES

Introduction to Nutrition Vampires

1. Fullerton DT, Getto CJ, Swift WJ, Carlson IH. 1985 Jun;14(6):673-80. "Sugar, opioids and binge eating." *Brain Res Bull*. https://www.ncbi.nlm.nih.gov/pubmed/3161588#.
2. "Highly processed foods dominate U.S. grocery purchase", Science Daily, 29 March 2015, https://www.sciencedaily.com/releases/2015/03/150329141017.htm.
3. Bleich, Sara N, and Kelsey A Vercammen. "The negative impact of sugar-sweetened beverages on children's health: an update of the literature." *BMC obesity* vol. 5 6. 20 Feb. 2018, doi:10.1186/s40608-017-0178-9.
4. *Children's Mental Health, Data and Statistics*, CDC, Centers for Disease Control and Prevention, 2019, https://www.cdc.gov/childrensmentalhealth/data.html.
5. McCarthy, Claire, "More than half of today's children will be obese adults", Harvard Health Publishing, 05 December, 2017, https://www.health.harvard.edu/blog/more-than-half-of-todays-children-will-be-obese-adults-2017120512879.
6. https://www.bbc.com/news/magazine-28191865
7. Gray, Laura, "Will today's children die earlier than their parents?", 08 July 2014, BBC News, https://www.bbc.com/news/magazine-28191865.

Lesson: Too Much Sugar

1. "Effects of Consuming Too Much Sugar." *Mercola.com*, articles.mercola.com/sugar-side-effects.aspx.
2. Children's Health Team. "Sugar: How Bad Are Sweets for Your Kids?" *Health Essentials from Cleveland Clinic*, Health Essentials from Cleveland Clinic, 21 Feb. 2019, health.clevelandclinic.org/sugar-how-bad-are-sweets-for-your-kids/.
3. Levy, Jillian. "Added Sugars Increase the Risk of Breast Cancer and Metastasis to the Lungs." *Dr. Axe*, 21 June 2017, draxe.com/hidden-sugar-foods/.
4. Doheny, Kathleen. "CDC Report: Kids Still Eat Too Much Added Sugar." *WebMD*, WebMD, 29 Feb. 2012, www.webmd.com/children/news/20120229/cdc-report-kids-still-eat-too-much-added-sugar#2.
5. "How Much Sugar Should a Teen Have a Day?" *LIVESTRONG.COM*, Leaf Group, www.livestrong.com/article/478658-how-much-sugar-should-a-teen-have-a-day/.
6. "Fast Facts | Fact Sheets | CDC." *Centers for Disease Control and Prevention*, Centers for Disease Control and Prevention, www.cdc.gov/tobacco/data_statistics/fact_sheets/fast_facts/index.htm.
7. Lustig, R., Schmidt, L. & Brindis, C. The toxic truth about sugar. Nature 482, 27–29 (2012). https://doi.org/10.1038/482027a.
8. "Your Leaky Gut May Be Caused by Excessive Grain Consumption." *Mercola.com*, articles.mercola.com/sites/articles/archive/2012/01/21/grains-causing-gut-leaks.aspx.
9. "5 Steps to Kill Hidden Bad Bugs in Your Gut That Make You Sick." *Dr. Mark Hyman*, 8 May 2017, drhyman.com/blog/2010/09/27/5-steps-to-kill-hidden-bad-bugs-in-your-gut-that-make-you-sick/.
10. Volk, Katrina M et al. "High-Fat, High-Sugar Diet Disrupts the Preovulatory Hormone Surge and Induces Cystic Ovaries in Cycling Female Rats." *Journal of the Endocrine Society* vol. 1,12 1488-1505. 2 Nov. 2017, doi:10.1210/js.2017-00305.
11. Johnson, Richard J, et al. "Attention-Deficit/Hyperactivity Disorder: Is It Time to Reappraise the Role of Sugar Consumption?" *Postgraduate Medicine*, U.S. National Library of Medicine, Sept. 2011, www.ncbi.nlm.nih.gov/pmc/articles/PMC3598008/.
12. Avena, Nicole M et al. "Evidence for sugar addiction: behavioral and neurochemical effects of intermittent, excessive sugar intake." *Neuroscience and biobehavioral reviews* vol. 32,1 (2007): 20-39. doi:10.1016/j.neubiorev.2007.04.019
13. Johnson RK, Appel LJ, Brands M, et al. Dietary sugars intake and cardiovascular health: a scientific statement from the American Heart Association. Circulation. 2009;120:1011-20.
14. Amanda. "1 In 3 Americans Will Have Diabetes by 2050, CDC Says." *LiveScience*, Purch, 22 Oct. 2010, www.livescience.com/10195-1-3-americans-diabetes-2050-cdc.html.
15. How Much Sugar Do You Eat? You May Be Surprised." NH DHHS-DPHS-Health Promotion in Motion, www.dhhs.nh.gov/dphs/nhp/documents/sugar.pdf.

Lesson: Nutrition Vampires and FDA Approval

1. "Overview of Food Ingredients, Additives, and Colors", FDA, April 2010, https://www.fda.gov/food/food-ingredients-packaging/overview-food-ingredients-additives-colors.

INTRODUCTION TO PHYSICAL ACTIVITIES

1. *"Grounding the Human Body: The Healing Benefits of Earthing."* Clint Ober and Gaetan Chevalier and Martin Zucker Chopra Center https://chopra.com/articles/grounding-the- human-body-the-healing-benefits-of-earthing.
2. *The biologic effects of grounding the human body during sleep as measured by cortisol levels and subjective reporting of sleep, pain, and stress.* Ghaly M, Teplitz D. J Altern Complement Med. 2004 Oct;10(5):767-76.
3. *Earthing: health implications of reconnecting the human body to the Earth's surface electrons.* Chevalier G, Sinatra ST, Oschman JL, Sokal K, Sokal P. J Environ Public Health. 2012;2012:291541. Doi: 10.1155/2012/291541. Review.

Yoga

1. Schiffman, Erich. *Yoga, The Spirit and Practice of Moving Into Stillness.* Pocket Books, 1996.
2. Stewart, Mary. *Yoga for Children,* Simon & Schuster, Inc., 1992.

Mindfulness Activities

1. Frontiers in Psychol. 2018; 9: 1034. Published online 2018 Jun 21. Doi: PMCID: PMC6021542 Effects of Mindfulness-Based Stress Reduction on Depression in Adolescents and Young Adults: A Systematic Review and Meta-Analysis, Xinli Chi,[1,2] Ai Bo.
2. Proc Natl Acad Sci U S A. 2015 Feb 17; 112(7): 1977–1982.
3. Psychological and Cognitive Sciences, Neuroscience. Self-affirmation alters the brain's response to health messages and subsequent behavior change, Emily B. Falk, a,[1] Matthew Brook O'Donnell,

ACTIVITIES; ARTS, CRAFTS, AND SCIENCE EXPERIMENTS

Indian Corn Jewelry

1. "Native American history of corn." Native Tech: Native American Technology and Art. 1994.
2. http://www.nativetech.org/cornhusk/cornhusk.html.

RECIPES

1. Dragaonwagon, Crescent, "Passionate Vegetarian", Workman Publishing Company, Inc. 2002.

CALCULATIONS

Macronutrient Calorie, Percentage, and Gram Calculations

1. Bauman, Ph.D., Edward, "Nutrition Educator Student Handbook", 2005, Bauman College Holistic Nutrition and Culinary Arts.

Water calculations

1. Daniels, Melissa C, and Barry M Popkin. "Impact of water intake on energy intake and weight status: a systematic review." *Nutrition reviews* vol. 68,9 (2010): 505-21. doi:10.1111/j.1753-4887.2010.00311.x.
2. Mitchel, H. H. et al. *The Chemical Composition Of The Adult Human Body And Its Bearing On The Biochemistry Of Growth.* Division of Animal Nutrition, and the Departments of Physiology and Animal Husbandry, University of Illinois, Urbana, February 15, 1945.

BMI & BMR

1. "Evidence Report of Clinical Guidelines on the Identification, Evaluation, and Treatment of Overweight and Obesity in Adults."1998. NIH/National Heart, Lung, and Blood Institute (NHLBI).
2. "Body Mass Index (BMI) | Healthy Weight | CDC." *Centers for Disease Control and Prevention*, Centers for Disease Control and Prevention, www.cdc.gov/healthyweight/assessing/bmi/index.html.
3. "About Child & Teen BMI | Healthy Weight | CDC." *Centers for Disease Control and Prevention*, Centers for Disease Control and Prevention, www.cdc.gov/healthyweight/assessing/bmi/childrens_bmi/about_childrens_bmi.html.

APPENDIX

The Food Tree Nutrient Scroll

1. "Listing of vitamins", Harvard Health Publishing, 14 Nov. 2018, https://www.health.harvard.edu/staying-healthy/listing_of_vitamins.

ABOUT THE AUTHOR

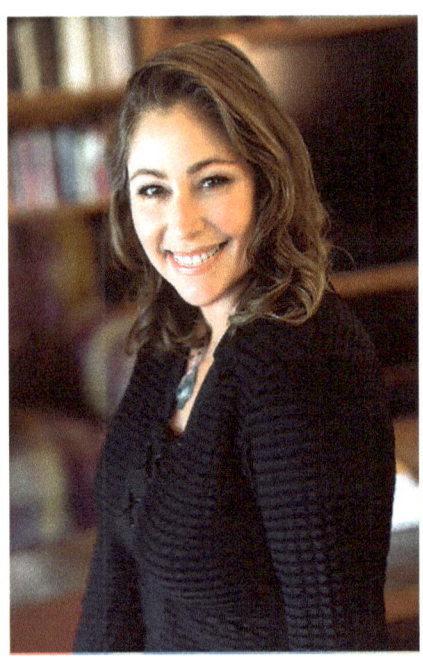

Jill Troderman is an award-winning Certified Holistic Nutritionist and Nutrition Educator specializing in family and child nutrition. Jill's mission is to educate, empower, and inspire people to navigate towards their ultimate health goals by utilizing holistic mind, body, and soul-based health and wellness practices. She is an advocate of eating plant-based nutrient-dense foods, using nutraceuticals and herbs, and practicing a mindful lifestyle.

She is passionate about all thing's wellness. Her love of plants and the powerful healing to be found from them is one of the core reasons she began on the path of learning about natural medicine and the positive force holistic, integrative healing, and mindfulness can bring to people. She is the creator of The Food Tree Guide, The Food Tree Magnetic Boards, and enjoys crafting herbal tea blends. When she is not in the garden, she provides nutrition counseling, teaches workshops on holistic nutrition, healthy cooking, and organic gardening. Jill is a certified Julia Ross Amino Acid and First Line Therapy practitioner and a member of the National Association of Nutrition Professionals. She is the mother of two grown sons and lives in Santa Cruz, California.

www.ingramcontent.com/pod-product-compliance
Lightning Source LLC
Chambersburg PA
CBHW061123070526
44584CB00033B/4207